AF616057

Fibrinolysis

Editors

Daniel L. Kline, Ph.D.
Professor and Director
Department of Physiology
University of Cincinnati
College of Medicine
Cincinnati, Ohio

K. N. N. Reddy, Ph.D.
Assistant Professor
Department of Physiology
University of Cincinnati Medical Center
Cincinnati, Ohio

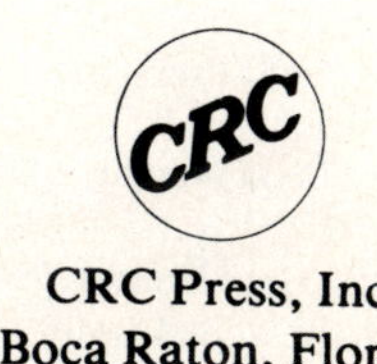

CRC Press, Inc.
Boca Raton, Florida

Library of Congress Cataloging in Publication Data
Main entry under title:

Fibrinolysis.

Bibliography: p.
Includes index.
1. Fibrinolysis. I. Kline, Daniel Louis, 1917— II. Reddy, K. Nagendra N.
QP93.5.F52 612'.115 79-20639
ISBN 0-8493-5425-0

Direct all inquiries to CRC Press, 2000 N.W. 24th Street, Boca Raton, Florida, 33431.

International Standard Book Number 0-8493-5425-0

Library of Congress Card Number 79-20639
Printed in the United States

INTRODUCTION

The modern era of fibrinolysis began about 50 years ago with the discovery that the culture media of certain strains of streptococci contained a substance which produced the rapid dissolution of human blood clots. It was soon demonstrated that the bacterial protein, now called streptokinase, acts indirectly by converting plasminogen, a plasma protein, to the active fibrinolytic enzyme, plasmin. Plasminogen and endogenous plasminogen activators were shown to be present in a wide variety of tissues and body fluids. Of special interest was the discovery of a plasminogen activator in urine, urokinase. The development of a reliable procedure for the partial purification of plasminogen opened the way to biochemical studies of all aspects of the fibrinolytic system including inhibitors. Animal and clinical studies showed that plasmin is an ineffective thrombolytic agent and that activators offered the most promising therapeutic approach. Extensive clinical trials have been carried out with highly purified streptokinase and urokinase.

Two mechanisms have been described which lead to the activation of plasminogen within the blood stream: (1) the release of plasminogen activator(s) from the walls of blood vessels under a wide variety of physiological and pharmacological stimuli and (2) the appearance of plasmin activity following the activation of Factor XII (Hageman Factor), the initial step in the so-called contact activation system.

Current research involves the elucidation of the structures of plasminogen, plasmin and some of the activators, particularly streptokinase and urokinase. The mechanism of activation by various activators is also being studied at a molecular level. Of particular interest is the interaction of streptokinase with plasminogen which involves the formation of a complex and is of interest not only in fibrinolysis but as a tool to study the activation of proteolytic enzymes at a fundamental level. Rapid advances are being made in the understanding of the plasma inhibitors of both plasmin and plasminogen activators and the physiological role of the inhibitors. Small molecular weight substances which induce fibrinolytic activity in the blood are being studied for possible clinical use and the action of plasmin on its natural substrate, fibrin, is under intensive investigation.

The aim of this book is to present the most important aspects of our current knowledge of fibrinolysis with sufficient background and clarity so that a reader can understand the developments in each area which led up to the present state of our knowledge. We hope the reader with either a basic or a clinical viewpoint will gain a dynamic picture of the developments in a field, become acquainted with the most recent advances and will be in a position to understand (and contribute to) further progress.

Since plasminogen and plasminogen activators have been found in many tissues and fluids in the body and interrelationships have been found between the fibrinolytic system, blood coagulation, inflammatory reactions and the complement system, it is important to keep in mind that clot-dissolving may prove to be the most obvious but not the only function of the fibrinolytic system.

Daniel L. Kline
Cincinnati, Ohio
July 1, 1979

THE EDITORS

Daniel L. Kline, Ph.D., is Professor and Chairman of the Department of Physiology, University of Cincinnati College of Medicine, Cincinnati.

Dr. Kline received his B.S. from Purdue University in 1942 and his Ph.D. in physiology from Columbia University College of Physicians and Surgeons in 1946. From 1949 to 1966 he held various posts in the Department of Physiology of the Yale University School of Medicine, rising to the position of Associate Professor. He has been at the University of Cincinnati since 1966.

Dr. Kline is a member of the International Society of Thrombosis and Haemostasis, the American Heart Association Council on Thrombosis, the American Physiological Society, the American Federation of Scientists and the American Association for the Advancement of Science, as well as other professional and honorary organizations.

He was a National Research Council and John Simon Guggenheim Fellow. He has served on the editorial boards of the *American Journal of Physiology* and the *Journal of Applied Physiology* and is presently a consulting editor of *Science*.

Dr. Kline has participated in many conferences and contributed to many publications chiefly in the field of fibrinolysis.

K. N. N. Reddy, Ph.D., is Assistant Professor of Physiology, University of Cincinnati Medical Center, Cincinnati. Dr. Reddy received his M.Sc. in organic chemistry from the University of Saugor, India, in 1959, and his Ph.D. in Biochemistry from the Indian Institute of Science in 1971. From October 1968 to June 1973 he was a Research Associate in the Department of Experimental Biology, Roswell Park Memorial Institute, Buffalo, New York and from July 1973 to August 1975 he was a Senior Research Associate in the Department of Physiology, University of Cincinnati Medical Center.

Dr. Reddy is the recipient of a Research Career Development Award from the National Institutes of Health. He is a member of the American Chemical Society and the American Society of Biological Chemists. His research publications are in the field of fibrinolysis.

CONTRIBUTORS

Désiré Collen, M.D., Ph.D.
Docent
Faculty of Medicine
University of Leuven
Leuven, Belgium

Ulla Hedner, M.D.
Coagulation Laboratory
Allmänna Sjukhuset
Malmö, Sweden

Robert F. Highsmith, Ph.D.
Associate Professor of Physiology
University of Cincinnati
College of Medicine
Cincinnati, Ohio

Allen P. Kaplan, M.D.
Professor of Medicine
State University of New York at Stony Brook
Stony Brook, New York

Inga Marie Nilsson, M.D.
Professor
Coagulation Laboratory
Allmänna Sjukhuset
Malmö, Sweden

Maurizio Pandolfi, M.D.
Professor
Department of Ophthalmology
Allmänna Sjukhuset
Malmö, Sweden

Marc Verstraete, M.D.
Professor of Medicine
Director
Center for Thrombosis and Vascular Research
University of Leuven
Leuven, Belgium

Kurt N. von Kaulla, M.D.
Professor Emeritus of Medicine
Formerly Director of Coagulation Laboratories
University of Colorado Medical Center
Denver, Colorado

Per Wallén, M.D.
Associate Professor
Department of Medical Chemistry
Faculty of Medicine
University of Umeå
Umeå, Sweden

George D. Wilner, M.D.
Director of Laboratory Medicine
Associate Professor of Pathology
Assistant Professor of Medicine
The Jewish Hospital of St. Louis
St. Louis, Missouri

Lewis D. Yecies, M.D.
Assistant Professor of Medicine
State University of New York at Stony Brook
Stony Brook, New York

TABLE OF CONTENTS

Chapter 1

BIOCHEMISTRY OF PLASMINOGEN

Per Wallén

TABLE OF CONTENTS

I. INTRODUCTION

Fibrinolysis has been known as a phenomenon for about 200 years. During the 19th century, it was discovered that fibrinolysis is a proteolytic process and that proteolytic activity leading to fibrinolysis is found in blood in certain conditions, such as stress and hemorrhagic shock. Studies on the biochemical mechanism behind the fibrinolytic process started about 40 years ago.

The finding, during the 1930s, that certain strains of streptococci release an exotoxin which specifically induces lysis of fibrin clots led to an increasing interest in fibrinolysis. This was presumably due to the feeling that the streptococcal factor could be of practical value for thrombolytic therapy. In parallel there was an increase in the understanding of the biochemical background to fibrinolysis. It soon became evident that the streptococcal factor per se was not a fibrinolytic agent, but required a plasma factor for activity. In some brilliant studies, Christensen and Kaplan showed that the serum factor was a proenzyme, which was activated to a proteolytic enzyme.[1,2] The proenzyme was named "plasminogen", and the enzyme was named "plasmin".[3] When it was realized that the central reaction in the fibrinolytic system is the conversion of plasminogen to plasmin, it became of great interest to isolate and characterize plasminogen. Certain features of plasminogen, however, proved to be quite annoying for those working with its purification. In fact it took more than 20 years before a plasminogen which with certainty could be regarded as native was isolated.

Our knowledge about plasminogen (its chemistry and interactions) has increased to a great extent during the last 10 years. Studies on the structure of plasminogen and plasmin which eventually have led to the elucidation of the complete primary structure of these proteins have been prerequisites for this development. They have made it possible to elucidate phenomena, such as activation of plasminogen and inhibition of plasmin at the molecular level. Another advance is the growing realization that the activation of plasminogen is not a separate process, but is influenced by other reactions in blood coagulation. Thus, fibrin itself seems to be of great importance for the localization and regulation of the fibrinolytic process.

II. PURIFICATION OF PLASMINOGEN

Remmert and Cohen were among the first to make serious efforts to purify plasminogen by conventional techniques.[4] One of their findings was that plasminogen has a marked tendency to stick to other plasma proteins and was distributed in several fractions with only slight purification. Attempts were made to circumvent this tendency to form complexes by making use of the rather high stability of plasminogen against treatment with acid and alkali. Thus, Kline obtained preparations of high purity by a technique in which the essential steps were extraction of plasma fractions with dilute sulfuric acid and dialysis against a phosphate buffer at pH 6.[5] This type of plasminogen was frequently used into the 1960s in studies on fibrinolysis. However, Alkjaersig has shown that the treatment of plasminogen with acid causes changes of the physicochemical properties. They occur at pH below pH 4.5 and include marked changes of the solubility characteristics and sedimentation behavior, indicating significant conformational changes.[6] It has been observed that native and acid-treated plasminogens differ in their interactions with antifibrinolytic amino acids in fibrinolytic systems and that acid treatment furthermore causes an increase in activability of native plasminogen.[7] This suggests that conformational changes similar to those observed on partial proteolytic degradation of native plasminogen (see Section V) may occur.

At the end of the 1950s, it was observed that low concentrations of ε-aminocaproic acid and lysine cause a marked increase in the solubility of plasminogen.[8,9] As discussed in a later section, these amino acids interact specifically with certain sites in the plasminogen molecule and seem to cause a marked decrease of the interaction between plasminogen with other proteins. This discovery has been of great importance for the development of techniques for the purification of plasminogen. The first application of these amino acids in purification of plasminogen was a chromatographic procedure which made use of the selective decrease of affinity of plasminogen towards anion exchangers (DEAE-cellulose) induced by these amino acids.[10] Subsequently several procedures were developed based on the extraction and precipitation in the presence of lysine or ε-aminocaproic acid or on chromatography on ion exchangers in presence of these amino acids. An extensive review of the earlier techniques for purification of plasminogen has been given by Heberlein and Barnhart.[11]

The presently most-used application of the antifibrinolytic amino acids to the purification of plasminogen is the affinity chromatographic technique of Deutsch and Mertz in which lysine coupled to Sepharose is used as adsorbant of plasminogen.[12] In the original method, crude plasma or serum was passed through a column of lysine Sepharose. After washing, the adsorbed plasminogen was eluted with 0.1 *M* ε-aminocaproic acid. Several modifications of this technique have subsequently been used for the purification of plasminogen from plasma and different crude plasma fractions. They have recently been reviewed by Chibber et al.[13] By using gradient elution with ε-aminocaproic acid, Brockway and Castellino succeeded in separating highly purified human plasminogen into two fractions with different electrophoretic mobilities.[14] They have been called plasminogens Type 1 and Type 2, according to the order in which they are eluted. They are discussed in more detail in Section V.C.

The efforts at purification and characterization of plasminogen have mainly been concentrated on human plasminogen. However, some studies on the purification of plasminogen from other species have been published. Ox plasminogen and dog plasminogen have earlier been isolated with conventional methods.[15,16] The affinity adsorbtion on lysine Sepharose has also been applied to plasminogen from other species. Plasminogen preparations from cat, rat, dog, sheep, horse, goat, monkey, and duck have been obtained using this technique.[14,17] All plasminogen preparations from mammalian species studied so far can be separated into two main types by chromatography on lysine Sepharose. The only bird plasminogen investigated, duck plasminogen, contained just one type.

A fact which has complicated the isolation of native plasminogen is its sensitivity for partial proteolytic degradation by traces of plasmin. There is a tendency for plasmin generation during the purification, especially at neutral pH and in the presence of antifibrinolytic amino acids, such as ε-aminocaproic acid. Using slightly acidic conditions (pH 4 to 5) throughout, preparations practically free from contaminating plasmin have been obtained,[18,19] possessing glutamic acid as NH_2-terminal amino acid.[20] Due to the acidic conditions, these preparations were, however, poorly soluble. In more recent procedures working at near neutral reaction, a low molecular weight inhibitor, aprotinin (Trasylol®), was used to neutralize contaminating plasmin in certain critical steps.[21,22] These preparations also contained glutamic acid in NH_2-terminal position, but were highly soluble. Plasminogen prepared from fresh plasma by affinity chromatography has been shown to contain mainly glutamic acid in NH_2-terminal position.[23]

Another type of plasminogen, containing mainly lysine in NH_2-terminal position, has been produced and characterized by Robbins et al.[24,25] It was contaminated with considerable amounts of plasmin. Using zymographic analysis after starch gel electrophoresis, it was demonstrated that the plasminogen, which has glutamic acid as NH_2-terminal amino acid is electrophoretically identical to the native plasminogen of fresh plasma, whereas the plasminogen forms with lysine or valine in NH_2-terminal position have significantly higher isoelectric points.[21,22,26] It has also been shown that NH_2-terminal glutamic acid plasminogen is converted to the NH_2-terminal lysine form by slight digestion with plasmin.[22,27] In the following presentation, these two types of plasminogen will be referred to as Glu-plasminogen and Lys-plasminogen, respectively.*

As will be discussed in later sections, Glu-plasminogen and Lys-plasminogen differ markedly from each other with regard to chemical and functional properties. It has furthermore been shown that the turnover rate of radiolabeled Lys-plasminogen is much faster than that of radiolabeled Glu-plasminogen (plasma half life less than 1 day and about 2 days, respectively).[30] In many experiments using highly purified plasminogen, it is therefore of importance to define whether Glu- or Lys-plasminogen is used. The affinity chromatography of fresh plasma according to Deutsch and Mertz yields mainly Glu-plasminogen, although small amounts of Lys-plasminogen are frequently present. However, plasminogen is often prepared from crude fractions obtained on large-scale purification of plasma proteins. Such fractions often contain a mixture of the two forms which do not separate by affinity chromatography on lysine Sepharose. Glu- and Lys-plasminogen can, however, be separated by ion exchange chromatography on DEAE-Sephadex.[22] Highly or partially purified preparations of plasminogen often contain trace amounts of contaminating plasmin. In order to avoid proteolytic degradation of Glu-plasminogen, it is therefore often necessary to inactivate or remove this contamination by treatment with inhibitors (in solution or insolubilized) before operations such as gel filtrations or long-time incubations are performed.

III. ENZYMATIC PROPERTIES OF PLASMIN — ASSAY OF PLASMIN AND PLASMINOGEN

A. Substrate Specificity of Plasmin

Plasmin is a proteolytic enzyme with a pH optimum of about 7, as measured with casein as substrate.[3] It is an endopeptidase with general proteolytic action and able to hydrolyze a great variety of proteins.[31] Plasmin resembles trypsin and thrombin in the sense that it splits synthetic esters and amides of the basic amino acids lysine and arginine.[32] This is in accordance with the fact that plasmin only cleaves lysyl and arginyl bonds in proteins.[33-36]

Studies on the degradation of fibrinogen demonstrate, however, marked differences between the three enzymes, plasmin, trypsin, and thrombin, as for their specific requirements. Thrombin has a very narrow specificity, cleaving only four arginyl bonds in the fibrinogen molecule. On the other hand, trypsin cleaves practically all lysyl and arginyl bonds, whereas plasmin being more restrictive only cleaves about 60% of them.[33] An illustrative example of the difference is the finding that the thrombin-sensitive arginyl-glycyl bonds in fibrinogen are very rapidly cleaved by trypsin, but resistant to digestion with plasmin.[37] Another feature of plasmin is its preferential specificity for lysyl side chains, as demonstrated by studies on fibrino- and fibrinogenolysis.[36,38] Thus, Weinstein and Doolittle have found that at the time a fibrin gel is just liquefied, about eight bonds per mole of fibrin are split, all of which are lysyl bonds when plasmin is used as enzyme. The liquification with trypsin requires the cleavage of 20 bonds per mole of fibrin, 6 of which are arginyl bonds.[38] On the basis of their analyses, they furthermore suggest that the cleavage of two pairs of lysylalanine and arginylmethion-

* It should be pointed out that the form named Lys-plasminogen is heterogeneous and that although lysine is the dominating NH_2-terminal amino acid, valine and often methionine occur in significant amounts. Other names that have been used are plasminogen A and B for Glu- and Lys-plasminogen, respectively.[28] The designation neoplasminogen K77/v78 has also been suggested for Lys-plasminogen.[29]

ine bonds symmetrically placed in the fibrin molecule plays a key role in the fibrinolytic process.

B. Synthetic Plasmin Inhibitors

Mounter and Shipley first demonstrated that diisopropylfluorophosphate (DFP) inactivates plasmin.[39] They also found that the concentration of DFP required is considerably higher for plasmin than for trypsin. These results suggested that plasmin like trypsin, chymotrypsin, and thrombin belong to the serine proteases. Using ^{32}P-DFP, Robbins and co-workers localized the serine of the catalytic site to the B- (light) chain of plasmin. They also were able to isolate and partially sequenate a peptide containing this seryl residue.[40,41]

Schoellmann and Shaw introduced a different series of serine protease inhibitors which inactivate the enzymes irreversibly by alkylating the histidyl residue of the catalytic site.[42,43] These compounds which are chloromethylketone derivatives of amino acids, such as phenylalanine and lysine, are more specific inhibitors than DFP due to their different interactions with the substrate binding pocket of the enzymes. Thus the chloromethylketone derivative of N-tosyl-L-phenylalanine (TPCK) inactivates chymotrypsin, whereas the corresponding derivative of N^{α}-tosyl-L-lysine (TLCK) inactivates trypsin. TLCK but not TPCK inactivates plasmin, and one histidine residue in B- (light) chain is alkylated in this reaction.[41,44]

TLCK acts slowly on plasmin and is not a suitable inhibitor if a very fast inactivation of the enzyme is required. For several years, Shaw and co-workers have been studying the effect of chloromethylketone derivatives of oligopeptides on several serine enzymes.[45] The amino acid residues penultimate to the C terminal amino acid moderate the binding of the compound to secondary binding sites in the enzyme and may increase both the activity and selectivity of the compounds. Thus, both the chloromethyl ketone derivatives of Ala-Phe-Lys and Phe-Ala-Lys are considerably better inhibitors of plasmin than TLCK. One of them, the Phe-Ala-Lys derivative, is also an inhibitor of a plasminogen activator from kidney cells, whereas the Ala-Phe-Lys derivative is not.[46]

Compounds, which form stable acyl complexes with the active site serine residue are effective inhibitors of serine proteases. The active site titrant *p*-nitrophenyl-*p*′-guanidinobenzoate (NPGB), introduced by Chase and Shaw, belongs to this category.[47,48] It reacts with trypsin-like enzymes. The initial step in which the guanidinobenzoyl-enzyme complex is formed and nitrophenol is released ("burst reaction") is very rapid and can be followed by measuring the change in absorbance at 405 nm. The deacylation of the acyl-enzyme complex is slow, but occurs with various rates for different enzymes. On comparison between the guanidinobenzoyl derivatives of trypsin, plasmin, and thrombin, the thrombin derivative is deacylated almost 200 times faster than the plasmin derivative and 25 times faster than the trypsin derivative. The high acylation rate and extremely slow deacylation rate ($t_{1/2}$ is about 1.5 days) make NPGB an excellent site titrant for plasmin, as well as a good inhibitor.

Schick and Castellino have prepared a similar radioactive compound [^{14}C]-*p*-nitrophenyl-*p*′-(amidino thiomethyl)benzoate suitable for radiolabeling of the active sites of serine enzymes.[49] They have used it to label the active site of the streptokinase-plasminogen complex.

C. Assay of Plasmin and Plasminogen

Plasminogen can be assayed indirectly by measuring plasmin activity after activation of plasminogen with urokinase or streptokinase or by using quantitative immunological techniques.

Casein was among the first protein substrates used for measurement of plasmin activity and is still frequently used.[4,50,51] Other substrates which have also been used are gelatin,[3] fibrin[52-56] and synthetic substrates, such as esters of arginine and lysine.[32,53,57] More recently, chromogenic substrates such as paranitroanilide derivatives of specific peptides have been used. A substrate of this type which is a very sensitive and a rather specific substrate for plasmin is H−D−Val−Leu−Lys−Nan (S-2251, KABI) which is easily split also by the streptokinase-plasmin (plasminogen) complex.[58-60]

A standard preparation obtained by autocatalytic activation of plasminogen in glycerol has been prepared by Sgouris et al.[61] It is provided by the National Institute for Biological Standards and Control, London, and has been checked by ten laboratories in an international collaborative study (see Kirkwood et al.).[62] It has been recommended by the International Committee on Thrombosis and Haemostasis for use as an international standard.

Assay of plasminogen as plasmin activity after activation has to be judged with caution, since the activation rate of different plasminogens varies considerably. Furthermore the results may be influenced by the fact that it is very difficult to achieve complete activation without losses due to plasmin autodigestion. These matters have been discussed in detail in a study by Gaffney et al.[63]

The determination of plasminogen in plasma as plasmin after activation is further complicated by the presence of plasmin inhibitors which have to be removed or destroyed. A method to inactivate inhibitors selectively by acidification of plasma have been elaborated by Alkjaersig et al.[64] In other methods, the plasminogen has been selectively precipitated by acetone or ammoniumsulfate.[55,65] It has been claimed that the ammoniumsulfate precipitation method compares rather well with immunochemical methods, whereas the acid inactivation technique shows less good correlation.[66]

Plasminogen and plasmin can also be measured as equimolar complexes with streptokinase, especially on synthetic substrates. It was originally demonstrated by Kline and Fishman that the plasmin-streptokinase complex largely retains the esterase activity of plasmin, whereas the activity against proteins such as fibrin or casein is poor.[67] Reddy and Markus have later shown that the same is applicable also to the plasminogen-streptokinase complex which is quite stable in the presence of synthetic substrates in sufficient concentrations. It was also shown that the activities of the plasminogen- or plasmin-streptokinase complexes are not inhibited by soybean trypsin inhibitor.[67,68] A method for determination of plasminogen in plasma based on assay of the plasminogen-streptokinase complex with the plasmin substrate H−D−Val−Leu−Lys−Nan (S-2251, KABI) has recently been worked out.[60] The physiological plasmin inhibitors of plasma do not seem to interfere with this assay.

Plasminogen determinations by immunochemical methods have the advantage that there is no need for removal or inactivation of inhibitors. However, like other immunological methods, they give no information about biological activity and cannot easily discriminate between plasminogen, plasmin, and plasmin-inhibitor complexes. In fibrinolytic conditions, therefore, the plasminogen level may be overestimated which may give rise to large errors, e.g., during thrombolytic therapy.[77] Among immunological techniques, the radial immunodiffusion[69,70] and electroimmunodiffusion[66,71] have been commonly used. A sensitive and accurate radioimmunoassay has also been worked out by Rabiner et al.[72]

Determinations of the plasminogen level in human plasma have given somewhat different results. Rabiner et al. have made determinations with a radioimmunoassay and found 206 ± 36 μg plasminogen per milliliter plasma and reported somewhat lower values for determinations with a caseinolytic assay.[72] Using a radial immunodiffusion technique, Storiko reported levels of 200 to 400 μg/mℓ in normal sera.[70] Sherry has found levels of 100 to 200 μg plasminogen per milliliter plasma, using a caseinolytic method on acid treated plasma.[73] Collen, also using a caseinolytic technique, found 203 ± 26 μg/mℓ.[74] However, on the basis of affinity chromatography studies in which the yield has been determined to greater than 90%, Collen claims that the plasminogen level would be about 120 μg/mℓ plasma and that the values obtained by applying the caseinolytic technique to plasma may be overestimated.

IV. THE PRIMARY STRUCTURE OF PLASMINOGEN AND PLASMIN

Native plasminogen consists of a single polypeptide chain composed of 790 amino acid residues and about 2% carbohydrate. The molecule has glutamic acid as single NH_2-terminal amino acid,[20,21,23] asparagine as COOH-terminal amino acid,[25] and is stabilized by 24 disulfide bridges. One of the greatest achievements in the field of fibrinolysis during the past 5 years is the determination of the complete amino acid sequence of human plasminogen. The studies behind this have been performed by several groups which will be referred to in the following. The structure is in Figure 1* which describes the complete amino acid sequence and disulfide bridge arrangement in plasminogen.**

From studies on the structure of Lys-plasminogen and on the plasmin obtained by activation of this type of plasminogen, Robbins et al. have shown that plasmin is formed by proteolytic cleavage of the single chain plasminogen molecule into two polypeptides of unequal size connected by disulfide bonding.[25] The large chain, heavy chain, or A-chain (mol wt about 60,000) is derived from the NH_2-terminal part of plasminogen and the small chain, light chain, or B-chain (mol wt about 25,000), is derived from its COOH-terminal part.[25] Robbins et al. furthermore suggested that the activation of plasminogen occurs by cleavage of a single arginyl-valine bond.[25,76] It has subsequently been shown that two types of plasmin may arise on activation of Glu-plasminogen. One of them, "Lys-plasmin", is identical to the one obtained from Lys-plasminogen, whereas the other one, "Glu-plasmin", contains an A-chain consisting of the complete NH_2-terminal part of Glu-plasminogen. The relationship between the different plasminogens and plasmins will be discussed in Section VI.A.

Lys-plasminogen is derived from the native plasminogen, Glu-plasminogen, by the release of peptides from the NH_2-terminal part of the molecule. As discussed in later sections, this transformation also occurs during in vitro activation of plasminogen and is then accompanied by significant changes of conformation and activation kinetics. It was therefore of obvious interest to examine the difference between these two types of plasminogen with regard to primary structure. Determinations of the primary structure of the 81 amino acid residues in the NH_2-terminal part of Glu-plasminogen were performed on peptides released during activation and by treatment with cyanogen-bromide.[78,79] This sequence overlapped the NH_2-terminal sequence of Lys-plasminogen which was known earlier.[80] The main NH_2-terminal residue of Lys-plasminogen was recognized as Lys_{77} in the sequence of Glu-plasminogen (Figure 2a).

It was of considerable interest for the understanding of plasminogen activation to determine the sequence of the region of plasminogen in which a proteolytic cleavage generates active plasmin. The amino acid sequence of the NH_2-terminal part of the B-(light) chain of plasmin was first studied.[80,81] By sequence studies of cyanogen bromide fragments or a chymotryptic fragment obtained from plasminogen and plasmin, Wiman and Wallén[82,83] and Sottrup-Jensen et al.[84] independently succeeded in deducing

* Figure 1 is the color plate following page 24.

** Residue Gln_{32} of this figure is probably not present in the structure. All numbers should therefore be reduced by one. This correction has been done when numbering the residues in the text. A disulfide bridge, Cys_{168}–Cys_{296}, connecting the second and third "kringle" structure is not indicated in the figure.

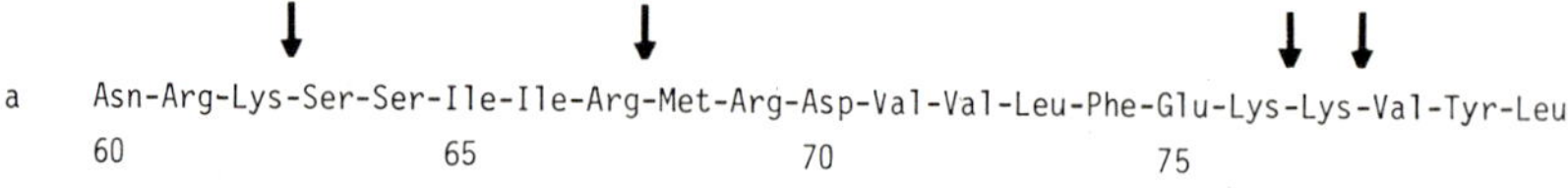

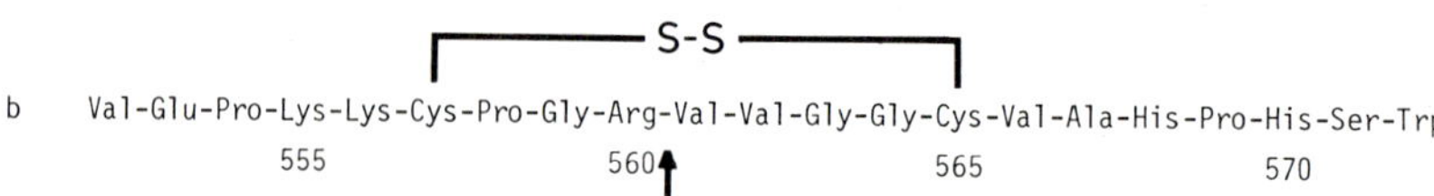

FIGURE 2. Sequences over the parts of Glu-plasminogen in which cleavages occur during activation. (a) Cleavages in the NH_2-terminal part of plasminogen, which result in the generation of Lys-plasminogen; the arrows indicate plasminsensitive peptide bonds, and (b) the cleavage resulting in generation of active plasmin; the arrow indicates the activatorsensitive bond.

the amino acid sequence on both sides of the urokinase-sensitive site (Figure 2b). These investigations on the structure of plasminogen and plasmin have confirmed the earlier suggestions by Robbins et al.[25] that the generation of the two-chain structure of plasmin follows the cleavage of a single arginyl-valine bond.

The amino acid sequence of the two regions in which proteolysis occurs during activation of plasminogen is in Figure 2. The conversion of Glu-plasminogen to Lys-plasminogen is accompanied by the cleavage of at least one of three bonds in the NH_2-terminal part of plasminogen leading to the appearance of Met_{68}, Lys_{77}, or Val_{78} as new NH_2-terminal amino acids (Figure 2a). As discussed below, these cleavages seem to be caused autocatalytically by plasmin. The urokinase-sensitive peptide bond, Arg_{560}−Val_{561} (Figure 2b), is situated in a narrow disulfide loop formed by the disulfide bridge Cys_{557}−Cys_{565}. This structure is probably of importance for the specific interaction with activators. Thus, the synthetic substrate Bz−Pro−Gly−Arg−Nan which is based on the sequence preceeding the bond attacked by the activators is cleaved by urokinase, but at a slow rate.[85] It has furthermore been observed that a peptic fragment obtained from plasminogen and containing this loop intact was a good substrate for plasminogen activators, whereas fragments with this disulfide bridge reduced and carboxymethylated are not.[29,83,84] After activation the disulfide bridge forming this loop becomes an interchain disulfide which in plasmin connects the COOH-terminal part of the A-chain with the NH_2-terminal part of the B-chain. This disulfide bridge is unique for plasmin. There is also a second interchain bridge, Cys_{547}−Cys_{665}, which according to the adjacent sequence in the B-chain corresponds to the single interchain disulfide bridge of chymotrypsin.[29,86]

The primary structure of the A- (heavy) chain part of plasminogen has to a large extent been clarified by Magnusson et al. The NH_2-terminal part of the fragment overlapping the A- (heavy) and the B- (light) chain parts of plasminogen showed a high degree of sequential homology with the two so called "kringle" structures of prothrombin.[84,85] The "kringle" structure is a characteristic triple disulfide structure originally discovered in the "pro"-fragment of prothrombin, where it occurs in two variants, one in the A-fragment and the other in the S-fragment. The detailed structural features of the "kringle" have been described by Magnusson et al.[85,87] The occurrence of sequence homologies between prothrombin and plasminogen has been confirmed by others.[83,88,89] Studies of the sequence of fragments obtained from plasminogen by proteolytic digestion suggested the presence of five mutually homologous "kringle" structures in the A-chain part of plasminogen (Figure 1). They have been numbered 1 to 5 (K-1, K-2, K-3, K-4, and K-5), as counted from the NH_2-terminal part of plasminogen.[85] This was confirmed by complete amino acid sequence studies of the A-chain of plasmin and by defining most of the disulfide bridges in this part of the plasminogen molecule.[29]

Plasminogen contains 2 to 3% carbohydrate, all of which is found in the A-chain of plasmin.[82,90] The oligosacharides seem to be bound to Asn_{280} and Thr_{345}.[29] The carbohydrate composition and its influence on the physicochemical properties of plasminogen will be discussed in Section V.C.

It has been shown by Robbins et al. that the serine and histidine of the catalytic site is localized to the B-chain of plasmin and furthermore that the amino acid sequences around these residues are homologous to corresponding parts of other serine proteases, such as chymotrypsin and trypsin.[41,44] The complete sequence of the B-chain has recently been determined independently by Wiman and Sottrup-Jensen et al.[86,91] The B-chain of plasmin is highly homologous to other pancreatic serine enzymes, especially chymotrypsin. The number and position of the intrachain disulfide bridges are exactly as in chymotrypsin. The catalytic site is formed by His_{605},Asp_{645}, and Ser_{740}. As in other serine proteases with specificity towards basic amino acids, the bottom of the substrate binding pocket consists of the side chain of aspartic acid (Asp_{734}).

V. PHYSICOCHEMICAL PROPERTIES OF PLASMINOGEN AND PLASMIN

A. Hydrodynamic Properties and Molecular Weights of Plasminogen and Plasmin

The hydrodynamic properties of Glu-plasminogen, Lys-plasminogen, and plasmin as found by Sjöholm et al.[92] and Robbins et al.[93] are in Table 1. The values of sedimentation constant, partial specific volume, and frictional coefficient accord on the whole and agree also with findings in other laboratories.[6,94,95] These data give important information on the conformation of the different types of plasminogen and plasmin and will be discussed later on in this section. The values on molecular weights as determined by sedimentation equilibrium analysis differ, however, the values of Robbins et al.[93] in general being somewhat lower than those of Sjöholm et al.[92] A remarkable finding is the fact that the difference between the molecular weights of Glu-plasminogen and Lys-plasminogen as obtained by ultracentrifuge analysis is 1000 to 2000 *Mr* in both laboratories, whereas the difference calculated from the known amino acid sequence of the two plasminogen forms is almost 9000 *Mr*. The latter value is in better agreement with the determinations of molecular weights based on sodium dodecylsulfate polyacrylamide gel electrophoresis (Table 1).[27,81,92,94] It is likely that the anomalous values obtained from hydrodynamic studies are due to a change to a more hydrated and/or asymmetric form on the transformation of Glu-plasminogen to Lys-plasminogen. This assumption is supported by the fact that Lys-plasminogen elutes earlier than Glu-plasminogen on gel filtration[22] which is furthermore in agreement with more thorough physicochemical studies showing that Stokes' radius is larger for Lys-plasminogen than for Glu-plasminogen.[92] Ultracentrifuge analysis of both the plasminogen forms under denaturating conditions (6 *M* guanidiniumhydrochloride) has furthermore shown that the sedimentation coefficient is clearly lower for Lys-plasminogen than for Glu-plasminogen, indicating a significant difference in molecular weight.[92] According to circular dichroism measurements in the far UV range (200 to 250 nm), Glu-plasminogen contains no α-structure and only about 20% β-structure. Thus, the greater part of plasminogen has a random structure.[92] Measurements of Lys-plasminogen and DFP-treated plasmin in the same wavelength interval gave similar results, indicating

TABLE 1

The Hydrodynamic Properties of Glu-plasminogen, Lys-plasminogen, and Lys-plasmin

	Sedimentation constant		Partial specific volume		Frictional ratio		Molecular weight			
							Sedimentation equilibrium		SDS-PAG[a]	
	c	d	c	d	c	d	c	d	d	Calculated[b]
Glu-plasminogen	5.0	5.1	0.709	0.706	1.54	1.50	83800	92000	93000	90600
Lys-plasminogen	4.4	4.8	0.714	0.709	1.63	1.56	82400	90000	86000	81900
Lys-plasmin	4.3	4.3	0.714	0.713	1.64	1.55	76500	81000	—	81900

[a] Sodium dodecylsulphate-polyacrylamide electrophoresis. Sjöholm, I., Wiman, B., and Wallén, P., *Eur. J. Biochem.*, 39, 471, 1973.

[b] Calculated from the known amino acid sequences and corrected for a carbohydrate content of 2.5%.

[c] Robbins, K. C., Boreisha, J. G., Arzadon, L., Summaria, L., and Barlow, G. H., *J. Biol. Chem.*, 250, 4044, 1975.

[d] Sjoholm, I., Wiman, B., and Wallén, P., *Eur. J. Biochem.*, 39, 471, 1973.

small, if any, differences in α- and β-structures between the different forms of plasminogen and plasmin. Circular dichroism measurements performed in the near UV range (250 to 308 nm) indicated, however, significant changes in conformation during the transformation of Glu-plasminogen to Lys-plasminogen and additional changes on the conversion of Lys-plasminogen to plasmin.[92] Of interest is that ε-aminocaproic acid and lysine in concentrations of 0.01 and 0.1 *M*, respectively, induced a change of the circular dichroism pattern of a Glu-plasminogen solution similar to that observed on conversion to plasmin.

The alteration in structure caused by the release of NH_2-terminal peptide material from native plasminogen seems to be partially reversible. Addition of an excess of the NH_2-terminal peptide isolated from an activation mixture to a solution of Lys-plasminogen restored to a large extent the conformation of the native plasminogen as measured by spectropolarimetry.[92] These results indicate that an intramolecular noncovalent interaction, in which the NH_2-terminal part of the molecule participates, is important for the conformation of the native plasminogen and that a disruption of this bond with accompanying conformational change may be effected either by proteolysis or interaction with antifibrinolytic amino acids, e.g., ε-aminocaproic acid. Such an interaction has in fact been demonstrated by adsorption of NH_2-terminal peptides, Glu_1–Lys_{62} and Ala_{44}–Lys_{50}, isolated from plasmic and tryptic digests of Glu-plasminogen to insolubilized Lys-plasminogen.[96] Elution was performed with 5 m*M* ε-aminocaproic acid, indicating that a lysine binding site (see Section V.B.) may be involved in this interaction.

B. Interaction of Plasminogen with the Antifibrinolytic Amino Acids. Lysine Binding Sites

The discovery by Okamoto et al.[97] of the antifibrinolytic effect of ε-aminocaproic acid (ε-ACA, 6-aminohexanoic acid) has been of great importance in clinical practice and for many studies of the fibrinolytic enzyme system. Subsequently the search for more potent antifibrinolytic substances has resulted in the development and use of compounds, such as *trans*-aminomethyl cyclohexane-1-carboxylic acid (*t*-AMCHA, tranexamic acid) and *p*-aminobenzoic acid (PAMBA).[98,99] Lysine belongs also to these compounds, although it has a much weaker effect than the former compounds. The common feature for these substances is that they possess a basic and an acidic group within a certain distance from each other (about 0.7 nm). In spite of an extensive literature on the subject, the background to the effects of these compounds on the fibrinolytic system is still not fully understood. It has been shown that ε-aminocaproic and aminomethylcyclohexanoic acid are weak competitive inhibitors to urokinase-catalyzed hydrolysis of synthetic substrates.[100] It has also been claimed that the antifibrinolytic amino acids exert their effect by interaction with fibrin. Other studies have failed to demonstrate such an interaction.[101] There are good reasons to believe that the main target for these amino acids in the fibrinolytic system is plasminogen itself.

It is now well established that lysine and the antifibrinolytic amino acids interact specifically with one or more binding sites in plasminogen. Such sites are in the following named "lysine binding sites" (LBS). These interactions are important for the effects of the antifibrinolytic amino acids in fibrinolysis. This section will mainly deal with the effect of these compounds on the physicochemical properties of plasminogen. As first demonstrated by Alkjaersig, the presence of ε-aminocaproic acid in a solution of plasminogen causes a change in sedimentation behavior consisting of a significant decrease of sedimentation coefficient from about 5 to 4.3 S.[6] This change is reversible, and it was proposed that it is due to a conformational alteration of the plasminogen molecule. Similar results have been obtained by others (see Abiko et al. and Brockway and Castellino).[14,102,103] Further support for conformational changes induced by antifibrinolytic amino acids have been given by gel filtration,[22] circular dichroism,[92] and rotational diffusion measurements.[104] The data suggest an increase of Stokes' radius, indicating that the antifibrinolytic amino acids cause an "opening" of the structure. The effects are only observed when Glu-plasminogen is studied, whereas the conformation of Lys-plasminogen seems to be very little affected by the antifibrinolytic amino acids.[92,103] Of considerable interest is that the physicochemical effects of the amino acids are very similar to the effects observed on transformation of Glu-plasminogen to Lys-plasminogen and plasmin. In both cases, there are a decrease of sedimentation constant, an increase of Stokes' radius, and a similar change of circular dichroism pattern in the near UV range.[22,92,103] As discussed in Section V.A. the changes of conformation underlying these effects may be largely explained by the dissociation of an intramolecular noncovalent interaction involving the NH_2-terminal part of native plasminogen and a lysine binding site.

The studies by Abiko et al. indicated that the antifibrinolytic amino acids form a stoichiometric 1:1 complex with plasminogen.[102] The dissociation constants for the assumed stoichiometric complexes between plasminogen and *trans*-aminomethylcyclohexanoic acid and ε-aminocaproic acid or lysine have been determined to about 0.08, 0.45, and 68 m*M*, respectively.[14] More recent studies have indicated that plasminogen contains more than one lysine binding site. Thus, determinations of Iwamoto have indicated a binding ratio of 2 mol aminomethylcyclohexanoic acid per mole plasminogen and plasmin.[101] A direct evidence for more than one lysine binding site in plasminogen was also given by Paoni and Castellino, who showed that two large fragments obtained by digestion of sheep plasminogen with plasmin both were adsorbed on lysine Sepharose.[105] Sottrup-Jensen et al. succeeded to cleave human plasminogen with elastase into three main types of fragments, two of which both originating from the A- (heavy) chain part of the molecule were adsorbed to lysine Sepharose.[29] By using an ultrafiltration technique, Markus et al. recently gave evidence for the presence of between five or six binding sites for ε-aminocaproic acid in human Glu-plasminogen. One of these sites seemed to have high affinity for ε-aminocaproic acid, the dissociation constant being 9 μ*M*, which is considerably lower than the earlier reported value.[106] The dissociation constants for the weaker sites were about 5 m*M*. Studies on Lys-plasminogen showed that the proteolytically modified plasminogen possesses the same number of lysine binding sites, although the affinity for ε-aminocaproic acid had decreased somewhat for the strong binding site (dissociation constant 35 μ*M*) and increased for one of the weak sites (dissociation constants 0.26 m*M*).[107] Evidence for a high-affinity lysine binding site in plasmin has also been given by the fact that the rate of the first reversible step in the interaction between plasmin and antiplasmin which is dependent on a lysine binding site in plasmin is effectively decreased to 50% by ε-aminocaproic acid in a concentration of 20 μ*M*.[108]

Some knowledge of localization and structure of the lysine binding site(s) of plasmin and plasminogen has recently been acquired. Using affinity chromatography on lysine Sepharose of partially reduced plasmin, Rickli and Otavsky have shown that the association of the antifibrinolytic amino acids is confined to the heavy chain of plasmin.[109] One lysine binding site has been found in a chymotryptic fragment from the plasmin A-chain originating from the first kringle situated in the NH_2-terminal part of the A-chain.[110] One of the two fragments with affinity for lysine Sepharose isolated by Sottrup-Jensen et al. from elastase digests of human plasminogen contained the three NH_2-terminal kringles (K-1, K-2, and K-3) and the other, one kringle (K-4).[29] Preliminary studies indicate that also the COOH-terminal kringle (K-5) has a weak affinity to lysine.[111] Thus, it may be speculated that the kringles bear the structural elements responsible for the affinity between plasminogen and the antifibrinolytic amino acids and that the binding sites have been more or less preserved during the multiple gene-duplication which is assumed to have occurred during the evolution of the A-chain part of plasminogen.

C. The Microheterogeneity of Plasminogen

Electrophoresis on starch and polyacrylamide gels as well as isoelectric focusing have revealed a pronounced heterogeneity of highly purified plasminogen. This was first observed on starch block electrophoresis of highly purified human plasminogen at pH 4.0 in which two fractions were obtained. These fractions could also be separated by chromatography on CM-cellulose.[19] A similar separation has more recently been obtained by affinity chromatography on Sepharose lysine (Castellino et al.).[14] The latter separation has been used in several studies on the microheterogeneity of plasminogen. These two plasminogen fractions will in the following be designated plasminogen Type 1 and plasminogen Type 2.

A more complicated pattern is obtained on electrophoresis at weakly alkaline conditions (pH 8.5 to 9.5), using starch or polyacrylamide gels as supporting media. Between four and ten bands may appear depending on the species and type of plasminogen applied.[12,18,19,112,113] As first demonstrated in the rabbit, each of plasminogen Type 1 and 2 can be subdivided into about five fractions. Thus, at least ten forms of plasminogen may exist in rabbit blood.[114] Similarly the occurrence of about 12 forms of human Glu-plasminogen have been demonstrated, 6 from each of the plasminogen Types 1 and 2.[115] In accordance with these findings, Glu-plasminogen has been separated into about a dozen fractions by isoelectric focusing with isoelectric points in the range from pH 6 to about pH 7.[107] Another family of plasminogen forms range under Lys-plasminogen. These may as expected also be divided into about 12 forms by affinity chromatography on Sepharose lysine, electrophoresis in alkaline pH, and by isoelectric focusing.

Knowledge of the structure of plasminogen is still insufficient to explain in full the chemical background to the microheterogeneity. Some conclusions may, however, be drawn from studies performed in the last few years. Thus, it has been demonstrated that plasminogen Type 1 in rabbit, as well as in human plasminogen, contains 1 mol sialic acid more per mole proenzyme than Type 2.[115,116] On removal of the sialic acid, the charge difference between the two types decreases, whereas the difference in affinity to Sepharose lysine is retained. The carbohydrate composition of different forms of rabbit plasminogen has been studied by Hayes et al.[117] All carbohydrate was localized to the A-chain part of plasminogen, whereas the B-chain was devoid of carbohydrate ligands. Plasminogen Type 1 had a considerably higher content of carbohydrate than Type 2. Still more remarkable, however, was the qualitative difference between the two forms; Type 1 contained glucosamine, galactosamine, mannose, and galactose, whereas Type 2 contained galactosamine and galactose, but lacked glucosamine and mannose.

Two sites for attachment of oligosaccharides have been found in the structure of human plasminogen.[29] One of them containing glucosamine was linked to Asn_{288} situated in kringle 3, and the other one containing galactosamine was linked to Thr_{345}. The Asn_{288}-linked glucosamine containing oligosaccharide seems to be missing in a part of plasminogen which could then be the background to the properties of plasminogen Type 2. There is also evidence that variations in the composition of the oligosaccharide substituted on Thr_{345} may be the chemical background to other heterogeneous forms.[29] Thus, variations in the structure of the oligosaccharide ligands seem to be mainly responsible for the occurrence of different molecular forms of plasminogen. Other causes for the microheterogeneity, however, can not be excluded. Reports have appeared on the occurrence of several forms of fragments of plasminogen which seem not to contain carbohydrates. Thus, the B-chain and a COOH-terminal fragment of the A-chain of plasmin have been separated into several components by electrophoresis.[82,113] The structural cause of this microheterogeneity, however, has not been elucidated.

VI. ACTIVATION OF PLASMINOGEN

Activation of plasminogen is effected in vivo by several activators. The mode of action of these activators is somewhat different. However, the structural changes in the plasminogen molecule seem to be about the same.[76] The commercially available activator, urokinase, which can be obtained in highly purified state is one of the most commonly used activators in studies on plasminogen activation. In the studies reviewed in the following section, urokinase has, in general, been used as the activator.

A. Changes of the Primary Structure of Plasminogen During Activation

As discussed above (see the section entitled The Primary Structure of Plasminogen and Plasmin), early studies by Robbins and co-workers showed that the activation of Lys-plasminogen to plasmin is achieved by the cleavage of a single peptide bond (Arg−Val), generating the A- and B-chains of plasmin.[25,76] The finding of Wallén and Wiman that Lys-plasminogen is generated from the native plasminogen, Glu-plasminogen, by a release of peptides from the NH_2-terminal part of the molecule and that this degradation will cause marked changes of the properties of plasminogen[22,92] made it necessary to reinvestigate the structural changes on activation of plasminogen. Preliminary investigations indicated that plasmin obtained by activation of Glu-plasminogen in vitro was identical with plasmin generated from Lys-plasminogen.[118] This indicated that a cleavage in the NH_2-terminal part occurred in addition to the one demonstrated by Robbins et al.

In the past years, there has been much discussion about the structural changes occurring in plasminogen during activation. The questions at issue have mainly been centered around two problems. One is whether both sensitive sites in Glu-plasminogen are attacked by the activators or if the cleavage in the NH_2-terminal part of the molecule is effectuated autocatalytically by plasmin. The other question is whether the activation is a two-step reaction in which Lys-plasminogen in the first step is formed as an intermediary compound by release of NH_2-terminal material from Glu-plasminogen or if the cleavages at the two different parts of plasminogen occur at random. The structural relation between different possible types of plasminogen and plasmin, Glu-plasminogen, Lys-plasminogen, Glu-plasmin, and Lys-plasmin is in Figure 3.

Analysis of different derivatives of plasminogen appearing in the course of activation of Glu-plasminogen showed in addition to unmodified plasminogen, Lys-plasminogen and Lys-plasmin (see Wiman and Wallén).[118] The experimental conditions were designed to minimize eventual autocatalytic degradation, and there was no evidence for the generation of Glu-plasmin. Mainly based on these experiments, it was suggested that the activation of native plasminogen occurs in two consecutive steps, both catalyzed by the activator. Glu-plasminogen in the first step is converted to Lys-plasminogen which in the second step is transformed to active plasmin, Lys-plasmin, by cleavage of a single peptide bond. Using other techniques, Rickli and Otavsky and Walther et al. draw the same conclusions.[119,120]

Castellino et al.[121] and Robbins et al.[122] performed activation experiments of human and rabbit Glu-plasminogen with urokinase in the presence of aprotinin (Trasylol®) which effectively inhibits plasmin, but has no inhibitory effect towards urokinase. The inactive plasmin inhibitor complex formed under these conditions contained a heavy chain with the same NH_2-terminal sequence as Glu-plasminogen. Thus, no NH_2-terminal peptide was released, suggesting that urokinase does not cleave peptide bonds

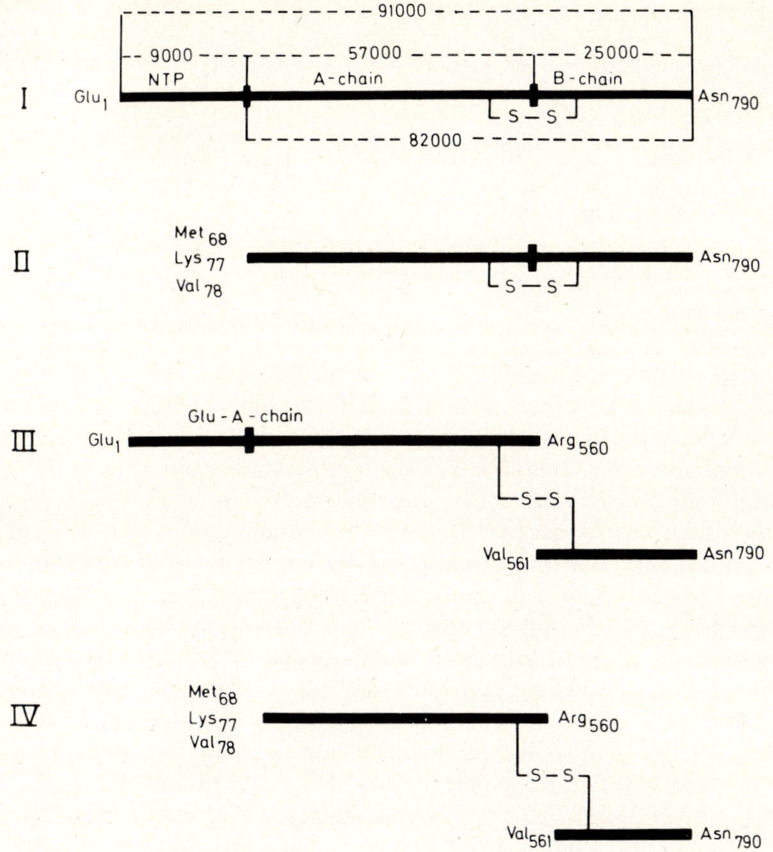

FIGURE 3. Arrangements of chains in different types of plasminogen and plasmin. (I) Glu-plasminogen, (II) Lys-plasminogen, (III) Glu-plasmin, and (IV) Lys-plasmin.

in the NH_2-terminal part of Glu-plasminogen. It was also shown that plasmin rapidly releases the NH_2-terminal peptide(s) from the A-chain of plasmin in complex with inhibitor, whereas urokinase does not.[123] These results have recently been confirmed by experiments on native Glu- A-chain obtained after partial reduction of a Glu-plasmin Trasylol® complex and isolated by affinity chromatography on lysine Sepharose®.[109] Neither urokinase nor tissue activator cleaved this derivative, whereas plasmin readily released peptide material from its NH_2-terminal part.[124] Violand and Castellino have found small amounts of Glu-plasmin in very early stages of activation of plasminogen by urokinase in the absence of inhibitors. Plasminogen, however, was very soon converted to Lys-plasminogen or Lys-plasmin in the activation process, and it was claimed that this transformation is accompanied by cleavages of a few plasmin-sensitive bonds.[125] Two pathways for activation of Glu-plasminogen were suggested by Violand and Castellino, both proceeding in two steps (Figure 4). In one of the pathways supposed to be the minor one, the first step is a conversion of Glu-plasminogen to Glu-plasmin by cleavage of a single bond, and the second step is the release of peptide(s) from the NH_2-terminal part of the heavy chain by autocatalytic degradation. In the other pathway, the first step is a conversion of Glu-plasminogen to Lys-plasminogen by the release of peptide(s) from the NH_2-terminal part of Glu-plasminogen. The Lys-plasminogen is activated in the second step to Lys-plasmin. By following the appearance of intermediate products during activation of human Glu-plasmin-

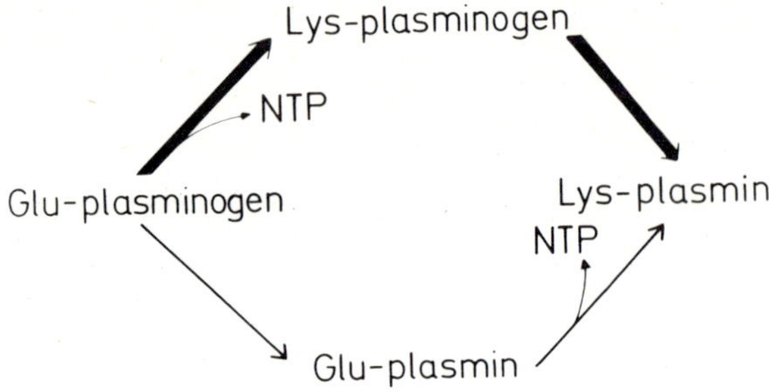

FIGURE 4. Possible pathways for the activation of Glu-plasminogen to Lys-plasmin.

ogen, Violand and Castellino concluded that the latter pathway is predominant, especially at low concentrations of urokinase.

Based on data now available, it seems justified to state that (the) specific plasminogen activators, e.g., urokinase, act by cleaving one bond ($Arg_{560}-Val_{561}$) in the plasminogen molecule. The release of NH_2-terminal peptides, which may occur during the activation process and which as discussed below has a profound effect on activation kinetics, may be caused by a plasmin "feedback" mechanism in which a few very plasmin-sensitive peptide bonds are cleaved. This proteolysis is strongly stimulated by low concentrations of antifibrinolytic amino acids. All discussions on structural changes of plasminogen during activation are based so far on experiments in pure systems. Interactions with other components present in the blood clot, such as fibrin and plasmin inhibitors, have not been taken into account. At present it is unclear whether Lys-plasmin or Glu-plasmin is the physiological thrombolytic enzyme.

B. Kinetics of the Activation of Plasminogen — Influence of Partial Proteolysis and Antifibrinolytic Amino Acids on the Activation

As mentioned earlier, the proteolytic release of NH_2-terminal peptides from native plasminogen, Glu-plasminogen, will cause a change of the gross conformation which seems to be very similar to the change of conformation induced by certain concentrations of antifibrinolytic amino acids. The structural changes may be explained in both cases by the dissociation of a noncovalent interaction between the NH_2-terminal part of plasminogen and one of the lysine binding sites in the A-chain part of the molecule. These alterations of the structure, whether they are brought about by proteolysis or by the influence of antifibrinolytic amino acids, have marked effects on the activation with urokinase.

Comparative studies have shown that urokinase activates Lys-plasminogen considerably faster (10 to 20 times) than Glu-plasminogen.[94,126,127] This suggests that the conformational change induced by the dissociation of the noncovalent bond referred to above makes the $Arg_{560}-Val_{561}$ bond more easily accessible for cleavage by urokinase.

Recently Christensen and Müllertz performed thorough kinetic analyses of the activation of both Glu-plasminogen and Lys-plasminogen by urokinase.[128,129] Their data indicate that the generation of plasmin from both these types of plasminogen follows the Michaelis-Menten equation. It was also found that the Michaelis constants are similar for both types of plasminogen (K_m for Glu-plasminogen was 23 μM and for Lys-plasminogen was 40 μM). These data do not indicate any significant difference in affinity of urokinase for Glu- or Lys-plasminogen. They found, however, that the catalytic constant for the activation reaction is about ten times higher for Lys-plasminogen than for Glu-plasminogen (k_c for Glu-plasminogen was 0.26 s^{-1} and for Lys-plasminogen was 2.6 s^{-1}).

The activation of the fibrinolytic enzyme system is strongly influenced by the antifibrinolytic amino acids. Dependent on the conditions, both inhibiting and stimulating effects are observed. Using a clot lysis time method, Thorsen et al. found that the effect of antifibrinolytic amino acids on urokinase activation of plasminogen is highly dependent on the concentration of the amino acids.[7,130] Thus, an inhibition of fibrinolysis was observed in the presence of ε-aminocaproic acid in concentrations between 10^{-5} and 10^{-3} *M*. An increase of the concentration to between 10^{-3} and 10^{-2} *M* caused a significant increase of the fibrinolytic activity, whereas further increase to more than 10^{-4} *M* again led to a marked decrease. In agreement with these findings and by using fibrin-free systems, it has been shown that the presence of between 10^{-3} and 10^{-2} *M* ε-aminocaproic acid markedly stimulates the activation rate of Glu-plasminogen which approaches that of Lys-plasminogen.[94,107,126,127] The activability of Lys-plasminogen is not enhanced under the same conditions. Similar effects are observed with AMCHA and lysine, although in concentrations which are about tenfold lower and higher, respectively. Addition of 0.1 *M* lysine causes a significant increase of the catalytic constant for the reaction between Glu-plasminogen and urokinase, whereas the Michaelis constant remains about the same (k_c 1.5 s^{-1} and K_m 35 μM in the presence and k_c0.26s^{-1} and K_m 32 μM in the absence of lysine).[129] Thus, the changes in the kinetics of activation induced by antifibrinolytic amino acids are very similar to those observed on transformation of Glu-plasminogen to Lys-plasminogen. The effects of the antifibrinolytic amino acids in the fibrinolytic system can largely be explained by their interactions with plasminogen and plasmin. The finding by Markus et al.[106] of five or six lysine binding sites with different affinities for ε-aminocaproic acid offers an explanation for the fact that different concentrations of the amino acid may cause either inhibition or stimulation of the plasminogen activation rate. Thus, the inhibitory action at very low concentrations of ε-aminocaproic acid (10^{-5} to 10^{-3} *M*) observed by Thorsen et al.[7,130] may be explained by saturation of the single "strong" binding site. It appears from all studies so far performed that the stimulating effect on plasminogen activation and on fibrinolysis of ε-aminocaproic acid in the concentration range 1 to 10 m*M* is due to the change of the gross conformation induced by binding of the amino acid to one or more of the "weak" binding sites (K_d about 5 m*M*) defined by Markus et al. It is also very likely that the primary structural event is the dissociation of an intramolecular noncovalent interaction leading to these conformational changes and that the same effects are achieved by partial proteolysis in the NH_2-terminal part of plasminogen as described in earlier section.

VII. INTERACTION OF PLASMINOGEN AND PLASMIN WITH COMPONENTS OF THE FIBRINOLYTIC ENZYME SYSTEM

As a pure enzyme, plasmin is a rather aggressive protease capable of degrading a great variety of proteins (see Section III.A). In vivo, however, plasmin is acting largely as a fibrinolytic enzyme. The regulation behind this restricted proteolysis is not fully understood, although the research in this field during the last few years has given some valuable ideas about possible mechanisms. In broad outline, two main processes are in balance during fibrinolysis, the activation of plasminogen and the inhibition of excess plasmin. Fibrin itself may have an important function as regulator of these processes.

It was early noticed that fibrin is degraded much faster than fibrinogen in spontaneously fibrinolytic blood and that plasminogen, as well as plasminogen activators, are adsorbed to the fibrin in clotted blood. These effects of fibrin were regarded as physicologically important for the localization and acceleration of the fibrinolytic process (see Astrup and Sherry et al.).[31,131] It was suggested by Alkjaersig et al.[132] that thrombolysis is achieved by activation of plasminogen firmly bound to the fibrin by activators diffusing into the thrombus. This would allow the fibrinolytic process to take place in an environment in which the concentration of inhibitors is low. Small, if any, differences have been found between the plasminogen concentration of plasma and serum samples, and the amounts of added plasminogen adsorbed to plasma clots have varied between practically 0 and 30% in different reports (see Hedner et al. and Thorsen).[133,134] These discrepancies between different studies can at least be explained by interesting observations by Thorsen.[134] He showed that the native Glu-plasminogen has a very low affinity for fibrin. Only about 5% of the plasminogen was adsorbed to the fibrin in a clot prepared from purified fibrinogen and plasminogen in approximately the same concentrations as in normal plasma. However, if Glu-plasminogen was replaced with Lys-plasminogen, as much as 50% of the modified plasminogen was adsorbed to the fibrin. It was also shown that the binding between fibrin and plasminogen is effectively prevented by ε-aminocaproic acid in concentrations higher than 10^{-4} *M* and that most of the adsorbed plasminogen was recovered by extractions with ε-aminocaproic acid. It has been shown that chymotryptic fragments from plasminogen with molecular weights down to 7000 and with affinity for lysine Sepharose also have affinity for fibrin, indicating that one or several of the lysine binding sites are involved in this interaction.[110] Using ^{125}I-labeled Glu-plasminogen and Lys-plasminogen, Rakoczi et al. have recently shown that in plasma Lys-plasminogen has a higher affinity for fibrin than Glu-plasminogen, although the difference is smaller than reported by Thorsen.[134,135] About 5% of Glu-plasminogen and 10% of Lys-plasminogen were adsorbed to the fibrin formed in plasma which should mean that approximately 1 or 2 out of 100 monomers in the fibrin matrix contain 1 molecule of plasminogen. It was further demonstrated that the presence of antiplasmin has no influence on the adsorption of plasminogen to fibrin which is in contrast to earlier suggestions.[136]

Whether plasmin is specifically adapted for cleavage of fibrin has been a matter of discussion. In an interesting paper Landmann has compared the caseinolytic and fibrinolytic activities of plasmin with other proteolytic enzymes.[137] Plasmin was by far the most potent fibrinolytic enzyme. It was followed in efficiency by trypsin, whereas other enzymes, such as chymotrypsin, subtilisin, and papain, had very weak fibrinolytic activity, as compared to their general proteolytic activity. Thus, cleavage of lysyl- or arginyl-bonds seems to be of special importance for the fibrinolysis. There was also evidence that digestion of fibrin with plasmin proceeds in two phases, the first of which is effectively inhibited by the antifibrinolytic amino acids, whereas the second is not. These findings suggest that plasmin is directed towards certain bonds of special importance for the liquification of the fibrin gel and that this occurs by the interaction between lysine binding site(s) of plasmin and certain regions in the fibrin monomer. When the strategically situated bonds are cleaved, which may occur after the dissolution of the fibrin, plasmin continues in the second phase as an ordinary trypsin-like enzyme.

It has been shown that tissue plasminogen activator is specifically bound to fibrin.[138,139] It has also been observed that the activation of plasminogen by this activator is strongly stimulated in the presence of fibrin, an effect which ceases when the fibrin is dissolved.[139,140] This effect is neutralized by ε-aminocaproic acid in low concentrations (about 1 m*M*), indicating that the binding of plasminogen to fibrin by means of the lysine binding site(s) is of importance also for the activation of plasminogen.

Another process in which the lysine binding sites may be of physiological importance, is the inactivation of plasmin by α_2-antiplasmin. As shown by Wiman and Collen,[108] this reaction is markedly retarded by ε-aminocaproic acid in low concentration,

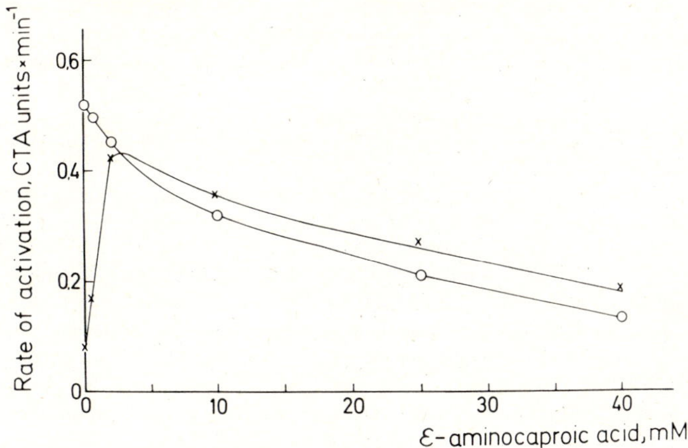

FIGURE 5. The effect of the concentration of ε-aminocaproic acid on the initial rate of plasmin generation from Glu-plasminogen (-x-x-x-) and Lys-plasminogen (-o-o-o-).

indicating that one or several lysine binding sites participate in the binding of α_2-antiplasmin to plasmin. It has also been suggested that the same lysine binding site(s) is involved in the binding of plasmin to fibrin.[141] This would prevent the inhibitor from reacting with plasmin in the presence of fibrin until after dissolution of the fibrin.

REFERENCES

1. **Kaplan, M. H.**, Nature and role of lytic factor in hemolytic streptococcal fibrinolysis, *Proc. Soc. Exp. Biol. Med.*, 57, 40, 1944.
2. **Christensen, L. R.**, Streptococcal fibrinolysis: a proteolytic reaction due to a serum enzyme activated by streptococcal fibrinolysin, *J. Gen. Physiol.*, 28, 363, 1945.
3. **Christensen, L. R. and MacLeod, C. M.**, A proteolytic enzyme of serum: characterization, activation and reaction with inhibitors, *J. Gen. Physiol.*, 28, 559, 1945.
4. **Remmert, L. F. and Cohen, P.**, Partial purification and properties of a proteolytic enzyme of human serum, *J. Biol. Chem.*, 181, 431, 1949.
5. **Kline, D. L.**, Purification and crystallization of plasminogen (profibrinolysin), *J. Biol. Chem.*, 204, 949, 1953.
6. **Alkjaersig, N.**, The purification and properties of human plasminogen, *Biochem. J.*, 93, 171, 1964.
7. **Thorsen, S., Kok, P., and Astrup, T.**, Reversible and irreversible alterations of human plasminogen indicated by changes in susceptibility to plasminogen activators and in response to ε-aminocaproic acid, *Thromb. Diath. Haemorrh.*, 32, 325, 1974.
8. **Alkjaersig, N., Fletcher, A. P., and Sherry, G.**, ε-Aminocaproic acid: an inhibitor of plasminogen activation, *J. Biol. Chem.*, 234, 832, 1959.
9. **Ablondi, F. B., Hagan, J. J., Philips, M., and de Renzo, E. C.**, Inhibition of plasmin, trypsin and the streptokinase-activated fibrinolytic system by ε-aminocaproic acid, *Arch. Biochem. Biophys.*, 82, 153, 1959.
10. **Wallén, P. and Bergström, P.**, Purification of human plasminogen on DEAE-cellulose, *Acta Chem. Scand.*, 14, 217, 1960.
11. **Heberlein, P. J. and Barnhart, M. I.**, The purification of profibrinolysin and fibrinolysin, in *Thrombosis and Bleeding Disorders*, Bang, N. U., Beller, F. K., Deutsch, E., and Mammen, E. F., Eds., Academic Press, New York, 1971, 336.
12. **Deutsch, D. G. and Mertz, E. T.**, Plasminogen purification from human plasma by affinity chromatography, *Science*, 170, 1095, 1970.

13. **Chibber, B. A. K., Deutsch, D. G., and Mertz, E. T.**, Plasminogen, in *Methods of Enzymology*, Vol. 34, Jak-by, W. B. and Wilchek, M., Academic Press, New York, 1974, 424.
14. **Brockway, W. J. and Castellino, F. J.**, Measurement of the binding of antifibrinolytic amino acids to various plasminogens, *Arch. Biochem. Biophys.*, 151, 194, 1972.
15. **Bergström, K.**, Purification of bovine plasminogen, *Ark. Kemi*, 21, 517, 1963.
16. **Heberlein, P. J. and Barnhart, M. I.**, Canine plasminogen: purification and a demonstration of multimulecular forms, *Biochim. Biophys. Acta*, 168, 195, 1968.
17. **Summaria, L., Arzadon, L., Bernabe, P., and Robbins, K. C.**, Isolation, characterization, and comparison of the S-carboxymethyl heavy (A) and light (B) chain derivatives of cat, dog, rabbit, and bovine plasmins, *J. Biol. Chem.*, 248, 6522, 1973.
18. **Wallén, P.**, Studies on the purification of human plasminogen. I. The preparations of a partially purified human plasminogen with low spontaneous activity, *Ark. Kemi*, 19, 451, 1962.
19. **Wallén, P.**, Studies on the purification of human plasminogen. II. Further purification of human plasminogen on cellulose ion exchangers and by means of gel filtration through Sephadex, *Ark. Kemi*, 19, 469, 1962.
20. **Bergström, K. and Wallén, P.**, Purification and properties of plasminogen, in *Proc. 9th Congr. Eur. Soc. Haematology, Lisbon 1963*, S. Karger, New York, 1963, 1325.
21. **Wallén, P. and Wiman, B.**, Characterization of human plasminogen. I. On the relationship between different molecular forms of plasminogen demonstrated in plasma and found in purified preparations, *Biochim. Biophys. Acta*, 221, 20, 1970.
22. **Wallén, P. and Wiman, B.**, Characterization of human plasminogen. II. Separation and partial characterization of different molecular forms of human plasminogen, *Biochim. Biophys. Acta*, 257, 122, 1972.
23. **Rickli, E. E. and Cuendet, P. A.**, Isolation of plasmin-free human plasminogen with N-terminal glutamic acid, *Biochim. Biophys. Acta*, 250, 447, 1971.
24. **Robbins, K. C., Summaria, L., Elwyn, O., and Barlow, G. H.**, Further studies on the purification and characterization of human plasminogen and plasmin, *J. Biol. Chem.*, 240, 541, 1965.
25. **Robbins, K. C., Summaria, L., Hsieh, B., and Shah, R.**, The peptide chains of human plasmin. Mechanism of activation of human plasminogen to plasmin, *J. Biol. Chem.*, 242, 2333, 1967.
26. **Summaria, L., Spitz, F., Arzadon, L., Boreisha, I. G., and Robbins, K. C.**, Isolation and characterization of the affinity chromatography forms of human Glu- and Lys-plasminogens and plasmins, *J. Biol. Chem.*, 251, 3693, 1976.
27. **Claeys, H., Molla, A., and Verstraete, M.**, Conversion of NH_2-terminal glutamic acid to NH_2-terminal lysine human plasminogen by plasmin, *Thromb. Res.*, 3, 315, 1973.
28. **Wallén, P. and Wiman, B.**, On the generation of intermediate plasminogen and its significance for activation, in *Proteases and Biological Control*, Reich, E., Rifkin, D. B., and Shaw, E., Eds., Cold Spring Harbor Laboratory, Cold Spring Harbor, N.Y., 1975, 291.
29. **Sottrup-Jensen, L., Claeys, H., Zajdel, M., Petersen, T. E., and Magnusson, S.**, The primary structure of human plasminogen: isolation of two lysine-binding fragments and one "mini"-plasminogen (MW 38000) by elastase-catalyzed-specific limited proteolysis, in *Progress in Chemical Fibrinolysis*, Vol. 3, Davidson, J. F., Rowan, R. M., Samama, M. M., and Desnoyers, P. C., Eds., Raven Press, New York, 1978, 191.
30. **Collen, D. and Verstraete, M.**, Molecular biology of human plasminogen. II. Metabolism in physicological and some pathological conditions in man, *Thromb. Diath. Haemorrh.*, 34, 403, 1975.
31. **Sherry, S., Fletcher, A., and Alkjaersig, N.**, Fibrinolysis and fibrinolytic activity in man, *Physiol. Rev.*, 39, 343, 1959.
32. **Troll, W., Sherry, S., and Wachman, J.**, The action of plasmin on synthetic substrates, *J. Biol. Chem.*, 208, 85, 1954.
33. **Wallén, P. and Iwanaga, S.**, Difference between plasmic and tryptic digests of human S-sulfo-fibrinogen, *Biochim. Biophys. Acta*, 154, 414, 1968.
34. **Iwanaga, S., Wallén, P., Grondahl, N. J., Henschen, A., and Blomback, B.**, Isolation and characterization of N-terminal fragments obtained by plasmin digestion of human fibrinogen, *Biochim. Biophys. Acta*, 147, 606, 1967.
35. **Groskopf, W. R., Hsieh, B., Summaria, L., and Robbins, K. C.**, The specificity of human plasmin on the B-chain of oxidized bovine insulin, *Biochim. Biophys. Acta*, 168, 376, 1968.
36. **Wallén, P.**, Plasmic degradation of fibrinogen, in *Scand. J. Haematol. Suppl.*, 13, 3, 1971.
37. **Wallén, P. and Bergstrom, K.**, Action of thrombin on plasmindigested fibrinogen, *Acta Chem. Scand.*, 12, 574, 1958.
38. **Weinstein, M. J. and Doolittle, R. F.**, Differential specificities of thrombin, plasmin and trypsin with regard to synthetic and natural substrates and inhibitors, *Biochim. Biophys. Acta*, 258, 577, 1972.

39. **Mounter, L. A. and Shipley, B. A.**, The inhibition of plasmin by toxic phosphorous compounds, *J. Biol. Chem.*, 231, 855, 1958.
40. **Summaria, L., Hsieh, B., Groskopf, W. R., and Robbins, K. C.**, The isolation and characterization of the S-carboxymethyl β (light) chain of human plasmin, *J. Biol. Chem.*, 242, 5046, 1967.
41. **Groskopf, W. R., Summaria, L., and Robbins, K. C.**, Studies on the active center of human plasmin. Partial amino acid sequence of a peptide containing the active center serine residue, *J. Biol. Chem.*, 244, 3590, 1969.
42. **Schoellmann, G. and Shaw, E.**, Direct evidence for the presence of histidine in the active center of chymotrypsin, *Biochemistry*, 2, 252, 1963.
43. **Shaw, E., Mares-Guia, M., and Cohen, W.**, Evidence for an active-center histidine in trypsin through use of a specific reagent 1-chloro-3-tosylamido-7-amino-2-heptanon the chloromethyl ketone derived from N^{α}-tosyl-L-lysine, *Biochemistry*, 4, 2219, 1965.
44. **Groskopf, W. R., Hsieh, B., Summaria, L., and Robbins, K. C.**, Studies on the active center of human plasmin. The serine and histidine residues, *J. Biol. Chem.*, 244, 359, 1969.
45. **Shaw, E.**, Progress in designing small inhibitors which discriminate among trypsin-like enzymes, in *Proteinase Inhibitors (Bayer-Symposium V)*, Fritz, H., Tschesche, H., Greene, L. J., and Truscheit, E., Eds., Springer-Verlag, Berlin, 531, 1974.
46. **Shaw, E.**, Synthetic protease inhibitors acting by affinity labeling, in *Proteases and Biological Control*, Reich, E., Rifkin, D. B., and Shaw, E., Eds., Cold Spring Harbor Laboratory, Cold Spring Harbor, N.Y., 1975, 455.
47. **Chase, T., Jr. and Shaw, E.**, Comparison of the esterase activities of trypsin, plasmin and thrombin on guanidinobenzoate esters. Titration of the enzymes, *Biochemistry*, 8, 2213, 1969.
48. **Chase, T., Jr. and Shaw, E.**, Titration of trypsin, plasmin and thrombin with *p*-nitrophenyl *p*′-guanidinobenzoate HCl, *Methods of Enzymology*, Vol. 19, Perlmann, G. E. and Lorand, L., Eds., Academic Press, New York, 1970, 20.
49. **Schick, L. A. and Castellino, F. J.**, Direct evidence for the generation of an active site in the plasminogen moiety of the streptokinase-human plasminogen activator complex, *Biochem. Biophys. Res. Commun.*, 57, 47, 1974.
50. **Müllertz, S.**, Formation and properties of the activator of plasminogen and of human and bovine plasmin, *Biochem. J.*, 61, 424, 1955.
51. **Johnson, A. J., Kline, D. L., and Alkjaersig, N.**, Assay methods and standard preparations for plasmin, plasminogen and urokinase in purified systems, *Thromb. Diath. Haemorrh.*, 21, 259, 1969.
52. **Nilsson, I. M., Skanse, B., and Gydell, K.**, Fibrinolysis in Boeck's sarcoid, *Acta Med. Scand.*, 159, 463, 1957.
53. **Lassen, M.**, The estimation of fibrinolytic components by means of the lysis tissue method, *Scand. J. Clin. Lab. Invest.*, 10, 384, 1958.
54. **Kowalski, E., Kopec, M., and Niewiarowski, S.**, An evaluation of the euglobin method for the determination of fibrinolysis, *J. Clin. Pathol.*, 12, 215, 1959.
55. **Brakman, P.**, A Standardized Fibrin Plate Method and a Fibrinolytic Assay of Plasminogen, Ph.D. thesis, University of Amsterdam, Scheltema and Holkema, Amsterdam, 1967.
56. **Vignal, A., Blatrix, C., and Steinbuch, M.**, Fibrinogen free of plasminogen as substrate for fibrinolytic assays, *Nature (London)*, 193, 693, 1962.
57. **Kline, D. L. and Fishman, J. B.**, The humoral protease, *Ann. N.Y. Acad. Sci.*, 68, 25, 1957.
58. **Claeson, G., Aurell, L., Karlsson, G., and Friberger, P.**, Substrate structure and activity relationships, in *Progress in Chemical Fibrinolysis and Thrombolysis*, Vol. 3, Davidson, J. F., Rowan, R. M., Samama, M. M., and Desnoyers, P. C., Eds., Raven Press, New York, 1978, 299.
59. **Soria, J., Soria, C., and Samama, M.**, A plasminogen assay using a chromogenic synthetic substrate: results from clinical work and from studies of thrombolysis, in *Progress in Chemical Fibrinolysis and Thrombolysis*, Vol. 3, Davidson, J. F., Rowan, R. M., Samama, M. M., and Desnoyers, P. C., Eds., Raven Press, New York, 1978, 337.
60. **Friberger, P., Knös, M., Gustavsson, S., Aurell, L., and Claeson, G.**, Methods for determination of plasmin, antiplasmin and plasmin by means of substrate S-2251, *Haemostasis*, 7, 138, 1978.
61. **Sgouris, J. T., Inman, J. K., McCall, K. B., Heyndman, L. A., and Anderson, H. D.**, The preparation of human fibrinolysine (plasmin), *Vox Sang.*, 5, 357, 1960.
62. **Kirkwood, T. B. L., Campbell, P. J., and Gaffney, P. J.**, A standard for human plasmin, *Thromb. Diath. Haemorrh.*, 34, 20, 1975.
63. **Gaffney, P. J., Brasher, M., Lord, K., and Kirkwood, T. B. L.**, Activation of plasminogen as a feature in its assay, *Haemostasis*, 6, 72, 1977.
64. **Alkjaersig, N., Fletcher, A. P., and Sherry, S.**, The mechanism of clot dissolution by plasmin, *J. Clin. Invest.*, 38, 1086, 1959.
65. **Hedner, U., Nilsson, I., and Robertson, B.**, Determination of plasminogen in clots and thrombi, *Thrombos. Diathes. Haemorrh.*, 16, 38, 1966.

66. **Ganrot, P. O. and Nilehn, J. E.,** Immunochemical determination of human plasminogen, *Clin. Chim. Acta,* 22, 335, 1968.
67. **Kline, D. L. and Fishman, J. B.,** Proactivator function of human plasmin as shown by lysine esterase assay, *J. Biol. Chem.,* 236, 2807, 1961.
68. **Reddy, K. N. N. and Markus, G.,** Esterase activities in the zymogen moiety of the streptokinase-plasminogen complex, *J. Biol. Chem.,* 249, 4851, 1974.
69. **Mancini, G., Carbonara, A. O., and Heremans, J. F.,** Immunological quantitation of antigens by single radial immunodiffusion, *Immunochemistry,* 2, 235, 1965.
70. **Störiko, K.,** Normal values for 23 different human plasma proteins determined by single radioimmunodiffusion, *Blut,* 16, 200, 1968.
71. **Laurell, C. B.,** Quantitative estimation of proteins by electrophoresis in agarose gel containing antibodies, *Anal. Biochem. Exp. Med.,* 15, 45, 1966.
72. **Rabiner, S. F., Goldfine, I. D., Hart, A., Summaria, L., and Robbins, K. C.,** Radioimmunoassay of human plasminogen and plasmin, *J. Lab. Clin. Med.,* 74, 265, 1969.
73. **Sherry, S.,** Fibrinolysis, *Annu. Rev. Med.,* 19, 243, 1968.
74. **Collen, D.,** Plasminogen and Prothrombin Metabolism in Man, Ph.D. thesis, University of Leuven, Belgium, 1974, 37.
75. **Wiman, B.,** Biochemistry of the plasminogen to plasmin conversion, in *Fibrinolysis. Current Fundamental and Clinical Concepts,* Gaffney, P. J. and Balkuv-Ulutin, S., Eds., Academic Press, London, 1978, 47.
76. **Summaria, L., Hsieh, B., and Robbins, K. C.,** The specific mechanism of activation of human plasminogen to plasmin, *J. Biol. Chem.,* 242, 4279, 1967.
77. **Kok, P.,** personal communication.
78. **Wiman, B.,** Primary structure of peptides released during activation of human plasminogen by urokinase, *Eur. J. Biochem.,* 39, 1, 1973.
79. **Wiman, B. and Wallén, P.,** Structural relationship between "glutamic acid" and "lysine" forms of human plasminogen and their interaction with the NH_2-terminal activation peptide as studies by affinity chromatography, *Eur. J. Biochem.,* 50, 489, 1975.
80. **Robbins, K. C., Bernabe, L. A., and Summaria, L.,** The primary structure of human plasminogen. I. The NH_2-terminal sequence of human plasminogen and the S-carboxymethyl heavy (A) and light (B) chain derivatives of plasmin, *J. Biol. Chem.,* 247, 6757, 1972.
81. **Walther, P. J., Steinman, H. M., Hill, R. L., and McKee, P. A.,** Activation of human plasminogen by urokinase. Partial characterization of a preactivation peptide, *J. Biol. Chem.,* 249, 1173, 1974.
82. **Wiman, B. and Wallén, P.,** On the primary structure of human plasminogen and plasmin. Purification and characterization of cyanogen-bromide fragments, *Eur. J. Biochem.,* 57, 387, 1975.
83. **Wiman, B. and Wallén, P.,** Amino acid sequence of the cyanogen-bromide fragment from human plasminogen that forms the linkage between the plasmin chains, *Eur. J. Biochem.,* 58, 539, 1975.
84. **Sottrup-Jensen, L., Zaidel, M., Claeys, H., Petersen, T. E., and Magnusson, S.,** Amino-acid sequence of activation cleavage site in plasminogen: Homology with "pro" part of prothrombin, *Proc. Natl. Acad. Sci. U.S.A.,* 72, 2577, 1975.
85. **Magnusson, S., Sottrup-Jensen, L., Petersen, T. E., Dudek-Wojciechowska, G., and Claeys, H.,** Homolgous "kringle" structures common to prothrombin and in *Proteolysis and Physiological Regulation,* Ribbons, D. W. and Brew, K., Eds., Academic Press, New York, 203, 1976.
86. **Wiman, B.,** Primary structure of the B-chain of human plasmin, *Eur. J. Biochem.,* 76, 129, 1977.
87. **Magnusson, S., Petersen, T. E., Sottrup-Jensen, L., and Claeys, H.,** Complete primary structure of prothrombin: isolation, structure and reactivity of ten carboxylated glutamic acid residues and regulation of prothrombin activation by thrombin, in *Proteases and Biological Control,* Reich, E., Rifkin, D. B., and Shaw, E., Cold Spring Harbor Laboratory, Cold Spring Harbor, N.Y., 1975, 123.
88. **Rickli, E. E., Lergier, W., and Gillessen, D.,** Investigations on the primary structure of human plasminogen. Further evidence for sequence homology, *Biochim. Biophys. Acta,* 439, 47, 1976.
89. **Lee, H. and Laursen, R. A.,** The primary structure of human plasminogen: characterization and alignment of the cyanogen bromide peptides, *FEBS Lett.,* 67, 113, 1976.
90. **Collen, D. and De Maeyer, L.,** Molecular biology of human plasminogen. I. Physicochemical properties and microheterogeneity, *Thromb. Diath. Haemorrh.,* 34, 396, 1975.
91. **Sottrup-Jensen, L.,** personal communication.
92. **Sjöholm, I., Wiman, B., and Wallén, P.,** Studies on the conformational changes of plasminogen induced during activation to plasmin and by 6-aminohexanoic acid, *Eur. J. Biochem.,* 39, 471, 1973.
93. **Robbins, K. C., Boreisha, I. G., Arzadon, L., Summaria, L., and Barlow, G. H.,** Physical and chemical properties of the NH_2-terminal glutamic acid and lysine forms of human plasminogen and their derived plasmins with an NH_2-terminal lysine heavy (A) chain, *J. Biol. Chem.,* 250, 4044, 1975.
94. **Claeys, H. and Vermylen, J.,** Physicochemical and proenzyme properties of NH_2-terminal glutamic acid and NH_2-terminal lysine human plasminogen. Influence of 6-aminohexanoic acid, *Biochim. Biophys. Acta,* 342, 351, 1974.

95. **Violand, B. N. and Castellino, F. J.,** Mechanism of the urokinase-catalyzed activation of human plasminogen, *J. Biol. Chem.,* 251, 3906, 1976.
96. **Wiman, B. and Wallén, P.,** Structural relationship between "Glutamic acid" and "Lysine" forms of human plasminogen and their interaction with the NH_2-terminal activation peptide as studied by affinity chromatography, *Eur. J. Biochem.,* 50, 489, 1975.
97. **Okamoto, S., Nakajima, T., Okamoto, U., Watonabe, H., Iguchi, Y., Igawa, T., Ching, C. C., and Hayashi, T.,** A suppressing effect of E-aminocaproic acid on the bleeding of dogs produced with the activation of plasmin in the circulatory blood, *Keio J. Med.,* 8, 247, 1959.
98. **Okamoto, S. and Okamoto, U.,** Amino-methyl-cyclohexane-carboxylic acid: AMCHA, a new potent inhibitor of the fibrinolysis, *Keio J. Med.,* 11, 105, 1962.
99. **Lohmann, K., Markwardt, F., and Landmann, H.,** Zusammenhange zwischen Konstitution und Wirkung bei Hemmstoffen der Fibrinolyse, *Thromb. Diath. Haemorrh.,* 10, 424, 1964.
100. **Walton, P. L.,** The hydrolysis of α-*N*-acetylglycyl-L-lysine methyl ester by urokinase, *Biochim. Biophys. Acta,* 132, 104, 1967.
101. **Iwamoto, M.,** Plasminogen-plasmin system. IX. Specific binding of tranexamic acid to plasmin, *Thromb. Diath. Haemorrh.,* 33, 573, 1975.
102. **Abiko, Y., Iwamoto, M., and Tomikawa, M.,** Plasminogen-plasmin system. V. A stoichiometric equilibrium complex of plasminogen and a synthetic inhibitor, *Biochim. Biophys. Acta,* 185, 424, 1969.
103. **Violand, B. N., Sodetz, J. M., and Castellino, F. J.,** The effect of ε-aminocaproic acid on the gross conformation of plasminogen and plasmin, *Arch. Biochem. Biophys.,* 170, 300, 1975.
104. **Castellino, F. J., Brockway, W. J., Thomas, J. K., Liao, H., and Rawitch, A. B.,** Rotational diffusion analysis of the conformational alterations produced in plasminogen by certain antifibrinolytic amino acids, *Biochemistry,* 12, 2787, 1973.
105. **Paoni, N. F. and Castellino, F. J.,** Isolation of a low molecular weight form of plasminogen, *Biochem. Biophys. Res. Commun.,* 65, 757, 1975.
106. **Markus, G., De Pasquale, J. L., and Wissler, F. C.,** Quantitative determination of the binding of ε-aminocaproic acid to native plasminogen, *J. Biol. Chem.,* 253, 727, 1978.
107. **Markus, G., Evers, J. L., and Hobika, G. H.,** Comparison of some properties of native (Glu) and modified (Lys) human plasminogen, *J. Biol. Chem.,* 253, 733, 1978.
108. **Wiman, B. and Collen, D.,** On the kinetics of the reaction between human antiplasmin and plasmin, *Eur. J. Biochem.,* 84, 573, 1978.
109. **Rickli, E. E. and Otavsky, W. I.,** A new method of isolation and some properties of the heavy chain of human plasmin, *Eur. J. Biochem.,* 59, 441, 1975.
110. **Wiman, B. and Wallén, P.,** The specific interaction between plasminogen and fibrin. A physiological role of the lysine binding site in plasminogen, *Thromb. Res.,* 10, 213, 1977.
111. **Boman, L., Wallén, P., and Wiman, B.,** unpublished results.
112. **Barlow, W. F., Jr., Boggiano, E., and De Renzo, E. C.,** Starch gel electrophoretic analysis of highly purified human plasminogen, *Biochim. Biophys. Acta,* 104, 470, 1965.
113. **Summaria, L., Arzadon, L., Bernabe, P., and Robbins, K. C.,** Studies on the isolation of the multiple molecular forms of human plasminogen and plasmin by isoelectric phocusing methods, *J. Biol. Chem.,* 247, 4691, 1972.
114. **Sodetz, J. M., Brockway, W. J., and Castellino, F. J.,** Multiplicity of rabbit plasminogen. Physical characterization, *Biochemistry,* 11, 4451, 1972.
115. **Collen, D. and DeMayer, L.,** Molecular biology of human plasminogen. I. Physicochemical properties and microheterogeneity, *Thromb. Diath. Haemorrh.,* 34, 396, 1975.
116. **Castellino, F. J., Siefring, G. E., Jr., Sodetz, J. H., and Bretthauer, R. K.,** Amino terminal amino acid sequences and carbohydrate of the two major forms of rabbit plasminogen, *Biochem. Biophys. Res. Commun.,* 53, 845, 1973.
117. **Hayes, M. L., Bretthauer, R. K., and Castellino, F. J.,** Carbohydrate compositions of the rabbit plasminogen isoenzyme, *Arch. Biochem. Biophys.,* 171, 651, 1975.
118. **Wiman, B. and Wallén, P.,** Activation of human plasminogen by an insoluble derivative of urokinase. Structural changes of plasminogen in the course of activation to plasmin and demonstration of a possible intermediate compound, *Eur. J. Biochem.,* 36, 25, 1973.
119. **Rickli, E. and Otavsky, W. I.,** Release of an N-terminal peptide from human plasminogen during activation with urokinase, *Biochim. Biophys. Acta,* 295, 381, 1973.
120. **Walther, P. J., Steinman, H. M., Hill, R. L., and McKee, P. A.,** Activation of human plasminogen by urokinase. Partial characterization of a preactivation peptide, *J. Biol. Chem.,* 249, 1173, 1974.
121. **Sodetz, J. M., Brockway, W. J., Mann, K. G., and Castellino, F. J.,** The mechanism of activation of rabbit plasminogen by urokinase. Lack of a preactivation peptide, *Biochem. Biophys. Res. Commun.,* 60, 729, 1974.

122. **Summaria, L., Arzadon, L., Bernabe, P., and Robbins, K. C.**, The activation of plasminogen to plasmin by urokinase in the presence of the plasmin inhibitor Trasylol, *J. Biol. Chem.*, 250, 3988, 1975.
123. **Sodetz, J. M. and Castellino, F. J.**, The mechanism of activation of rabbit plasminogen by urokinase, *J. Biol. Chem.*, 250, 3041, 1975.
124. **Boman, L., Wallén, P., and Wiman, B.**, unpublished results.
125. **Violand, B. N. and Castellino, F. J.**, Mechanism of the urokinase-catalyzed activation of human plasmin, *J. Biol. Chem.*, 251, 3906, 1976.
126. **Wallén, P. and Wiman, B.**, On the generation of intermediate plasminogen and its significance for activation, in *Proteases and Biological Control*, Reich, E., Rifkin, D. B., and Shaw, E., Eds., Cold Spring Harbor Laboratory, Cold Spring Harbor, N.Y., 291, 1975.
127. **Walther, P. J., Hill, R. L., and McKee, P. A.**, The importance of the preactivation peptide in the two-stage mechanism of human plasminogen activation, *J. Biol. Chem.*, 250, 5926, 1975.
128. **Christensen, U. and Müllertz, S.**, Kinetic studies of the urokinase catalyzed conversion of NH_2-terminal lysine plasminogen to plasmin, *Biochim. Biophys. Acta*, 480, 275, 1977.
129. **Christensen, U.**, Kinetic studies of the urokinase-catalyzed conversion of NH_2-terminal glutamic acid plasminogen to plasmin, *Biochim. Biophys. Acta*, 481, 638, 1977.
130. **Thorsen, S. and Astrup, T.**, Biphasic inhibition of urokinase-induced fibrinolysis by ε-aminocaproic acid; distinction from tissue plasminogen activator, *Proc. Soc. Exp. Biol. Med.*, 130, 811, 1969.
131. **Astrup, T.**, Fibrinolysis in the organism, *Blood*, 11, 781, 1956.
132. **Alkjaersig, N., Fletcher, A. P., and Sherry, S.**, The mechanism of clot dissociation by plasmin, *J. Clin. Invest.*, 38, 1086, 1959.
133. **Hedner, U., Nilsson, I. M., and Robertson, B.**, Determination of plasminogen in clots and thrombi, *Thromb. Diath. Haemorrh.*, 16, 38, 1966.
134. **Thorsen, S.**, Differences in the binding to fibrin of native plasminogen and plasminogen modified by proteolytic degradation. Influence of ω-aminocarboxylic acids, *Biochim. Biophys. Acta*, 393, 55, 1975.
135. **Rakoczi, I., Wiman, B., and Collen, D.**, On the biological significance of the specific interaction between fibrin, plasminogen and antiplasmin, *Biochim. Biophys. Acta*, 540, 295, 1978.
136. **Moroi, M. and Aoki, N.**, Inhibition of plasminogen binding to fibrin by α_2-plasmin inhibitor, *Thromb. Res.*, 10, 851, 1977.
137. **Landmann, H.**, Studies on the mechanism of action of synthetic antifibrinolytics, *Thromb. Diath. Haemorrh.*, 29, 253, 1973.
138. **Thorsen, S., Glas-Greenwalt, P., and Astrup, T.**, Difference in the binding of fibrin of urokinase and tissue plasminogen, *Thromb. Diath. Haemorrh.*, 28, 65, 1972.
139. **Wallén, P.**, Activation of plasminogen with urokinase and tissue activator, in *Thrombosis and Urokinase*, Paoletti, R. and Sherry, S., Eds., Academic Press, London, 1977, 91.
140. **Camiolo, S. M., Thorsen, S., and Astrup, T.**, Fibrinogenolysis and fibrinolysis with tissue plasminogen activator, urokinase, streptokinase-activated human globulin and plasmin, *Proc. Soc. Exp. Biol. Med.*, 38, 277, 1971.
141. **Wiman, B. and Collen, D.**, Molecular mechanism of physiological fibrinolysis, *Nature (London)*, 272, 549, 1978.

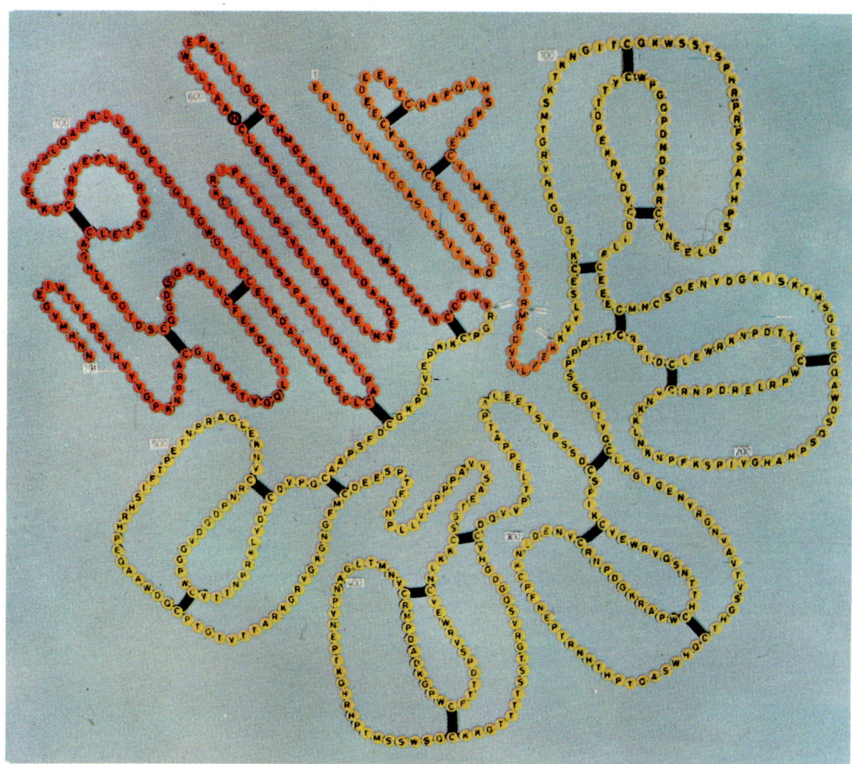

FIGURE 1. The primary structure of Glu-plasminogen. The fragments obtained on activation are indicated in different colors: the A-(heavy) chain, yellow; the B-(light) chain, red; the NH_2-terminal peptide(s) released on generation of Lys-plasminogen, orange. The arrows indicate peptide bonds cleaved during activation. With permission from Wiman, B., *Fibrinolysis, Current Fundamental and Clinical Concepts,* Gaffney, P. J. and Balkuv-Ulutin, S., Eds., Academic Press, London, 1978, 47. Copyright by Academic Press Inc. (London) Ltd.

Chapter 2

PLASMINOGEN ACTIVATORS

K. N. N. Reddy* and D. L. Kline**

TABLE OF CONTENTS

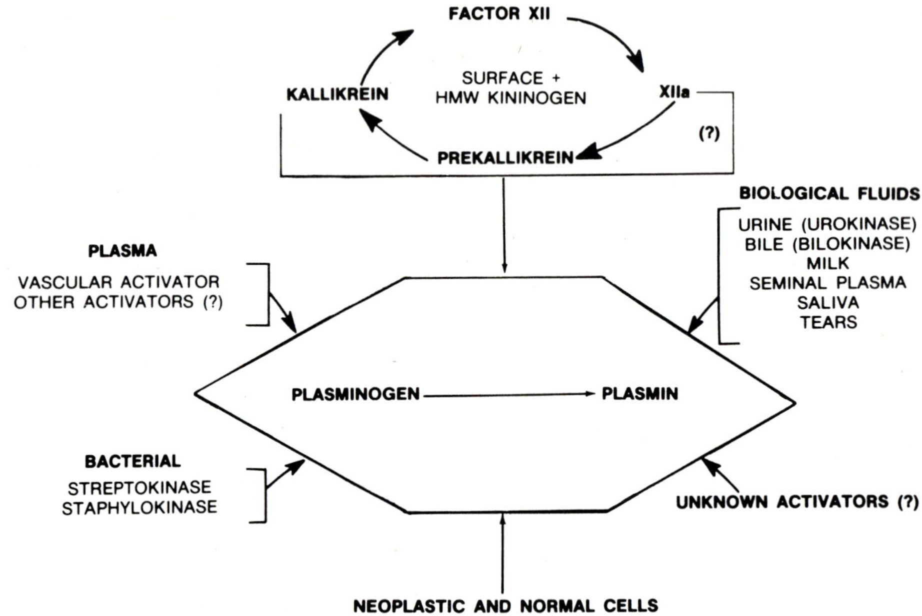

FIGURE 1. Contact activation.

I. INTRODUCTION

The enzyme plasmin, responsible for the dissolution of a fibrin clot, is found circulating in blood as the inactive zymogen plasminogen. The activation of plasminogen to plasmin involves the cleavage of a peptide bond in the plasminogen molecule. Plasminogen activators are known to be widely distributed in nature and can be found in microorganisms as well as in higher animals. The activators are present in many tissues (tissue activator), the circulating blood (blood activator), urine (urokinase), and in other body fluids (Figure 1). Recent studies on the production of plasminogen activators by various types of cells in culture indicate an important role for plasmin in cellular physiology.

II. BLOOD ACTIVATOR

It has been known for many years that blood obtained from victims of sudden or violent death did not clot at all, or if it did, the clots dissolved spontaneously within a short time. Müllertz[1] ascribed the lytic activity of cadaver blood to the presence of an activator of plasminogen. Biggs et al.[2] reported that fibrinolytic activity can also be found in healthy people, who were subjected to stress by severe exercise or by injecting adrenalin. Several investigators have confirmed that fibrinolytic activity appears in the blood of healthy individuals following various physiological and pharmacological stimuli. It is generally believed that this activity is due to the release of a plasminogen activator from the walls of the blood vessels. Fearnley and Tweed[3] reported that fibrinolytic activity is also present in the blood obtained from healthy people not subjected to any form of stress, indicating that a small amount of a plasminogen activator normally circulates in blood. Since the activator is present in very low amounts in normal blood, its determination requires very sensitive techniques. The circulating blood activator(s) has not been isolated and characterized.

Recent studies have shown that blood contains an elaborate system to generate plasmin. Activator of plasminogen appears in plasma when the clotting factor, Hageman Factor (Factor XII) is activated (see later). The fibrinolytic activity obtained by the Hageman Factor-dependent pathway is greater than that dependent on the circulating activator. Using a very sensitive method for the determination of plasmin, we found that in normal healthy individuals, the Hageman Factor-dependent pathway gave rise to 0.25 CTA units of plasmin activity per milliliter of plasma, while only 0.01 CTA units of plasmin activity could be generated by the circulating activator.[4]

Recently, Ogston et al.[5] have partially purified an activator of plasminogen from blood obtained after venous occlusion of the upper arm of healthy volunteers. It is very well known that increased fibrinolytic activity appears in blood following temporary venous stasis. Purification of the activator was carried out by column chromatography on Sephadex G-200 using phosphate-saline buffers. The activator preparation, although not homogeneous, was free from plasmin, plasminogen, C1-inactivator, α_1-antitrypsin, antithrombin III, α_2-macroglobulin, and Factors VIII, IX, and XII. Traces of Factor XI were present in the activator preparation. Although no activator could be found in nonocclusion plasma from rested volunteers (indicating that the activator which they partially purified may have been released from vessel walls), the authors did not rule out the possibility that the activator could have been formed via the Factor XII-dependent pathway.

III. HAGEMAN FACTOR-DEPENDENT PLASMINOGEN ACTIVATOR

Ratnoff and co-workers[6,7] were the first to describe the presence of an enzyme in precursor form in plasma, called Hageman Factor (Factor XII), which, when adsorbed to surfaces such as glass or kaolin, initiated a series of reactions leading to the clotting of blood. It was soon found that surface-dependent activation of Hageman Factor also results in the generation of fibrinolytic activity in normal plasma.[8-10] Ogston et al.[11] in a detailed investigation of the kaolin-induced generation of plasmin in normal plasma, found that plasmin formation required the presence of a surface, Hageman Factor, a factor called Hageman Factor cofactor, and an unidentified component in plasma. Activated Hageman Factor was also found to be involved in the conversion of prekallikrein to kallikrein, an enzyme in plasma which releases vasoactive peptides from kininogen.[12-14] Kallikrein was also found to activate plasminogen to plasmin.[15] Thus, Hageman Factor is involved in the mechanisms of blood clotting, fibrinolysis, and inflammation which Ratnoff recently described as being entwined in a "tangled web".[16] Over the last 10 years, investigations by various groups of workers have led to a better understanding of the complex interactions involved in these processes. (A detailed description of the Hageman Factor-dependent generation of plasmin in plasma can be found in Chapter 3.) These advances were made possible by the discovery that some individuals lack one of the factors, and consequently their plasmas exhibit defective clotting and fibrinolysis. From studies of such plasmas, it has been established that the following proteins participate in the generation of fibrinolytic activity:

1. Hageman Factor
2. Prekallikrein (Fletcher Factor)[17-20]
3. High molecular weight kininogen (Fitzgerald Factor,[21-23] Flaujeac Factor,[24] Williams Factor,[22] and contact activation cofactor[25])

Activation of Hageman Factor involves proteolytic cleavage of the native molecule into one or more active fragments. These fragments then activate prekallikrein to kallikrein which in turn activates plasminogen to plasmin. The surface and the heavy molecular weight kininogen participate in the reaction sequence by enhancing the rate of activation of Hageman Factor and its catalytic activity. It is not known at the present time how activation of Hageman Factor is initiated. Both plasmin and kallikrein are known to activate Hageman Factor, but they themselves exist in plasma as inactive precursors and require activated Hageman Factor for their activation.

While in normal plasma kallikrein has been shown to be an activator of plasminogen, plasma deficient in prekallikrein has been found to generate plasmin, albeit at a slow rate, indicating the presence of another pathway for the surface-mediated activation of plasminogen. Goldsmith et al. have recently suggested the possibility that activated Hageman Factor can activate plasminogen directly.[26]

The existence of pathways other than the Hageman Factor-dependent one in plasma has been suggested by some recent studies. Astrup and Rosa[27] found that while kaolin did not generate significant amounts of fibrinolytic activity in Hageman Factor-deficient plasma, addition of dextran sulfate to the same plasma gave normal levels of fibrinolytic activity. Schreiber and Austen[28] have also reported that fibrinolysis in normal plasma can occur independently of Hageman Factor, but requires the complement component C3. In addition, plasma may contain as yet unidentified activators of plasminogen present as such or derived from precursors involving different pathways.

Many questions remain to be answered before we can fully understand how plasminogen is activated to plasmin in its physiological milieu, plasma. The essential requirement for the occurrence of fibrinolysis in plasma, of course, is the cleavage of a peptide bond in the plasminogen molecule to give rise to the active enzyme plasmin. Since a protease is required to participate in this reaction, it is quite possible that many of the proteases present in plasma may be found to activate plasminogen to plasmin in vitro. However, whether these different activators do indeed participate in the in vivo activation of plasminogen will depend upon several factors, such as their kinetic properties, interaction with inhibitors present in plasma, and affinities for plasminogen and fibrin. Further work is necessary to find out whether nature has a single preferred pathway to generate plasmin in plasma or whether multiple pathways do exist so that the absence of a factor may not be of serious consequence for the normal functions of plasma in clotting and fibrinolysis.

IV. TISSUE ACTIVATORS

Astrup and co-workers have studied extensively the plasminogen activator of various tissues of the body, and the findings have been recently reviewed.[29] The distribution of plasminogen activator in tissues depends upon the organ and the species of animal from which the tissue is obtained. Thus, in the human, uterus, adrenals, lymph nodes, prostrate, thyroid, lung, ovary, pituitary, kidney, and skeletal muscle all exhibit activator activity, while little or no activity is found in the testes, spleen, and liver.[29] The activator activity of tissues from any organ in the same animal species (e.g., rabbit, ox, guinea pig, and cat) was found to be low, while in other species the same organs have very high activator activity. Thus, the pig heart and the lung of mouse and rat were found to be rich in plasminogen activator activity. Most of the tissue activator is strongly bound to cellular elements and can be extracted with strong agents, such as thiocyanate and urea, while a small amount of activator can be extracted with saline.

Todd[30] developed a sensitive histochemical technique for detecting fibrinolytic activity in tissues and found that the vascular endothelial cells were the source of plasminogen activator in tissues.[30] Plasminogen activator activity was also found in epithelial

* Supported by NIH Grant 1-K04-HL 00420-01 (RCDA).

** Supported by NIH Grant 2-R01-HL 11172-12.

cells from cornea, vagina, oviduct, and urinary excretory tract.[31] In studies on the location of plasminogen activator in subcellular fractions, both the lysosomal and microsomal fractions were reported to contain the activator. Ali and Lack, upon fractionation of rabbit kidney cells found the bulk of activator activity in the lysosomes.[32] On the other hand, Nakahara and Celander[33] reported that the microsomal fraction from bovine and porcine heart muscle contained the plasminogen activator.

The purification of plasminogen activator from pig heart has been carried out by several workers.[33-37] Cole and Bachman[38] recently achieved a purification of pig heart activator using buffers containing EDTA, cysteine, and 2,3-dimercaptopropanol-1 to remove contaminants from the crude extract in their purification procedure. Some of their preparations with specific activities of 200,000 CTA units per milligram of protein gave a single band on polyacrylamide gel electrophoresis. A molecular weight of 52,500 daltons was estimated for the activator from pig heart. The activity of the pig heart activator was found to be inhibited by the serine specific inhibitor diisopropyl fluorophosphate (DFP), but not by the histidine specific reagent tosyl lysine chloroketone.[36]

The partial purification of a plasminogen activator from pregnant hog ovaries has been reported by Kok and Astrup.[39] Gel filtration studies indicated a molecular weight of about 60,000 for this activator. Differences in the electrophoretic migration of the hog ovary activator and urokinase suggest that the two activators are chemically different. An activator of plasminogen has been partially purified from human myometrium.[40] Its size was estimated by gel filtration to be approximately 60,000, and its activity was found to be inhibited by ε-amino-*n*-caproic acid, soybean trypsin inhibitor, and Trasylol®.

Aoki has partially purified a vascular activator from the vascular trees of human cadavers.[41] While this activator did not have any protease activity, it exhibited esterase activity against the synthetic substrate acetyl glycyl lysine methyl ester. The molecular weight of the vascular activator was 80,000 by gel filtration studies. The requirement of high salt concentrations for the stability of the vascular activator, its molecular size, and its nonreactivity with a specific antiserum to human urokinase all indicate nonidentity between the vascular activator and urokinase.

Auerswald et al.[42] have fractionated the vascular plasminogen activator into three active fractions on Sephadex G-150 with molecular weights of 30,500, 61,000, and 120,000. Maximum activator activity was associated with the 61,000 fraction. They suggest that the higher molecular weight forms could be polymers of the 30,500 mol wt activator.

V. TISSUE CULTURE ACTIVATOR

The presence of a plasminogen activator in the growth medium of monkey kidney cell cultures was reported by Barnett and Baron.[43] Studies by Painter and Charles[44] showed that the activator obtained from kidney cell culture is closely related if not identical to urokinase, the activator of plasminogen found in urine. Biochemical[45] and immunological studies[46,47] showed identity between kidney cell culture activator and urokinase. Ali and Evans[48] have found very close similarity between human urokinase and an activator of plasminogen extracted from rabbit kidney. Bernik and Kwaan[49] have found the plasminogen activator in culture media of fetal lung and ureter and renal blood vessels of adults, indicating that the same urokinase-like activator may be produced by different tissues in the body.

VI. PLASMINOGEN ACTIVATORS IN NORMAL AND NEOPLASTIC CELLS

Recently, Reich and co-workers have shown that malignant cells in culture contained elevated levels of intracellular and extracellular activators of plasminogen. These and other studies, recently reviewed[50-55] suggest an important role for plasmin in cellular processes. Fibrinolytic activity was found in primary cultures of chemically induced mouse and rat tumors, a variety of human and animal tumor cell lines, and in mammalian and avian fibroblasts transformed to malignancy by chemical carcinogens or by oncogenic viruses. Thus, production of fibrinolytic activity appears to be independent of the nature of the transforming agent. The fibrinolytic activity found associated with transformed cells in culture was due to the release of an activator of plasminogen from the cells which acted upon the plasminogen present in the sera added to the growth medium.[56,57] Plasminogen activators have been partially purified from Rous sarcoma virus-transformed chick embryo fibroblasts, SV40-transformed hamster cells, R2426 rat breast carcinoma cells, human pancreatic carcinoma cells, murine sarcoma virus-transformed mouse embryo fibroblasts, simian virus-transformed 3T3 cells, and human melanoma cells.

The activator from transformed chick embryo fibroblasts[58] has been found to be an arginine-specific protease, inhibited by the active site-specific reagents *p*-nitrophenyl guanidinobenzoate and diisopropyl fluorophosphate, indicating that it is a serine protease. A molecular weight of 39,000 daltons was found for the activator, and the molecule appears to contain more than one polypeptide chain; reduction with mercaptoethanol gave a main polypeptide chain of 28,000 daltons, with a loss in activator activity.

Christman and Acs[59] achieved a 14,000-fold purification of plasminogen activator from SV-40-transformed hamster cells. The activator exhibited a single band on SDS-gel electrophoresis and had a molecular weight of 50,000. It had an isoelectric point of 9.5. The activator was found to be a serine protease containing two polypeptide chains joined by disulfide linkages. Labeled diisopropyl fluorophosphate incorporation studies showed the active site to be located on a polypeptide of approximately 25,000 daltons. The plasminogen activator produced by normal hamster lung cells and by SV40 virus-transformed hamster embryo cells has been found to be antigenically identical.[60]

Recently the plasminogen activator from human pancreatic carcinoma cell cultures has been purified.[61] A 7000-fold purification over conditioned serum-free medium was obtained by using a Sepharose-L--arginine methyl ester affinity column procedure in the presence of Triton X-100, followed by Sephadex G-200 filtration and isoelectric focusing steps. This activator had a molecular weight of 55,000 daltons, as determined by SDS-gel electrophoresis and by gel filtration methods. It exhibited esterase activity against tosyl-arginine methyl ester and *N*-acetyl lysine methyl ester and was inhibited by benzamidine and diisopropyl fluorophosphate, but not by pancreatic trypsin inhibitor or soybean trypsin inhibitor. It activated human plasminogen to plasmin in a manner similar to that of urokinase. Since the above-mentioned properties as well as the thermostability and pH stability of the pancreatic carcinoma activator appears to be similar to that of urokinase, it is suggested that this activator may be identical to urokinase. It is of interest to note in this connection that recently Astedt and Holmberg[62] reported immunologic identity between urokinase and a plasminogen activator from tissue cultures of ovarian carcinoma.

While the activators secreted by neoplastic cells from different sources were all found to be serine proteases, inhibited by diisopropyl fluorophosphate and *p*-nitrophenyl guanidino benzoate, and made up of more than one polypeptide chain, their molecular weights varied considerably, ranging from 38,000 daltons for the activator chick embryo fibroblasts to a molecular weight of 83,000 for an activator from mouse fibroblasts. The molecular weight of most activators from neoplastic mammalian cultures, however, was in the range of 48,000 to 50,000 daltons. The plasminogen activators exhibit species specificity. Thus, the activators from mammalian cells were found to activate dog, human, and fetal bovine plasminogens, but not chicken plasminogen. The avian plasminogen was activated only by the activator obtained from transformed chick fibroblast cultures.

The plasminogen activators appear to be associated with membrane structures of the cell. Christman et al.[51] found the activator from SV40-transformed hamster and mouse 3T3 cells to be concentrated in the membrane-rich fractions of cell homogenates. Similar localization of the activator from Rous sarcoma virus-transformed chick embryo fibroblasts has been reported by Quigley.[63]

While these studies clearly showed that the fibrinolytic activity associated with transformed cells is due to the activator-plasminogen system, Chen and Buchanan[64] reported the presence of a plasminogen-independent fibrinolytic activity in RSV-transformed chick embryo fibroblasts. Using plasminogen- free fibrin as the substrate, they observed release of fibrinopeptides by RSV-transformed chick embryo fibroblasts, but not by the untransformed fibroblasts. These results suggest that the plasminogen activator itself may possess fibrinolytic activity or that cells produce a fibrinolytically active protease. Wu et al.[65] have also found that cultured R2426 rat breast carcinoma cells secrete a fibrinolytic enzyme distinct from a plasminogen activator. This fibrinolysin was found to hydrolyze fibrinogen as well as the synthetic substrate tosyl arginine methyl ester, and its activity was inhibited by soybean trypsin inhibitor and ε-aminocaproic acid. The rat carcinoma cell fibrinolysin differed from human plasmin in its digestion of the fibrinogen molecule. Moreover, this fibrinolysin was found to be immunologically distinct from human, horse, and calf plasmin.[66]

The presence of fibrinogenolytic activity distinct from plasmin and plasminogen activator in human benign hyperplastic prostate tissue has been reported by Brassinne et al.[67] Upon gel filtration of a crude extract of the tissue, two fractions exhibiting fibrinogenolytic activity were obtained. The first fraction exhibited caseinolytic, fibrinogenolytic, and esterase activity towards tosyl arginine methyl ester. The second had no esterase activity and showed a higher fibrinogenolytic activity than caseinolytic activity. These proteases were inhibited by diisopropyl fluorophosphate and differed from plasmin in their cleavage of the fibrinogen molecule. These recent studies have clearly established the presence of fibrinolytic activity, whether due to plasminogen activators or to proteases similar to plasmin, in transformed cells. In view of the close association between fibrinolytic activity and cell transformation, it was suggested that increased levels of fibrinolytic activity could be a distinguishing property of neoplastic cells. Indeed, Pollack et al.[55] showed an association between tumorigenicity in vivo and high levels of plasminogen activator production. Laug et al.[68] found a correlation between the ability of a variety of human and animal cells to induce fibrinolysis and their ability to form tumors in immunosuppressed hosts. A close correlation between malignant behavior and the appearance of fibrinolytic activity in response to hormone stimulation in a murine mammary carcinoma (Shionogi SC-115) has been reported by Mak et al.[69] Physiological concentrations of dihydroxytestosterone rapidly induced the fibrinolytic activity in cell cultures of these carcinoma cells. However, whether fibrinolytic activity is a significant correlate of cell transformation has been questioned by many workers, since many normal cell types have been found to produce the plasminogen activator.

VII. FIBRINOLYTIC ACTIVITY IN NORMAL CELLS

Different laboratories have reported that fibrinolytic activity is associated with many normal cells,[70-73] activated macrophages,[74] embryonic cells during differentiation,[75,76] granulosa cells during ovulation,[77] and hormone-treated uterine cells.[78] An interesting finding is that rat liver cells from normal animals in primary culture showed high levels of fibrinolytic activity, while a malignant neoplasm of liver cells, the HTC cell line, had no fibrinolytic activity.[70] Moderate to high levels of plasminogen activator activity have been found in cell cultures of both normal mouse muscle and skin, as well as in several lines of transplanted sarcomas of mice.[71] High activator activities have been found in human fibroblasts W1-38 and W1-26, as well as in 3T3 cells.[72] Chou et al.[73] found that the expression of fibrinolytic activity in nontransformed 3T3 cell cultures depended upon the growth state of the cells. High levels of activator was exhibited by actively growing 3T3 cultures which decreased progressively as the cells became confluent and density inhibited. In contrast, dense cultures of SV40-virus transformed 3T3 cells continued to secrete large amounts of the activator. However, both subconfluent and confluent Swiss 3T3 cells were found to produce increasing amounts of activator when treated with high concentrations of calcium (3 to 4.9 m*M*, or in the presence of normal levels of calcium (1.8 m*M*) supplemented with the ionophore A 23187.[79]

Macrophages obtained from the peritoneal cavity of untreated mice do not normally produce plasminogen activator. However, induction of enzyme synthesis and secretion occurs following stimulation by thioglycollate, endotoxin, mineral oil, and asbestos.[80] Glucocorticoid hormones, cholera toxin, colchicine, vinblastine, and prostaglandins E_1 and E_2 have been found to inhibit the production of plasminogen activator by cultured macrophages.[81] It appears that macrophage plasminogen activator production may be regulated in part by lymphocytes, since normal macrophages cultured in the presence of conditioned medium from concavalin-A-stimulated spleen cells produced the activator.[82] Klimetzek and Sorg[83] have found that macrophages can also be stimulated to secrete plasminogen activator when exposed to lymphokine-rich lymphocyte culture supernates, while Nogueira et al.[84] have shown that normal unstimulated macrophages can be activated to secrete high levels of activator by a lymphocyte product(s) derived from the interaction of sensitized peritoneal or spleen cells with trypanosoma cruzi antigen. Soluble fibrin complexes have also been reported to induce secretion of activator by macrophages.[85]

Another example of plasminogen activator production by normal cells comes from studies on embryogenesis.[75,76] Plasminogen activator activity in cultured mouse embryos could first be detected by the sixth equivalent gestation day and followed a biphasic time course. The first phase of enzyme synthesis was by the trophoblast, and the second phase was due to parietal endoderm. The pattern of enzyme production by the trophoblast is closely correlated with the invasive period of these cells in vivo and implies that plasminogen activator is involved in embryo implantation.

The involvement of plasminogen activator in the process of ovulation has recently been studied.[77] It has been found that rat ovarian granulosa cells in vivo produce high levels of plasminogen activator as the time of ovulation approaches, and this activator is produced only by those cells obtained from follicles destined to ovulate. Inactive granulosa cells could be stimulated in vitro to produce the activator by exposure to gonadotropins. The stimulation of these cells to produce the activator appears to involve RNA and protein synthesis. In addition to the gonadotropins, cyclic AMP, dibutyryl cyclic AMP, and prostaglandins E_1 and E_2 were also found to stimulate the in vitro production of plasminogen activator.

Vascular endothelial cells from rabbit vena cava maintained in culture synthesized and secreted a plasminogen activator[86] with an approximate molecular weight of 50,000. The activator was found associated with a membrane fraction. Phorbol myristate ester induced increased production of the activator by these cells.

VIII. UROKINASE

In 1947 Macfarlane and Pilling reported the presence of fibrinolytic activity in normal urine.[87] It was soon established[88,89] that the fibrinolytic activity of urine was due to the presence of a plasminogen activator to which the name "urokinase" was given by Sobel and co-workers.[90]

The purification of urokinase from urine has been reported by many workers.[91-95] Lesuk et al. obtained urokinase in crystalline form.[96] Ogawa et al.[97] have reported the novel use of a polyacrylonitrile fiber to absorb urokinase from urine in their purification procedure. In recent years, affinity chromatography methods have been introduced to obtain highly purified preparations of urokinase.[98-100]

The existence of different molecular forms of urokinase has been established by various purification procedures[39,95,96,98,99] and by immunological methods.[101] One form of urokinase was found to have a molecular weight in the range of 47,000 to 54,000 daltons, while another form had a molecular weight of 31,000 to 34,000 daltons. It has been suggested that the lower molecular weight form may have been derived from the higher form as a result of proteolytic degradation during isolation procedures. Thus, Lesuk et al.[102] showed that trypsin can cleave the 54,000 dalton form to a fragment of 36,000 daltons retaining biological activity. Soberano et al.[103] found that the 54,000-dalton form of urokinase consisting of two polypeptide chains linked together by disulfide bonds was converted to a 33,100-dalton fragment containing a single polypeptide chain either by autocatalysis or by protease(s) contaminating the urokinase preparation. It is interesting that this conversion appears to involve extensive degradation of the light chain moiety of the 54,000 form of urokinase without a loss in biological activity. Although the 33,400 form of urokinase appears to consist of a single polypeptide chain as determined by sodium dodecyl sulfate-polyacrylamide gel electrophoresis, the presence of small peptide fragments of the light chain still attached to the heavy chain by disulfide bonds is quite possible.

The activation of human plasminogen by urokinase involves the cleavage of an arginyl-valyl peptide bond in the plasminogen molecule. Urokinase is a protease with trypsin-like specificity for substrate hydrolysis. Sherry et al.[104] studied the esterase activity of urokinase against a variety of arginine and lysine esters and found that the lysine esters were more susceptible to hydrolysis than the arginine derivatives. Substitution of the α-amino group in the lysine ester further enhanced the rate of hydrolysis by urokinase. Thus, *N*-acetyl lysine methyl ester[104] and *N*-acetyl glycyl lysine methyl ester[105] were found to be the most sensitive substrates of urokinase.

Although urokinase exhibits trypsin-like specificity, it does not react with pancreatic trypsin inhibitor and soybean trypsin inhibitor.[105] The presence of a urokinase inhibitor in plasma distinct from known protease inhibitors, such as C1-inactivator, α_1-antitrypsin, and antithrombin, has been reported.[106-108] Partial purification of an inhibitor of urokinase from human placenta has been recently reported.[109] The inhibitor, α_1-antitrypsin, was shown to inhibit urokinase by forming 1:1 and 2:1 molar enzyme-inhibitor complexes.

Active site studies revealed that a serine residue and a histidine residue on the urokinase molecule are involved in its catalytic action. Ong et al.,[111] using acetyl glycyl lysine chloroketone and norleucyl glycyl lysine chloroketone as active site specific reagents, found that the enzyme was rapidly inactivated as a result of alkylation of a single histidine residue in the enzyme. Tosyl lysine chloroketone which readily inactivates trypsin reacts incompletely with urokinase, indicating subtle differences in the active site region of the two proteases. The irreversible inactivation of urokinase by diisopropyl fluorophosphate and *p*-nitrophenyl guanidino benzoate[112] established the presence of a serine residue in the active site of the enzyme molecule.

Extensive studies by Kwaan and co-workers[46,49] using tissue culture methods revealed kidney as the major source for urokinase production. Immunologic identity between urokinase and the activator from kidney tissue culture has been demonstrated.[46,47] Further identity between urokinase and a plasminogen activator isolated from human embryo kidney cell cultures has been established based on biochemical evidence.[45] Thus, the esterase activity against acetyl glycyl lysyl methyl ester, pH dependence on electrophoretic mobilities, isoelectric focusing profiles, sedimentation coefficients, elution profiles on Sephadex G-200 column chromatography, and immunodiffusion analyses using rabbit antibody were all indistinguishable between the two activators.

IX. STREPTOKINASE

This activator of plasminogen found in streptococcal culture filtrates is of interest both from historical and biochemical points of view. It was the studies on the fibrinolytic activity of streptococcal culture filtrates that led to the identification of plasminogen in plasma as the fibrinolytic enzyme, its presence in normal plasma in an inactive precursor form, and its activation to plasmin as a prerequisite for fibrinolytic activity.

Unlike the activators of plasminogen described so far, streptokinase is not an enzyme, and yet its addition to plasminogen results in the conversion of plasminogen to plasmin involving a peptide bond cleavage. The mechanism by which streptokinase activates human plasminogen has been recently discovered by Reddy and Markus.[113] Briefly, it is as follows: streptokinase interacts with plasminogen to form a stoichiometric complex. As a result of this complex formation, a proteolytic active site appears in the plasminogen moiety of the complex which then catalyzes the peptide bond cleavage in the plasminogen molecule. For a detailed description of the interaction of streptokinase with plasminogen, the reader is referred to Chapter 4.

Streptokinase of varying purity is commercially available from several pharmaceutical companies. It is a protein consisting of a single polypeptide chain with a molecular weight of approximately 47,000 to 50,000 daltons.[114-116] It has an isoelectric point of pH 4.7 and a sedimentation value $S_{20} \cdot W$ of 3.15. A low hexose content of 0.2 g% and a hexosamine content of 0.1 g% was found in the streptokinase.[116] Isoleucine has been found as its amino terminal amino acid residue and lysine in the carboxyl terminal position.[117] No cysteine and cystine amino acids were found in the streptokinase molecule. Partial amino acid sequences of the peptides isolated from streptokinase by cyanogen bromide fragmentation has been determined.[117] Optical rotatory dispersion studies showed that streptokinase exists predominantly in random coil conformation.[116,118]

X. STAPHYLOKINASE

Staphylokinase is an extracellular protein produced by many strains of staphlococcus which activates human plasminogen to plasmin.[119,120] The only known biological activity of staphylokinase appears to be its ability to activate the fibrinolytic system. No definite correlation between the production of this activator and clinical virulence of staphylococci has been established.

Purification of staphylokinase from growth media gave three active protein fractions with isoelectric points ranging from 5.5 to 6.7.[121-123] The molecular weight of staphylokinase was found to be approximately 13,000 to 15,000 daltons.[122,123] Thus, the molecule of staphylokinase is smaller than another bacterial activator, streptokinase, which has a molecular weight of 47,000 daltons. The two bacterial activators share certain properties in common. Neither activator possesses proteolytic activity, and yet both are capable of activating human plasminogen to plasmin. They exhibit species

. ecificity in their activator activity,[124] both are unable to activate bovine plasminogen. A significant difference between staphylokinase and streptokinase is that while a mixture of streptokinase and human plasminogen activates bovine plasminogen, staphylokinase does not activate bovine plasminogen, even in the presence of human plasminogen.[125]

The mechanism of activation of human plasminogen by staphylokinase appears to be similar to that of streptokinase.[122] Studies with the active center specific reagent *p*-nitrophenyl-*p*-guanidino benzoate showed that the generation of an active site in the plasminogen molecule as a result of complex formation with staphylokinase was a slow process requiring several minutes. It is of interest to note here that active site generation in dog plasminogen with streptokinase also requires several minutes.[126] Kowalska-Loth and Zakrzewski have also found that the kinetics of activation of human plasminogen by staphylokinase follows a sigmoid pattern.[122] The lag period in the activation of plasminogen disappeared when plasmin was present in the activation mixture, indicating that faster activation was obtained by a complex of staphylokinase-plasmin than with the staphylokinase-plasminogen complex.

Stable complex formation between staphylokinase and human plasmin[122] and with dog plasmin[123] has been found to occur. Makino et al.[123] found that when the pH 6.3 isoelectric form of staphylokinase was incubated with dog plasminogen, it was converted to the pH 5.7 isoelectric form of staphylokinase. Bovine pancreatic trypsin has also been found to mediate this conversion.[127] These results suggest the possibility that the different isoelectric forms of staphylokinase obtained from culture media may represent proteolytically modified forms.

XI. LEUKOCYTE PLASMINOGEN ACTIVATOR

Several workers have found that leukocytes contain an activator of plasminogen. Kopitar et al. have isolated and characterized the plasminogen activator from pig leukocytes.[128] This activator was found to have a molecular weight of 28,000 to 30,500, as determined by the gel filtration method. The activator from human polymorphonuclear leukocytes has been found to have an approximate molecular weight of 60,000.[129] Human leukocytes in culture could be stimulated to secrete the plasminogen activator with concanavalin-A or phorbol myristate acetate, and secretion was inhibited by steroids.[129] Both RNA and protein synthesis are required for the synthesis and secretion of the plasminogen activator.

XII. ERYTHROCYTE PLASMINOGEN ACTIVATOR

Erythrokinase, an activator of plasminogen, has been partially purified from human erythrocytes.[130] This activator activated both human and bovine plasminogens equally well. Erythrokinase was found to be different from urokinase, since acrylamide gel electrophoresis pattern, kinetics of synthetic ester hydrolysis, and chromatographic elution profiles on DEAE-cellulose were all different for the two activators. However, both activators were inhibited by ε-aminocaproic acid and Trasylol®.

XIII. PLASMINOGEN ACTIVATOR IN BIOLOGICAL FLUIDS

Human and animal bile contains an activator of plasminogen. The activator from bovine bile named bilokinase has been purified.[131] It has a molecular weight of 58,000. Its amino acid composition, esterase activity towards acetyl glycyl lysine methyl ester, and immunological reaction were found to be different from urokinase.

Human colostrum was shown to contain an activator of plasminogen.[132] Interestingly, this activator was reported to exhibit protease activity against casein, as well esterase activity. Partial purification of plasminogen activators from human seminal plasma has been reported recently.[133] Two activators with molecular weights of 70,000 and 74,000 have been obtained by gel filtration and ion exchange chromatography which showed immunologic identity with urokinase.

An interesting activator of plasminogen has been isolated from vampire bat saliva.[134] This activator has a molecular weight of 150,000 and was quite stable to elevated temperatures at acid or neutral pH. Although DFP irreversibly inhibited the activator, it did not exhibit any proteolytic or esterolytic activities. Moreover, it did not activate pure plasminogen in solution, while it lysed fibrin plates and whole blood clots, indicating a requirement for the presence of fibrin for its action. It also exhibited species specificity in that it lysed clots from mammalian species while avian clots were resistent.

XIV. CONCLUSION

At the present time, our knowledge of plasminogen activators is very limited. It is only very recently that plasma and various types of cells have been subjected to intensive investigations. In the past, urokinase and streptokinase have been the subject of numerous investigations due to their potential as drugs for thrombolytic therapy. Since urokinase is found excreted in the urine, the question arose as to whether it was made in the kidneys or whether it was a metabolic product derived from the tissue, vascular, or plasma activators. Recent studies established kidney as the source of urokinase.

The question still remains whether the plasminogen activators found in various tissues and body fluids are different molecular species or whether they are structurally related to one another and to urokinase. As most of these activators have not been obtained in pure form, identity with urokinase was sought for on the basis of differences in molecular size, electrophoretic mobility, antigenic properties, substrate specificities, and inhibitor profiles. These comparative studies will be valuable and meaningful only if the proteins to be compared have been prepared with great care from their sources, since proteolytic modification of these molecules can occur during the isolation procedures.

Although plasmin is considered to be primarily a fibrinolytic enzyme, the wide distribution of activators in the body, and the fact that plasminogen is available to every part of the body from the circulating blood suggests that plasmin may also play a role in processes which require the action of a general protease. The findings presented in this chapter are just a prelude for the many exciting discoveries to be made in the future.

REFERENCES

1. **Müllertz, S.,** A plasminogen activator in spontaneously active human blood, *Proc. Soc. Exp. Biol. Med.,* 82, 291, 1953.
2. **Biggs, R., Macfarlane, R. G., and Pilling, J.,** Observations on fibrinolysis: experimental activity produced by exercise or adrenaline, *Lancet,* 1, 402, 1947.
3. **Fearnley, G. R. and Tweed, J. M.,** Evidence of an active fibrinolytic enzyme in the plasma of normal people with observations on inhibition associated with the presence of calcium, *Clin. Sci.,* 12, 81, 1953.
4. **Kline, D. L. and Reddy, K. N. N.,** Proactivator and activator levels of plasminogen in plasma as measured by caseinolysis, *J. Lab. Clin. Med.,* 89, 1153, 1977.

5. **Ogston, D., Bennett, B., and Mackie, M.**, Properties of a partially purified preparation of a circulating plasminogen activator, *Thromb. Res.*, 8, 275, 1976.
6. **Ratnoff, O. D. and Colopy, J. E.**, A familial haemorrhagic trait associated with deficiency of a clot promoting fraction of plasma, *J. Clin. Invest.*, 34, 602, 1955.
7. **Ratnoff, O. D. and Rosenblum, J.**, Role of Hageman Factor in the initiation of clotting by glass. Evidence that glass frees Hageman factor from inhibition, *Am. J. Med.*, 25, 160, 1958.
8. **Niewiarowski, S. and Prou-Wartelle, O.**, Role di facteur contact (facteur Hageman) dans la fibrinolyse, *Thromb. Diath. Haemorrh.*, 3, 593, 1959.
9. **Iatridis, S. G. and Ferguson, J. H.**, Effect of surface and Hageman factor on the endogenous or spontaneous activation of the fibrinolytic system, *Thromb. Diath. Haemorrh.*, 6, 411, 1961.
10. **Iatridis, S. G. and Ferguson, J. H.**, Active Hageman factor: a plasma lysokinase of the human fibrinolytic system, *J. Clin. Invest.*, 41, 1277, 1962.
11. **Ogston, D., Ogston, C. M., Ratnoff, O. D., and Forbes, C. D.**, Studies on a complex mechanism for the activation of plasminogen by kaolin and chloroform: the participation of Hageman factor and additional cofactors, *J. Clin. Invest.*, 48, 1786, 1969.
12. **Webster, M. E. and Ratnoff, O. D.**, Role of Hageman factor in the activation of vasodilator activity in human plasma, *Nature (London)*, 192, 180, 1961.
13. **Colman, R. W., Mattler, L., and Sherry, S.**, Studies on the kallikreinogen-kallikrein enzyme system of human plasma. I. Isolation and purification of plasma kallikreins, *J. Clin. Invest.*, 48, 11, 1969.
14. **Colman, R. W., Mattler, L., and Sherry, S.**, Studies on the kallikreinogen-kallikrein enzyme system of human plasma. II. Identification of the kaolin activated arginine esterase as plasma kallikrein, *J. Clin. Invest.*, 48, 23, 1969.
15. **Colman, R. W.**, Activation of plasminogen by human plasma kallikrein, *Biochem. Biophys. Res. Comm.*, 35, 273, 1969.
16. **Ratnoff, O. D.**, A tangled web. Interdependence of mechanisms of blood clotting, fibrinolysis, immunity and inflammation, *Thromb. Diath. Haemorrh. Suppl.* 45, 109, 1971.
17. **Laake, K. and Venneröd, A. M.**, Factor XII-induced fibrinolysis: studies on the separation of prekallikrein, plasminogen proactivator, and Factor XI in human plasma, *Thromb. Res.*, 4, 285, 1974.
18. **Saito, H., Ratnoff, O. D., and Donaldson, V. H.**, Defective activation of clotting, fibrinolytic, and permeability-enhancing systems in human Fletcher trait plasma, *Circ. Res.*, 34, 641, 1974.
19. **Weiss, A. S., Gallin, J. I., and Kaplan, A. P.**, Fletcher factor deficiency. A diminished rate of Hageman factor activation caused by absence of prekallikrein with abnormalities of coagulation, fibrinolysis, chemotactic activity, and kinin generation, *J. Clin. Invest.*, 53, 622, 1974.
20. **Wuepper, K. D.**, Prekallikrein deficiency in man, *J. Exp. Med.*, 138, 1345, 1973.
21. **Saito, H., Ratnoff, O. D., Waldmann, R., and Abraham, J. P.**, Fitzgerald trait. Deficiency of a hitherto unrecognized agent, Fitzgerald factor, participating in surface-mediated reactions of clotting, fibrinolysis, generation of kinins, and the property of diluted plasma enhancing vascular permeability (PF/Dil), *J. Clin. Invest.*, 55, 1082, 1975.
22. **Colman, R. W., Bagdasarian, A., Talamo, R. C., Scott, C. F., Seavey, M., Guimaraes, J. A., Pierce, J. V., and Kaplan, A. P.**, Williams Trait. Human kininogen deficiency with diminished levels of plasminogen proactivator and prekallikrein associated with abnormalities of the Hageman factor-dependent pathways, *J. Clin. Invest.*, 56, 1650, 1975.
23. **Donaldson, V. H., Glueck, H. I., Miller, M. A., Movat, H. Z., and Habal, F.**, Kininogen deficiency in Fitzgerald trait: role of high molecular weight kininogen in clotting and fibrinolysis, *J. Lab. Clin. Med.*, 87, 327, 1976.
24. **Wuepper, K. D., Miller, D. R., and Lacombe, M. J.**, FlauJeac trait: deficiency of human plasma kininogen, *J. Clin. Invest.*, 56, 1663, 1975.
25. **Schiffman, S. and Lee, P.**, Partial purification and characterization of contact activation cofactor, *J. Clin. Invest.*, 56, 1082, 1975.
26. **Goldsmith, G., Saito, H., and Ratnoff, O. D.**, The activation of plasminogen by Hageman factor and Hageman factor fragments, *Thromb. Haemostas.*, 38, 136, 1977.
27. **Astrup, T. and Rosa, A.T.**, A plasminogen proactivator system in human blood effective in absence of Hageman factor, *Thromb. Res.*, 4, 609, 1974.
28. **Schreiber, A. D. and Austen, K. F.**, Hageman factor-independent fibrinolytic pathway, *Clin. Exp. Immunol.*, 17, 587, 1974.
29. **Astrup, T.**, Tissue activators of plasminogen, *Fed. Proc. Fed. Am. Soc. Exp. Biol.*, 25, 42, 1966.
30. **Todd, A. S.**, Histological localization of fibrinolysin activator, *J. Pathol. Bacteriol.*, 78, 281, 1959.
31. **Astrup, T.**, Cell-induced fibrinolysis: a fundamental process, in *Proteases and Biological Control*, Vol. 2, Cold Spring Harbor Conferences on Cell Proliferation, Reich, E., Rifkin, D. B., and Shaw, E., Eds., Cold Spring Harbor Laboratory, Cold Spring Harbor, N.Y., 1975, 343.
32. **Ali, S. Y. and Lack, C. H.**, Studies on the tissue activator of plasminogen. Distribution of activator and proteolytic activity in the subcellular fractions of rabbit kidney, *Biochem. J.*, 96, 63, 1965.

33. **Nakahara, M. and Celander, D. R.**, Properties of microsomal activator of profibrinolysin found in bovine and porcine heart muscle, *Thromb. Diath. Haemorrh.*, 19, 483, 1968.
34. **Bachmann, F., Fletcher, A. P., Alkjaersig, N., and Sherry, S.**, Partial purification and properties of the plasminogen activator from pig heart, *Biochemistry*, 3, 1758, 1964.
35. **Rickli, E. E. and Zaugg, H.**, Isolation and purification of highly enriched tissue plasminogen activator from pig heart, *Thromb. Diath. Haemorrh*, 23, 64, 1970.
36. **Hijikata, A., Fugimoto, K., Kitaguchi, H., and Okamoto, S.**, Some properties of the tissue plasminogen activator from the pig heart, *Thromb. Res.*, 4, 731, 1974.
37. **McCall, D. C. and Kline, D. L.**, Mechanism of action and some properties of a tissue activator of plasminogen, *Thromb. Diath. Haemorrh.*, 14, 116, 1965.
38. **Cole, E. R. and Bachmann, F.**, Purification and properties of a plasminogen activator from pig heart, *J. Biol. Chem.*, 252, 3729, 1977.
39. **Kok, P. and Astrup, T.**, Isolation and purification of a tissue plasminogen activator and its comparison with urokinase, *Biochemistry*, 8, 79, 1969.
40. **Soszka, T.**, Partial purification and some properties of the tissue plasminogen activator from the human myometrium, *Thromb. Res.*, 10, 823, 1977.
41. **Aoki, N.**, Preparation of plasminogen activator from vascular trees of human cadavers. Its comparison with urokinase, *J. Biochem. (Tokyo)*, 75, 731, 1974.
42. **Auerswald, W., Binder, B., and Doleschel, W.**, Angiokinase-molecular weights of proteins representing a perivascular plasminogen activator, *Thromb. Diath. Haemorrh.*, 26, 411, 1971.
43. **Barnett, E. and Baron, S.**, An activator of plasminogen produced by cell culture, *Proc. Soc. Exp. Med.*, 102, 308, 1959.
44. **Painter, R. and Charles, A.**, Characterization of a soluble plasminogen activator from kidney cell culture, *Am. J. Physiol.*, 202, 1125, 1962.
45. **Barlow, G. H. and Lazer, L.**, Characterization of the plasminogen activator isolated from human embryo kidney cells: comparison with urokinase, *Thromb. Res.*, 1, 201, 1972.
46. **Kucinski, C. S., Fletcher, A. P., and Sherry, S.**, Effect of urokinase antiserum on plasminogen activators: demonstration of immunologic dissimilarity between plasma plasminogen activator and urokinase, *J. Clin. Invest.*, 47, 1238, 1968.
47. **Bernik, M. B., White, W. F., Oller, E. P., and Kwaan, H. C.**, Immunologic identity of plasminogen activator in human urine, heart, blood vessels, and tissue culture, *J. Lab. Clin. Med.*, 84, 546, 1974.
48. **Ali, S. Y. and Evans, L.**, Purification of rabbit kidney cytokinase and a comparison of its properties with human urokinase, *Biochem. J.*, 107, 293, 1968.
49. **Bernik, M. B. and Kwaan, H. C.**, Plasminogen activator activity in cultures from human tissues. An immunological and histochemical study, *J. Clin. Invest.*, 48, 1740, 1969.
50. **Reich, E.**, Plasminogen activator: secretion by neoplastic cells and macrophages, in *Proteases and Biological Control*, Vol. 2, Cold Spring Harbor Conferences on Cell Proliferation, Reich, E., Rifkin, D. B., and Shaw, E., Eds., Cold Spring Harbor Laboratory, Cold Spring Harbor, N.Y., 1975, 333.
51. **Christman, J. K., Acs, G., Silagi, S., and Silverstein, S. C.**, Plasminogen activator: biochemical characterization and correlation with tumorigenicity, in *Proteases and Biological Control*, Vol. 2, Cold Spring Harbor Conferences on Cell Proliferation, Reich, E., Rifkin, D. B., and Shaw, E., Eds., Cold Spring Harbor Laboratory, Cold Spring Harbor, N.Y., 1975, 827.
52. **Wigler, M., Ford, J. P., and Weinstein, I. B.**, Glucocorticoid inhibition of the fibrinolytic activity of tumor cells, in *Proteases and Biological Control*, Vol. 2, Cold Spring Harbor Conferences on Cell Proliferation, Reich, E., Rifkin, D. B., and Shaw, E., Eds., Cold Spring Harbor Laboratory, Cold Spring Harbor, N.Y., 1975, 849.
53. **Goldberg, A. P., Wolf, B. A., and Lefebvre, P. A.**, Plasminogen activators of transformed and normal cells, in *Proteases and Biological Control*, Vol. 2, Cold Spring Harbor Conferences on Cell Proliferation, Reich, E., Rifkin, D. B., and Shaw, E., Eds., Cold Spring Harbor Laboratory, Cold Spring Harbor, N.Y., 1975, 857.
54. **Roblin, R., Chou, I-N., and Black, P.**, Role of fibrinolysin T activity in properties of 3T3 and Sv 3T3 cells, in *Proteases and Biological Control*, Vol. 2, Cold Spring Harbor Conferences on Cell Proliferation, Reich, E., Rifkin, D. B., and Shaw, E., Eds., Cold Spring Harbor Laboratory, Cold Spring Harbor, N.Y., 1975, 869.
55. **Pollack, R., Risser, R., Conlon, S., Freedman, V., Shin, S-I., and Rifkin, D. B.**, Production of plasminogen activator and colonial growth in semi-solid medium or in vitro correlates of tumorigenicity in the immunedeficient nude mouse, in *Proteases and Biological Control*, Vol. 2, Cold Spring Harbor Conferences on Cell Proliferation, Reich, E., Rifkin, D. B., and Shaw, E., Eds., Cold Spring Harbor Laboratory, Cold Spring Harbor, N.Y., 1975, 885.
56. **Unkeless, J. C., Tobia, A., Ossowski, L., Quigley, J. P., Rifkin, D. B., and Reich, E.**, An enzymatic function associated with transformation of fibroblasts by oncogenic viruses. I. Chick embryo fibroblast cultures transformed by avian RNA tumor viruses, *J. Exp. Med.*, 137, 85, 1973.

57. **Ossowski, L., Unkeless, J. C., Tobia, A., Quigley, J. P., Rifkin, D. B., and Reich, E.,** An enzymatic function associated with transformation of fibroblasts by oncogenic viruses. II. Mammalian fibroblast cultures transformed by DNA and RNA tumor viruses, *J. Exp. Med.,* 137, 112, 1973.

58. **Unkeless, J. C., Danø, K., Kellerman, G. M., and Reich, E.,** Fibrinolysis associated with oncogenic transformation. Partial purification and characterization of the cell factor, a plasminogen activator, *J. Biol. Chem.,* 249, 4295, 1974.

59. **Christman, J. K. and Acs, G.,** Purification and characterization of a cellular fibrinolytic factor associated with oncogenic transformation: the plasminogen activator from SV-40 transformed hamster cells, *Biochim. Biophys. Acta,* 340, 339, 1974.

60. **Christman, J. K., Silverstein, S. C., and Acs, G.,** Immunological analysis of plasminogen activators from normal and transformed hamster cells. Evidence that the plasminogen activators produced by SV40 virus-transformed hamster embryo cells and normal hamster lung cells are antigenically identical, *J. Exp. Med.,* 142, 419, 1975.

61. **Wu, M-C., Arimura, G. K., and Yunis, A. A.,** Purification and characterization of a plasminogen activator secreted by cultured human pancreatic carcinoma cells, *Biochemistry,* 16, 1908, 1977.

62. **Astedt, B. and Holmberg, L.,** Immunological identity of urokinase and ovarian carcinoma plasminogen activator released in tissue culture, *Nature (London),* 261, 595, 1976.

63. **Quigley, J. P.,** Association of a protease plasminogen activator with a specific membrane fraction isolated from transformed cells, *J. Cell. Biol.,* 71, 472, 1976.

64. **Chen, L-B. and Buchanan, J. M.,** Plasminogen independent fibrinolysis by proteases produced by transformed chick embryo fibroblasts, *Proc. Natl. Acad. Sci. U.S.A.,* 72, 1132, 1975.

65. **Wu, M-C., Schultz, D. R., Arimura, G. K., Gross, M. A., and Yunis, A. A.,** Characteristics of fibrinolysin secreted by cultured rat breast carcinoma cells, *Exp. Cell. Res.,* 96, 37, 1975.

66. **Schultz, D. R., Wu, M-C., and Yunis, A. A.,** Immunologic relationship among fibrinolysins secreted by cultured mammalian tumor cells, *Exp. Cell Res.,* 96, 47, 1975.

67. **Brassinne, C., Coune, A., Nijs, M., and Tagnon, H. J.,** Characterization of two direct fibrinogenolytic activities and of one proteolytic inhibitor activity in the human prostate, *Thromb. Res.,* 8, 803, 1976.

68. **Laug, W. E., Jones, P. A., and Benedict, W. F.,** Relationship between fibrinolysis of cultured cells and malignancy, *J. Natl. Cancer Inst.,* 54, 173, 1975.

69. **Mak, T. W., Rutledge, G., and Sutherland, D. J. A.,** Androgen-dependent fibrinolytic activity in a murine mammary carcinoma (Shionogi SC-115 cells) in vitro, *Cell,* 7, 223, 1976.

70. **Laishes, B. A., Roberts, E., and Burrowes, C.,** Fibrinolytic activity of adult rat liver cells in primary culture and inhibition by glucocorticoids, *Biochem. Biophys. Res. Commun.,* 72, 462, 1976.

71. **Chibber, B. A., Niles, R. M., Prehn, L., and Sarof, S.,** High extracellular fibrinolytic activity of tumors and control normal tissues, *Biochem. Biophys. Res. Commun.,* 65, 806, 1975.

72. **Mott, D. M., Fabisch, P. H., Sani, B. P., and Sorof, S.,** Lack of correlation between fibrinolysis and the transformed state of cultured mammalian cells, *Biochem. Biophys. Res. Commun.,* 61, 621, 1974.

73. **Chou, I-N., O'Donnell, S. P., Black, P. H., and Roblin, R. O.,** Cell density-dependent secretion of plasminogen activator by 3T3 cells, *J. Cell. Physiol.,* 91, 31, 1977.

74. **Unkeless, J. C., Gordon, S., and Reich, E.,** Secretion of plasminogen activator by stimulated macrophages, *J. Exp. Med.,* 139, 834, 1974.

75. **Sherman, M. I., Strickland, S., and Reich, E.,** Differentiation of early mouse embryonic and teratocarcinoma cells in vitro: plasminogen activator production, *Cancer Res.,* 36, 4208, 1976.

76. **Topp, W., Hall, J. D., Marsden, M., Teresky, A. K., Rifkin, D., Levine, A. J., and Pollack, R.,** In vitro differentiation of teratomas and the distribution of creatine phosphokinase and plasminogen activator in teratocarcinoma-derived cells, *Cancer Res.,* 36, 4217, 1976.

77. **Strickland, S. and Beers, W. H.,** Studies on the role of plasminogen activator in ovulation. In vitro response of granulosa cells to gonadotropins, cyclic nucleotides, and prostaglandins, *J. Biol. Chem.,* 251, 5694, 1976.

78. **Katz, J., Troll, W., Adler, S., and Levitz, M.,** Antipain and leupeptin restrict uterine DNA synthesis and function in mice, *Proc. Natl. Acad. Sci. U.S.A.,* 74, 3754, 1977.

79. **Chou, I-N., Roblin, R. O., and Black, P. H.,** Calcium stimulation of plasminogen activator secretion production by Swiss 3T3 cells, *J. Biol. Chem.,* 252, 6256, 1977.

80. **Hamilton, J., Vassalli, J. D., and Reich, E.,** Macrophage plasminogen activator: induction by asbestos is blocked by anti-inflammatory steroids, *J. Exp. Med.,* 144, 1689, 1976.

81. **Vassalli, J. D., Hamilton, J., and Reich, E.,** Macrophage plasminogen activator: modulation of enzyme production by anti-inflammatory steroids, mitotic inhibitors and cyclic nucleotides, *Cell,* 8, 271, 1976.

82. **Vassalli, J. D. and Reich, E.,** Macrophage plasminogen activator: induction by products of activated lymphoid cells, *J. Exp. Med.,* 145, 429, 1977.

83. **Klimetzek, V. and Sorg, C.**, Lymphokine-induced secretion of plasminogen activator by murine macrophages, *Eur. J. Immunol.*, 7, 185, 1977.
84. **Noguerra, N., Gordon, S., and Cohn, Z.**, Trypanasoma cruzi: the immunological induction of macrophage plasminogen activator requires thymus-derived lymphocytes, *J. Exp. Med.*, 146, 122, 1977.
85. **Sherman, L. A., Lee, J., and Stewart, C. C.**, Release of fibrinolytic enzymes by macrophages to soluble fibrin, *Thromb. Haemostas.*, 38 (Abstr.), 46, 1977.
86. **Loskatoff, D. J. and Edgington, T. S.**, Characterization of the fibrinolytic components specified by vascular endothelial cells, *Thromb. Haemostas.*, 38 (Abstr.), 139, 1977.
87. **Macfarlane, R. G. and Pilling, J.**, Fibrinolytic activity of normal urine, *Nature (London)*, 159, 779, 1947.
88. **Astrup, T. and Sterndorff, I.**, An activator of plasminogen in normal urine, *Proc. Soc. Exp. Biol.*, 81, 675, 1952.
89. **Williams, J. R. B.**, The fibrinolytic activity of urine, *Br. J. Exp. Pathol.*, 32, 530, 1951.
90. **Sobel, G. W., Mohler, S. R., Jones, N. W., Dowdy, A. B. C., and Guest, M. M.**, Urokinase: an activator of plasma profibrinolysin extracted from urine, *Am. J. Physiol.*, 171, 768, 1952.
91. **von Kaulla, K. M.**, Urine adsorbate with fibrinolytic and thromboplastic properties, *J. Lab. Clin. Med.*, 44, 944, 1954.
92. **Ploug, J. and Kjeldgaard, N. O.**, Urokinase: an activator of plasminogen from human urine. I. Isolation and properties, *Biochim. Biophys. Acta*, 24, 278, 1957.
93. **Celander, D. R. and Guest, M. M.**, The biochemistry and physiology of urokinase, *Am. J. Cardiol.*, 6, 409, 1960.
94. **Sgouris, J. T., Storey, R. W., McCall, K. B., and Anderson, H. D.**, The purification, assay, sterilization, and removal of pyrogenicity of human urokinase, *Vox Sang.*, 7, 739, 1962.
95. **White, W. F., Barlow, G. H., and Mozen, M. M.**, The isolation and characterization of plasminogen activators (urokinase) from human urine, *Biochemistry*, 5, 2160, 1966.
96. **Lesuk, A., Terminiello, L., and Traver, J. H.**, Crystalline human urokinase: some properties, *Science*, 147, 880, 1965.
97. **Ogawa, N., Yamamoto, H., Katamine, T., and Tojima, H.**, Purification and some properties of urokinase, *Thromb. Diath. Haemmorh.*, 34, 194, 1975.
98. **Holmberg, L., Bladh, B., and Astedt, B.**, Purification of urokinase by affinity chromatography, *Biochim. Biophys. Acta*, 445, 215, 1976.
99. **Soberano, M. E., Ong, E. B., Johnson, A. J., Levy, M., and Schoellmann, G.**, Purification and characterization of two forms of urokinase, *Biochim. Biophys. Acta*, 445, 763, 1976.
100. **Maciag, T., Weibel, M. K., and Pye, E. K.**, Urokinase, *Methods Enzymol.*, 34, 451, 1974.
101. **Ball, A. P. and Day, E. D.**, Immunological identification of two urokinases, *Thromb. Diath. Haemorrh.*, 24, 475, 1970.
102. **Lesuk, A., Terminiello, L., Traver, J. H., and Geoff, J. L.**, Biochemical and biophysical studies of human urokinase, *Thromb. Diath. Haemorrh.*, 18, 293, 1967.
103. **Soberano, M. E., Ong, E. B., and Johnson, A. J.**, The effects of inhibitors on the catalytic conversion of urokinase, *Thromb. Res.*, 9, 675, 1976.
104. **Sherry, S., Alkjaersig, N., and Fletcher, A. P.**, Assay of urokinase preparation with the synthetic substrate acetyl-L-lysine methyl ester, *J. Lab. Clin. Med.*, 64, 145, 1964.
105. **Walton, P. L.**, The hydrolysis of α-*N*-acetylglycyl-L-lysine methyl ester by urokinase, *Biochim. Biophys. Acta*, 132, 104, 1967.
106. **Hedner, U.**, Studies on an inhibitor of plasminogen activation in human serum, *Thromb. Diath. Haemorrh.*, 30, 414, 1973.
107. **Beattie, A. G., Ogston, D., Bennett, B., and Douglas, A. S.**, Inhibitors of plasminogen activation in human blood, *Br. J. Haematol.*, 32, 135, 1976.
108. **Gallimore, M. J. and Hedner, U.**, Further evidence for the presence of two plasma inhibitors of fibrinolysis distinct from α_2-macroglobulin, *Thromb. Res.*, 11, 267, 1977.
109. **Kawano, T., Morimoto, K., and Uemura, Y.**, Partial purification and properties of urokinase inhibitor from human placenta, *J. Biochem. (Tokyo)*, 67, 333, 1970.
110. **Clemmensen, I. and Christensen, F.**, Inhibition of urokinase by complex formation with human α_1-antitrypsin, *Biochim. Biophys. Acta*, 429, 591, 1976.
111. **Ong, E. B., Johnson, A. J., and Schoellmann, G.**, Identification of an active site histidine in urokinase, *Biochim. Biophys. Acta*, 429, 252, 1976.
112. **Landmann, H. and Markwardt, F.**, Irreversible synthetische inhibitoren der urokinase, *Experientia*, 26, 145, 1970.
113. **Reddy, K. N. N. and Markus, G.**, Mechanism of activation of human plasminogen by streptokinase. Presence of active center in streptokinase-plasminogen complex, *J. Biol. Chem.*, 247, 1683, 1972.
114. **Fletcher, A. P. and Johnson, A. J.**, Methods employed for purification of streptokinase, *Proc. Soc. Exp. Biol. Med.*, 94, 233, 1957.

115. **DeRenzo, E. C., Siiteri, P. K., Hutchings, B. I., and Bell, P. H.**, Preparation and certain properties of highly purified streptokinase, *J. Biol. Chem.*, 242, 533, 1967.
116. **Taylor, F. B., Jr. and Botts, J.**, Purification and characterization of streptokinase with studies of streptokinase activation of plasminogen, *Biochemistry*, 7, 232, 1968.
117. **Morgan, F. J. and Henschen, A.**, The structure of streptokinase, cyanogen bromide fragmentation, amino acid composition and partial amino acid sequences, *Biochim. Biophys. Acta*, 181, 93, 1969.
118. **Loch, T., Bilinski, T., and Zakrzewski, K.**, Studies on streptokinase. The conformation, *Acta Biochim. Pol.*, 15, 129, 1968.
119. **Lack, C. H.**, Staphylokinase: an activator of plasma protease, *Nature (London)*, 161, 559, 1948.
120. **Gerheim, E. B., Ferguson, J. H., Travis, B. L., Johnson, C. L., and Boyles, P. W.**, Staphylococcal fibrinolysis, *Proc. Soc. Exp. Biol. Med.*, 68, 246, 1948.
121. **Vesterberg, K. and Vesterberg, O.**, Studies on staphylokinase, *J. Med. Microbiol.*, 5, 441, 1972.
122. **Kowalska-Loth, B. and Zakrzewski, K.**, The activation by staphylokinase of human plasminogen, *Acta Biochim. Pol.*, 22, 327, 1975.
123. **Makino, T., Fujimura, S., and Hayashi, T. T. A.**, Studies on staphylokinase, *Zentrabl. Bakteriol. Parasitenkd. Infektionskr. Hyg., Abt. 1, Suppl.*, 5, 539, 1976.
124. **Lewis, J. H. and Ferguson, J. H.**, A proteolytic enzyme system of the blood. Activation of dog serum profibrinolysin by staphylokinase, *Am. J. Physiol.*, 166, 594, 1952.
125. **Davidson, F. M.**, The activation of plasminogen by staphylokinase: comparison with streptokinase, *Biochem. J.*, 76, 56, 1960.
126. **Reddy, K. N. N.**, Kinetics of active center formation in dog plasminogen by streptokinase and activity of a modified streptokinase, *J. Biol. Chem.*, 251, 6624, 1976.
127. **Makino, T.**, Proteolytic modification of staphylokinase, *Biochim. Biophys. Acta*, 522, 267, 1978.
128. **Kopitar, M., Stegnar, M., Accetto, B., and Lebez, D.**, Isolation and characterization of plasminogen activator from pig leucocytes, *Thromb. Diath. Haemorrh.*, 31, 72, 1974.
129. **Granelli-piperno, A., Vassalli, J. D., and Reich, E.**, Secretion of plasminogen activator by human polymorphonuclear leucocytes. Modulation by glucocorticoids and other effectors, *J. Exp. Med.*, 146, 1603, 1978.
130. **Semar, J., Skoza, L., and Johnson, A. J.**, Partial purification and properties of a plasminogen activator from human erythrocytes, *J. Clin. Invest.*, 48, 1777, 1969.
131. **Oshiba, S. and Ariga, T.**, Purification and characterization of bilokinase, a biliary plasminogen activator, *Thromb. Diath. Haemorrh.*, 34, 319, 1975 (Abs).
132. **Nagamatsu, Y., Horie, N., Yamamoto, J. I., and Okamoto, U.**, Studies of a plasminogen activating system in human milk. II. Some properties of milk plasminogen activator, *Acta Haematol. Jpn.*, 38, 157, 1975.
133. **Propping, D., Tauber, P. F., Zaneveld, L. J. D., and Schumacher, G. F. B.**, Purification and characterization of plasminogen activator from human seminal plasma, *Fed. Proc. Fed. Am. Soc. Exp. Biol.*, 33 (Abstr.), 289, 1974.
134. **Cartwright, T.**, The plasminogen activator of vampire bat saliva, *Blood*, 43, 317, 1974.

Chapter 3

INITIATION OF HAGEMAN FACTOR-DEPENDENT FIBRINOLYSIS

Allen P. Kaplan and Lewis D. Yecies

TABLE OF CONTENTS

I. INTRODUCTION

A. Identification of Critical Plasma Factors Required for Hageman Factor-Dependent Fibrinolysis

Toward the end of the 19th century, Denys and de Marbaix[1] made the observation that canine fibrin dissolved rapidly in serum that had been treated with either chloroform or ether, indicating the presence of a fibrinolysin. Soon thereafter, it was shown that fibrin would gradually dissolve when incubated in its own serum, even in the absence of an organic solvent, although the process was considerably slower.[2] It appeared that the addition of chloroform hastened the formation of an enzyme that could also digest gelatin or casein.[3] This enzyme was shown to be a euglobulin[4] and was given the name plasmin[5] or fibrinolysin[6] and was found in freshly drawn blood as an inert precursor called plasminogen or profibrinolysin. Lewis and Ferguson separated dog plasma into two fractions, one containing plasminogen and the other containing one or more additional plasma factors necessary for the generation of fibrinolytic activity.[7] Upon mixing the fractions, fibrinolytic activity gradually evolved, while the separate fractions generated no fibrinolytic activity when incubated under identical conditions.

In 1955, Ratnoff and Colopy described a patient named Hageman,[8] who had a markedly prolonged partial thromboplastin time (PPT) and appeared to lack a plasma factor, designated Hageman factor, which bound to surfaces and was active at the initiating step of the coagulation cascade.[9] When a euglobulin suspension prepared from normal plasma was incubated at 37°C, an increase in plasminogen-activating activity was observed, while similar incubation of the euglobulin suspension from Hageman factor-deficient plasma did not generate such activity.[10,11] Hageman factor-deficient plasma was then shown to possess a profound abnormality of surface-dependent fibrinolysis[12-14] and generated no bradykinin upon incubation with glass beads or kaolin.[15-17] However, activated Hageman factor did not appear to directly convert plasminogen to plasmin.[13] Thus, other plasma proteins appeared to participate in the Hageman factor-dependent fibrinolytic pathway.

In 1965, a new coagulation abnormality was discovered in a family named Fletcher[18] which was characterized as having a prolonged PPT which autocorrected as the time of incubation with surfaces was increased.[18,19] This latter property suggested that it possessed an abnormal rate of contact activation. The abnormality could be corrected upon addition of small quantities of normal plasma, and the factor was partially purified.[20] Subsequently Wuepper identified the Fletcher factor to be prekallikrein.[21] A detailed analysis of the functional abnormalities associated with prekallikrein deficiency revealed a diminished rate of Hageman factor-dependent fibrinolysis[22-24] which was also corrected upon prolonged incubation with surfaces[23] and an inability to generate any bradykinin, regardless of the incubation time. Weiss et al.[23] observed that the addition of preparations of activated Hageman factor to prekallikrein-deficient plasma corrected the diminished rate of intrinsic coagulation and fibrinolysis, suggesting that the deficient plasma possessed a subnormal rate of formation of activated Hageman factor. The autocorrection with time in the absence of prekallikrein suggested that a slower, alternative mechanism existed that could lead to the formation of activated Hageman factor. Thus, Hageman factor and prekallikrein are plasma proteins required for (1) the initiation of fibrinolysis, (2) the intrinsic coagulation pathway, and (3) the generation of bradykinin.

The next development in the identification of the plasma factors required for contact activation were observations by Webster and Pierce[25] and Schiffman et al.[26] which indicated that the combination of a surface, Hageman factor, and prekallikrein was not sufficient to initiate kinin generation or Factor XI activation. Evidence that an additional plasma factor is required was presented, and the latter workers called it the "contact activation cofactor". Soon thereafter, three different patients possessing unique abnormalities of contact activation were reported; two of these patients (named Williams and Fitzgerald, respectively) were reported at an international "kallikrein-kinin" meeting[27,28] and the third patient (named Flaujeac) was reported at a coagulation meeting in France.[29] Each plasma was shown to possess a markedly prolonged PTT which did not autocorrect with time, diminished surface-dependent fibrinolysis, and absence of kinin formation.[27,29-31] Flaujeac trait plasma was shown to possess only 8% of normal plasma kininogen, the precursor of kinins, and the functional abnormalities were each corrected upon addition of plasma fractions containing high molecular weight kininogen (HMW-kininogen).[32,33] Williams-trait plasma was found to be completely devoid of functional or antigenic kininogen,[27,34] and the abnormality was attributed at first to a new coagulation factor[34] that was later identified to be HMW-kininogen.[35] These observations were confirmed when Fitzgerald trait was identified as HMW-kininogen deficiency in a fourth patient (Washington), who possessed the identical functional abnormalities.[36] HMW-kininogen was also shown to be the same protein whose function had been observed earlier in partially purified plasma fractions,[25,26] and the contact activation cofactor was shown to be lacking in Fitzgerald-trait plasma[37] and was then found to be identical to HMW-kininogen.[27,38]

Factor XI is also a substrate of activated Hageman factor,[39] however, its role in Hageman-Factor dependent fibrinolysis is not yet clear; this is discussed in the last section. A time course of surface-dependent activation of the fibrinolytic pathway is in Figure 1 and demonstrates the marked abnormality present in both Hageman factor-deficient plasma and HMW-kininogen-deficient plasma, as well as the abnormal rate of activation of prekallikrein deficient plasma. The interactions of these three plasma proteins which leads to the generation of a plasminogen activator will be described herein.

B. Interaction of Prekallikrein, Factor XI, and HMW-Kininogen in Plasma

It is clear that Hageman factor, prekallikrein, HMW-kininogen, Factor XI, and plasminogen are intimately related in their functions, but they clearly represent different plasma proteins that are antigenically unrelated and are represented in the genome by distinct structural genes. However, reports suggesting that kallikrein can be purified as a complex with another plasma protein[40] and that prekallikrein appears to circulate in plasma as a complex[41] prompted the studies of Mandle et al.[42] and Thompson et al.[43] in which prekallikrein and Factor XI were each shown to circulate bound to HMW-kininogen.

When normal human plasma was fractionated on Sephadex G-200, the apparent molecular weight of each of the above proteins could be determined. As in Figure 2, Factor XI was found at a molecular weight of 380,000, prekallikrein was found at 260,000, Hageman factor was found at 115,000, and plasminogen was found at 95,000. However, when the molecular weights of purified Factor XI and prekallikrein were assessed by gel filtration, values of 175,000 and 100,000, respectively, were obtained — a discrepancy of approximately 200,000. Purified Hageman factor and plasminogen fractionated at the same position as they did when whole plasma was assessed, and therefore did not appear to circulate as part of a complex. When the molecular weight of prekallikrein and Factor XI was determined in plasma deficient in HMW-kininogen, Factor XI was found at 175,000 and prekallikrein was found at 100,000, suggesting that each protein normally circulates bound to HMW-kininogen. Reconstitution of HMW-kininogen deficient plasma with purified HMW-kininogen followed by fractionation by Sephadex G-200 gel filtration reproduced the chromatographic pattern of Factor XI and prekallikrein that is found in normal plasma.[42,43] In addition, direct

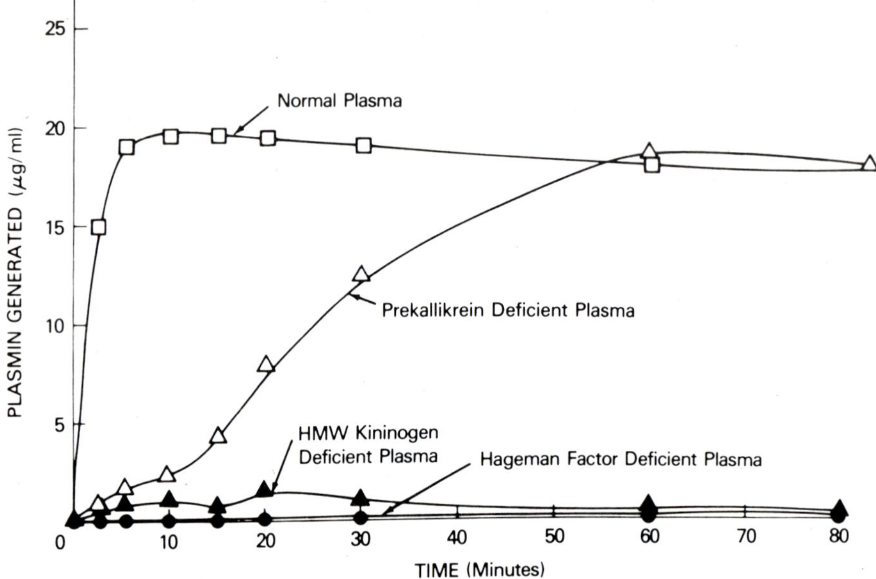

FIGURE 1. Time course of activation of the Hageman factor-dependent coagulation and fibrinolytic pathways.

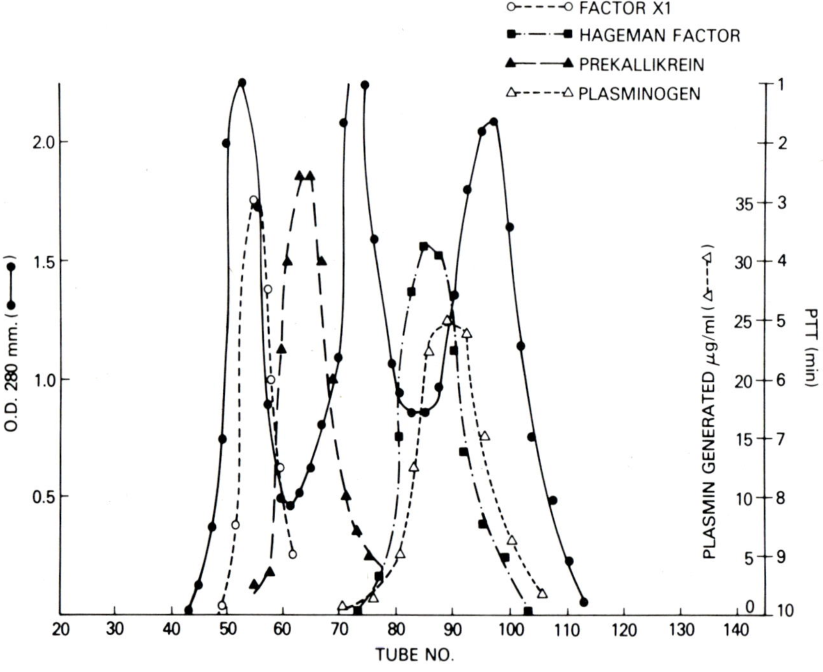

FIGURE 2. Sephadex® G-200 gel filtration of 4.0 mℓ of normal plasma, indicating the relative position of the Factor XI-HMW-kininogen complex, the prekallikrein-HMW-kininogen complex, Hageman factor, and plasminogen.

binding of purified prekallikrein to HMW-kininogen[42] and direct binding of partially purified Factor XI to HMW-kininogen[43] have been demonstrated. When a tenfold excess of purified HMW-kininogen was incubated with partially purified Factor XI

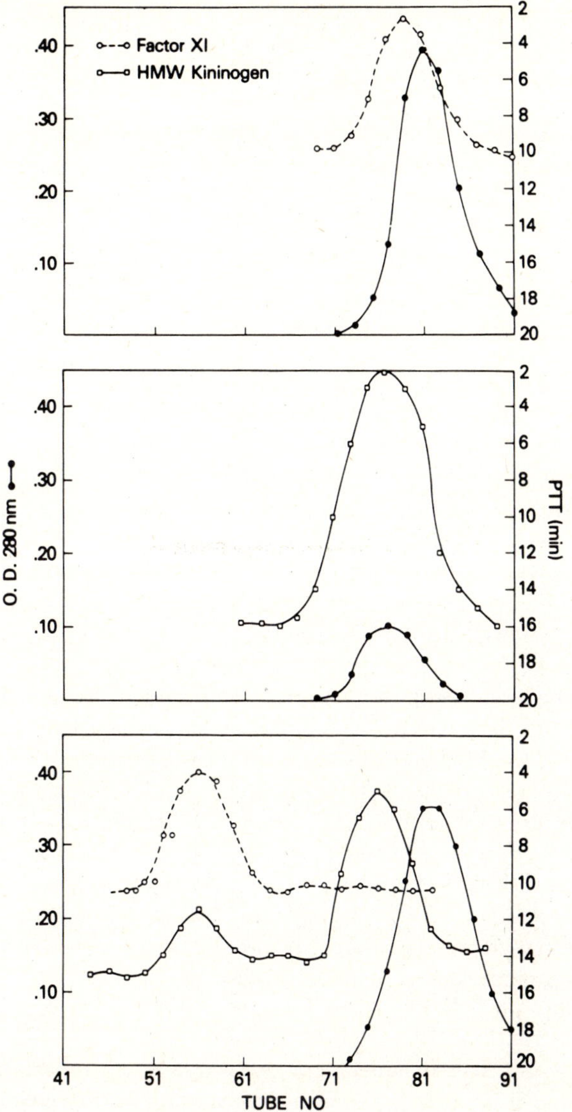

FIGURE 3. Sephadex® G-200 gel filtration of 2.0 mℓ of Factor XI (5 units/mℓ) (upper panel), 2.0 mℓ of purified HMW-kininogen (50 units/mℓ) (center panel), and a mixture of 2.0 mℓ Factor XI plus 2.0 mℓ HMW-kininogen (bottom panel). Buffer was added so that a total of 4.0 mℓ was applied to the column in each case.

for 10 min at 23°C and then fractionated on Sephadex G-200, the pattern in Figure 3 was observed. The Factor XI preparation had an apparent molecular weight of 175,000 (contaminating IgG is seen at 160,000), purified HMW-kininogen was found at a molecular weight of 210,000, and the mixture of Factor XI and HMW-kininogen yielded a peak of activity at 380,000, containing all of the Factor XI and approximately 10% of the HMW-kininogen. Normal plasma contains approximately twice the concentration of HMW-kininogen as the sum of the Factor XI and prekallikrein concentrations; thus, after complete binding of Factor XI and prekallikrein, the major peak of HMW-kininogen seen represents uncomplexed protein.[42] No complex has been observed containing prekallikrein, Factor XI, and HMW-kininogen as a single entity; prekallikrein and Factor XI appear to circulate as different complexes with HMW-kininogen. Binding to HMW-kininogen thus appears to be a specific property of the Hageman factor substrates, and the complexes of prekallikrein-HMW-kininogen and Factor XI-HMW-kininogen each adsorb to surfaces where they then interact with surface-bound Hageman factor.

II. HAGEMAN FACTOR

A. Purification and Properties Human Hageman Factor

The first partial purification of human Hageman factor was accomplished by Ratnoff and Davie, using a combination of chromatography on DEAE cellulose, CM cellulose, and gel filtration.[44] Similar procedures were subsequently reported[45-47] in which hexadimethrine bromide was added to the starting plasma in order to inhibit Hageman factor activation; plastic columns and test tubes were utilized in order to minimize interaction with surfaces, and alternative ion exchanges, such as QAE Sephadex A-25 and SP Sephadex C-25 were used to increase the yield as well as the purity. Nevertheless the purification of Hageman factor remained particularly difficult because it became activated and fragmented during the various procedures. Thus, the yield was low (about 5%), and the best preparations were contaminated with traces of other β globulins. Revak et al.[48] reported a similar procedure with the addition of two chromatographic steps on anion exchangers; the first was a salt gradient similar to that routinely utilized, and the second was a pH gradient. This latter step appeared to improve the stability of the Hageman factor, although it contributed little to the specific activity of the preparation. It is possible that small quantities of contaminating prekallikrein/kallikrein or Factor XI/Factor XIa were removed in the above modification, since neither protein adheres appreciably to anion exchangers. The purity of the resulting preparation was sufficient to determine its molecular weight with SDS gel electrophoresis, and, utilizing ^{125}I-Hageman factor, the pattern of cleavage could be followed.[48] Nevertheless this procedure proved to be variable in both yield and purity, and further improvements in methodology were sought.

Meier and Kaplan[49,50] reported a method for the isolation of Hageman factor in which plasma was fractionated on QAE-Sephadex A25 and SP-Sephadex and then passed over two immunoadsorbants. The first was a combined immunoadsorbant which included lysine Sepharose® to remove plasminogen and plasmin, and sheep IgG antibody to human IgG, prekallikrein, and Factor XI. In this fashion, traces of plasmin, kallikrein, and Factor XIa, each of which was known to activate and fragment Hageman factor, were removed. The second adsorbant was an antiHageman factor immunoadsorbant. Sheep antihuman Hageman factor was adsorbed with Hageman factor-deficient plasma, and a 45% ammonium sulfate fraction of the adsorbed antiserum was coupled to Sepharose. The solution of Hageman factor was passed over the column which was then washed extensively, and the Hageman factor was eluted with 1.0 *M* potassium thiocyanate. This procedure resulted in the rapid isolation of highly purified Hageman factor (2500-fold), however, the yield remained low at 5 to 10%; elution of Hageman factor from the adsorbant was variable, and sheep proteins were sometimes detected as trace contaminants in the sample. Chan and Movat[51] reported a four-step chromatographic procedure for the isolation of unactivated Hageman factor following adsorption of plasma with aluminum hydroxide and polyethylene glycol precipitation. An immunoadsorbant column was used as the final step in order to remove trace contaminants. A highly purified preparation resulted, with a yield varying from 8 to 16%. This represented a significant improvement over an earlier report from this laboratory in which a seven-step chromatographic procedure resulted in a 1% recovery of Hageman factor.[52]

The most recently published procedure for the isolation of human Hageman factor was reported by Griffin and Cochrane.[53] This method utilized succinate buffers with benzamidine hydrochloride added to inhibit contaminating proteases. A lysine Sepharose step was included to remove plasminogen and plasmin, and ammonium sulfate precipitation was utilized to concentrate the Hageman factor. The chromatographic steps included a salt gradient on DEAE Sephadex A-50, a pH-gradient on DEAE-Sephadex, and a salt gradient on SP Sephadex. We have utilized this procedure and have found it to improve the yield of Hageman factor to 15 to 25%, the resulting preparation was over 95% pure, and the purification factor was approximately 2500-fold. Although the chromatographic steps are similar to those reported previously, a number of important modifications have improved the yield and purity. Ammonium sulfate precipitation of plasma had previously been found to accelerate Hageman factor activation, and its use as a concentration step was abandoned. However, in the presence of inhibitors such as benzamidine, ammonium sulfate precipitation can be utilized to further purify and concentrate partially purified preparations. This eliminates the use of ultrafiltration which is slow, results in considerable loss by adsorption, and does not increase the specific activity of the material. In addition the Hageman factor appears to be particularly stable in the buffer system used by Griffin and Cochrane.

Hageman factor was found to be a single-chain β globulin of mol wt 80,000 and is present in plasma at concentrations ranging from 23 to 47 $\mu g/m\ell$ (mean 29 $\mu g/m\ell$).[48] The chief isoelectric point of human Hageman factor was reported to be between 6.1 and 6.5; however, considerable charge heterogeneity was observed with a pH range of 5.9 to 7.0.[46]

B. Initiation of Hageman Factor-Dependent Fibrinolysis: The Role of the Surface, Hageman Factor, HMW-Kininogen, and Prekallikrein

1. Role of the Hageman Factor

The activation of Hageman factor differs from that observed with the other proenzymes to be described because a two-step process is observed; the first consists of an initial cleavage without fragmentation, and the second consists of a cleavage which liberates one or more active fragments. The discovery of the active fragments of Hageman factor by Kaplan and Austen[54] provided the first evidence that activation could involve an enzymatic step.[55] The final product, a prealbumin fragment observed as two closely migrating bands upon alkaline disc gel electrophoresis, functioned as a potent prekallikrein activator, but retained only 2 to 5% of the coagulant activity of the unfragmented Hageman factor. Subsequently, plasmin was shown to be capable of directly digesting Hageman factor to yield these fragments.[55] Similar prealbumin activities described in the rabbit,[56] guinea pig,[57] and man[58,59] were subsequently shown to be derived from Hageman factor,[47,60] and the ability of plasmin to activate and fragment Hageman factor was confirmed.[61] Although not purified, an activated preparation of Hageman factor was also described whose molecular weight upon gel filtration (115,000) was identical to that of unactivated Hageman factor, yet it readily clotted Hageman factor-deficient plasma in the absence of kaolin. This preparation was designated intact activated Hageman factor.[55] In addition, at least two active fragments were described whose molecular weights were intermediate between those of the prealbumin fragments and the unfragmented active molecule.[55] In summary by gel filtration, active species were detected at molecular weights of 115,000, 90,000, 60,000, and 40,000,[46] and each of the first three species could be converted to the 40,000-mol wt prealbumin fragment.[46,55]

2. Role of Kallikrein in Activation of the Hageman Factor

The discovery of prekallikrein-deficient plasma led to an examination of the ability of kallikrein to activate and fragment Hageman factor. Kallikrein was found to function in a manner similar to plasmin; however, it was approximately ten times as effective[62] and could act upon either surface-bound or fluid-phase Hageman factor. When Hageman factor was iodinated, digested by trypsin plasmin and kallikrein, and examined by SDS gel electrophoresis, similar fragmentation patterns were found.[48] The molecular weight of Hageman factor was 90,000 in unreduced gels and 80,000 after reduction; upon digestion it was converted to a 28,000 active fragment which corresponded to the stable prealbumin fragment previously described (40,000 by gel filtration), and a 50,000-dalton fragment remained. Further digestion converted the 50,000-dalton fragment to fragments of 40,000 and 10,000. However, the formation of an active, unfragmented form of Hageman factor was not detected. The 50,000-dalton fragment was subsequently shown to be the portion of the molecule that binds to surfaces.[63] In Figure 4, the pattern of ^{125}I-Hageman factor digestion upon incubation with 2% (by weight) kallikrein for 30 min at 37°C is shown. The starting material, seen at 80,000 daltons, was converted to 50,000- and 28,000-dalton fragments. In the insert is an alkaline disc gel electrophoresis of Hageman factor before (left) and after (center) digestion with plasma kallikrein. When the digested product was incubated with kaolin, centrifuged, and the supernatant subjected to alkaline disc gel electrophoresis (right), only the active prealbumin fragments were seen. Bagdasarian and Colman investigated the cleavage of Hageman factor with kallikrein or plasmin[64] and observed that cleavage with kallikrein routinely generated the prealbumin fragments, while plasmin digestion could yield a larger active fragment[65] which appeared to resist further digestion to the prealbumin fragments. This cleavage product may be identical to one of the intermediate-sized active fragments described earlier;[55] however, the inability to further digest it to the prealbumin fragment has not yet been confirmed.

3. Role of Kininogen in Contact Activation

With the discovery of HMW-kininogen deficiency, it became clear that a reciprocal mechanism in which activated Hageman factor converts prekallikrein to kallikrein and kallikrein in turn activates the Hageman factor was an oversimplification. For example, addition of activated Hageman factor to Hageman factor-deficient plasma initiates coagulation and fibrinolysis in the absence of a foreign surface such as kaolin by activation of Factor XI and prekallikrein. Addition of Factor XIa to Factor XI-deficient plasma causes coagulation in the absence of kaolin by activation of Factor IX. However, addition of kallikrein to prekallikrein-deficient plasma in the absence of a surface does not result in appreciable coagulation.[50] Thus, the surface appeared to be required for this function of kallikrein to be expressed. Furthermore, the addition of activated Hageman factor to HMW-kininogen-deficient plasma, even in the presence of a surface, did not significantly shorten the partial thromboplastin time of the deficient plasma.[66,67] Thus, HMW-kininogen appeared to be required for the activation of Hageman factor and/or the expression of Hageman factor activity. When the role of HMW-kininogen was further examined, it was found to enhance both the function of activated Hageman factor and the formation of activated Hageman factor.[66-74]

Figure 5 shows that HMW-kininogen can augment the ability of surface-bound Hageman factor to activate prekallikrein, Factor XI, and initiate the conversion of plasminogen to plasmin. For a fixed quantity of surface-bound Hageman factor, the subsequent activation of each Hageman factor substrate was proportional to the quantity of HMW-kininogen added.[66,68,69,73] Such an experiment demonstrates the effect of HMW-kininogen upon the system, but does not distinguish between an effect upon the function of already activated Hageman factor from an effect on the formation of

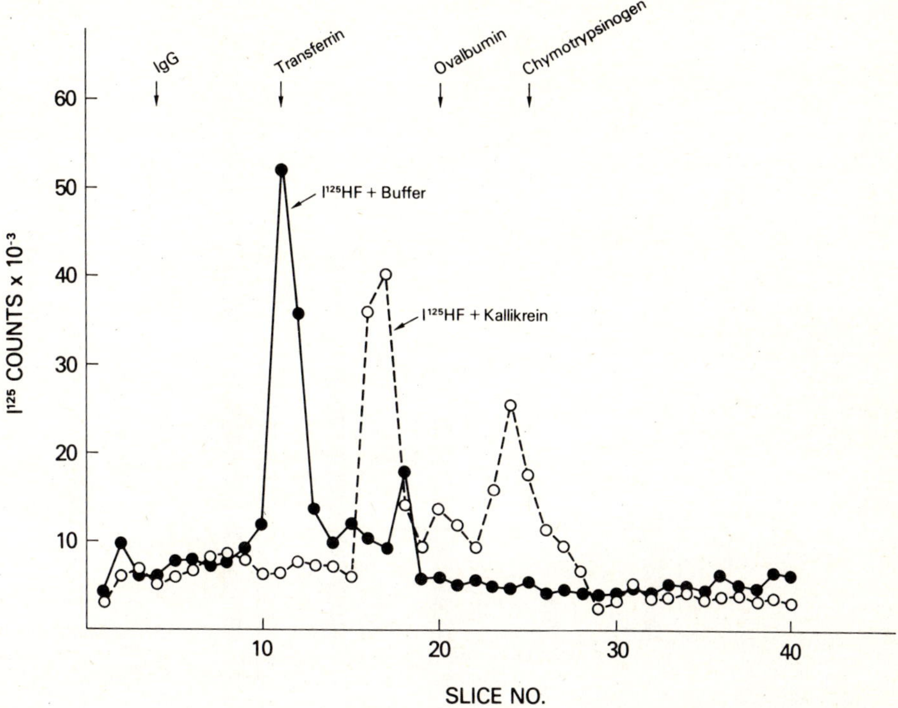

FIGURE 4. SDS gel electrophoresis of ^{125}I-Hageman factor before and after digestion with plasma kallikrein. The gels were sliced, each slice eluted, and the eluate counted. Conversion of ^{125}I Hageman factor seen at 80,000-, 52,000-, and 28,000-dalton fragments was observed. In the insert is an alkaline disc gel electrophoresis of Hageman factor (left gel), Hageman factor that has been digested with kallikrein (center gel), and the supernatant obtained from kallikrein-digested Hageman factor after adsorption with kaolin. The preparation demonstrates heterogeneity upon alkaline disc gel electrophoresis (left gel) and after digestion yields a series of bands at the center of the gel and prealbumin bands at the anode. After adsorption with kaolin (right gel), only the prealbumin bands remain.

activated Hageman factor. However, augmentation of the ability of Hageman factor fragments to convert prekallikrein to kallikrein in the absence of a surface has been reported.[67,71,72] In this case, the Hageman factor utilized is already active; thus the effect observed is upon its function. Furthermore, addition of Hageman factor fragments to HMW-kininogen-deficient plasma failed to yield the predicted activation of either prekallikrein or Factor XI, and this abnormality was corrected upon reconstitution with HMW-kininogen.[72] Alternatively, limited trypsin treatment of surface-bound Hageman factor could be utilized to achieve activation, and the enhancing effect of HMW-kininogen upon the subsequent activation of prekallikrein or Factor XI could then be observed.[68,69] Figure 6 shows a dose response of the ability of HMW-kininogen to augment the function of surface-bound Hageman factor, as assessed by prekallikrein activation. The reaction appeared stoichiometric[69,73] in that the activity observed was proportional to the HMW-kininogen input. There appeared to be an optimal concentration of HMW-kininogen that could be used and excess HMW-kininogen was inhibitory.[73] A similar dose-response curve profile has been found for the effect of HMW-kininogen upon the function of the Hageman factor fragments;[72] however, the cause of this inhibition is not known. To perform these assays, the Hageman factor was first adsorbed to the surface in the presence or absence of HMW-kininogen, centrifuged, and the pellet was extensively washed. The pellet was then incubated with the Hageman factor substrates in order to assay for the presence of activated Hageman

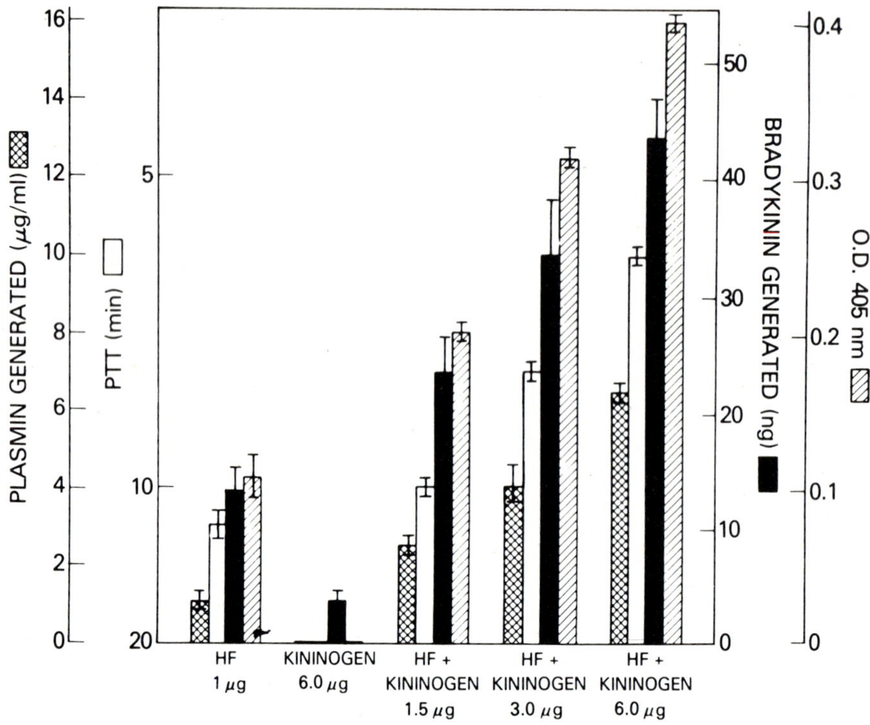

FIGURE 5. The effect of increasing quantities of HMW-kininogen upon the ability of Hageman factor to activate prekallikrein, Factor XI, and generate plasminogen activating activity.

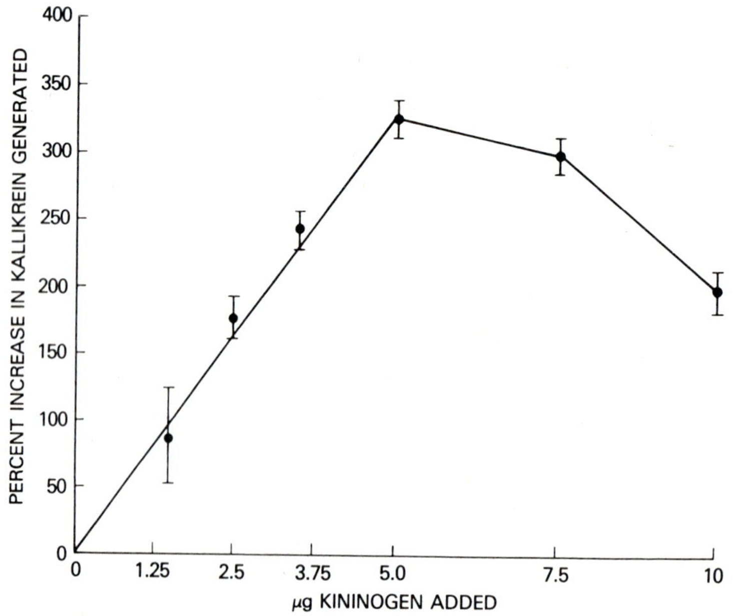

FIGURE 6. Enhancement of the activity of surface-bound Hageman factor upon prekallikrein as a function of the HMW-kininogen added.

factor. Critical to the interpretation of these experiments is a determination of whether HMW-kininogen affects binding of Hageman factor to surfaces. When this was examined, no effect was found.[73] Furthermore, any activated Hageman factor detected in the second step of the assay was firmly adsorbed to the surface, suggesting that the molecular form of activated Hageman factor detected was not the prealbumin fragments, since these fragments lack the binding site for the surface (Figure 4). The initial cleavage of human Hageman factor has been reported to occur within a disulfide bridge without fragmentation of the starting material.[74] A second cleavage external to the disulfide bond liberated the 28,000-dalton fragment which is found in the surrounding fluid rather than on the surface.

Although these data demonstrate an effect of HMW-kininogen upon the function of activated Hageman factor, they do not preclude an effect upon the activation of Hageman factor. Griffin and Cochrane reported that the rate of cleavage of Hageman factor by kallikrein appeared to be enhanced by HMW-kininogen,[69] suggesting an effect upon Hageman factor activation. Meier et al. assessed this reaction functionally and demonstrated that the ability of kallikrein to activate Hageman factor was markedly augmented by HMW-kininogen.[73] Figure 7 is a demonstration of the ability of kallikrein to activate DFP-treated Hageman factor, as assessed in the same two-stage assay described above. Unactivated Hageman factor and kallikrein were adsorbed to the surface in the presence or absence of HMW-kininogen. The mixture was centrifuged, the pellet was washed, and the washed pellet then assayed for its ability to convert prekallikrein to kallikrein. Activation of Hageman factor during the initial incubation with kallikrein was observed only in the presence of HMW-kininogen and the active moiety generated was bound to the surface. In Table 1 the incorporation of ^{3}H-DFP into the surface-bound reactants is shown. Nonspecific uptake of 7200 counts by the surface was observed. However, incubation of kaolin with Hageman factor alone or with Hageman factor plus HMW-kininogen did not yield a significant further uptake of radioactivity. There was no evident activation of the Hageman factor upon binding to surface, and HMW-kininogen did not activate the Hageman factor. However, incubation with kallikrein did activate the Hageman factor, as indicated by the additional incorporation of 6000 counts (the kallikrein alone could only incorporate 500 counts). However, the function of these additional sites produced by kallikrein would not be fully expressed in the absence of HMW-kininogen.[66,68,69,73] Incubation of surface-bound Hageman factor with kallikrein and HMW-kininogen followed by incubation with ^{3}H-DFP led to incorporation of an additional 34,000 counts. Thus, HMW-kininogen augmented the activation of Hageman factor by kallikrein when the presence of activated Hageman factor was assessed functionally[73] (Figure 6) or when the formation of new active sites was determined. In the presence of HMW-kininogen, the function of each of these sites could then be fully expressed. Figure 8 is a schematic diagram of this reciprocal interaction of surface-bound Hageman factor and prekallikrein, indicating that the reaction rate in each direction is augmented by HMW-kininogen. It should be emphasized that a surface and the active site of kallikrein were required for this activation of Hageman factor[71,73] to proceed. Thus, kallikrein did not correct prekallikrein-deficient plasma in the absence of a surface,[50,73] DFP-kallikrein did not correct prekallikrein deficient plasma in the presence of a surface,[71,73] and DFP-kallikrein would not activate purified surface-bound Hageman factor[73] (Table 1). The surface has been estimated to augment the rate of cleavage of bound Hageman factor 10- to 20-fold,[75] and when activation of Hageman factor was examined by incorporation of ^{3}H-DFP, no activation of Hageman factor by the surface was observed in the absence of prekallikrein and HMW-kininogen.

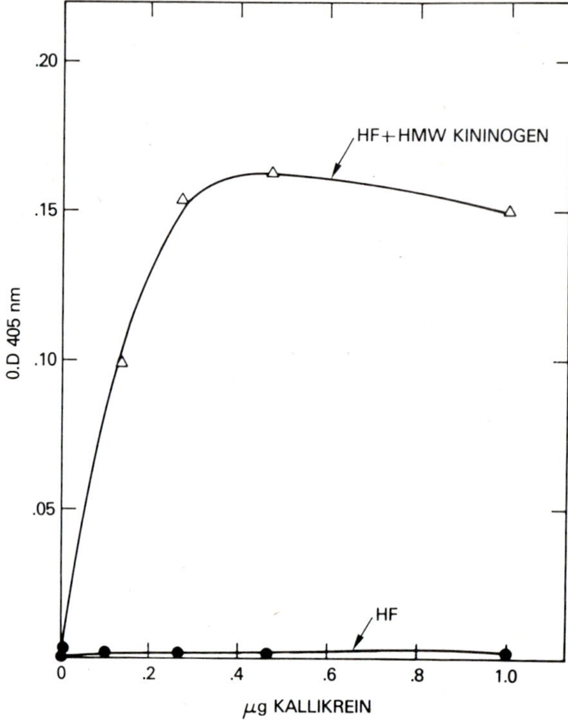

FIGURE 7. Dose response of the activation and function of surface-bound Hageman factor upon prekallikrein as a function of the HMW-kininogen added.

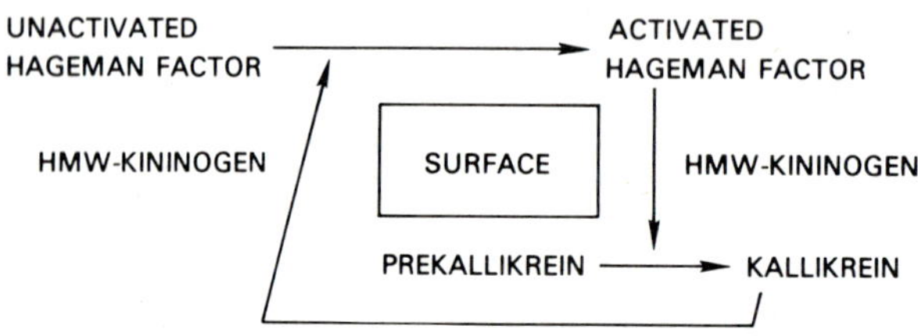

FIGURE 8. Schematic diagram of the reciprocal activation of surface-bound Hageman factor and prekallikrein that is catalyzed by HMW-kininogen.

4. Role of the Surface

The surface appears to augment the rate of interaction of the reactants and in particular render the Hageman factor a better substrate for plasma kallikrein. The ability of HMW-kininogen to augment the function of activated Hageman factor has been estimated to be 3- to 4-fold, while its effect upon the activation of Hageman factor yields a 40-fold enhancement.[73] When combined with the surface, the rate is augmented over 1000-fold. The major theoretical consideration that is not yet resolved is whether some combination of the surface, Hageman factor, prekallikrein, and HMW-kininogen generates an active site on the Hageman factor or prekallikrein or whether trace quantities of one of the plasma enzymes normally circulates in an active form. In the latter case, binding to the surface in the presence of HMW-kininogen might augment the reaction rate sufficiently to initiate the cascade. A recent report of con-

TABLE 1

Incorporation of ^{3}H-DFP by Surface-Bound Hageman Factor, HMW Kininogen, and Kallikrein

Proteins Added to Surface	^{3}H-DFP (cpm)
—	7,240 ± 442
Hageman factor	7,924 ± 438
HMW kininogen	7,635 ± 480
Hageman factor + HMW kininogen	8,081 ± 505
Kallikrein	8,426 ± 470
Kallikrein + HMW kininogen	8,269 ± 498
Kallikrein + Hageman factor	14,175 ± 770
Kallikrein + Hageman factor + HMW kininogen	34,395 ± 1,123
DFP kallikrein + Hageman factor + HMW kininogen	9,230 ± 521

formational changes observed upon binding of Hageman factor to surfaces or ellagic acid[76] may relate to the increased rate of cleavage of Hageman factor rather than the generation of a new active site in the Hageman factor.

C. Alternative Mechanisms of Hageman Factor Activation

Since the major activator of Hageman factor is kallikrein, it is likely that one or more enzymes present in active form in small concentration accounts for the gradual activation of Hageman factor observed in prekallikrein deficient plasma. Both plasmin and Factor XIa have been shown to be capable of activating and cleaving Hageman factor in the fluid phase,[55,62] and the ability of both of these enzymes to activate surface-bound Hageman factor has been investigated.[77] At ratios of enzyme to Hageman factor of 1:50, both plasmin and Factor XIa activated Hageman factor, as assessed by the subsequent ability of the surface-bound Hageman factor to convert prekallikrein to kallikrein. Plasmin was approximately one tenth as effective an activator as kallikrein, and in contrast to kallikrein, no augmentation by HMW-kininogen was evident. When Factor XIa was assayed, it was also about one tenth as potent a Hageman factor activator as kallikrein; however, Hageman factor activation, as assessed by the subsequent conversion of prekallikrein to kallikrein, was augmented 2- or 3-fold in the presence of HMW-kininogen (HMW-kininogen augmented the ability of kallikrein to activate Hageman factor 40-fold). The gradual activation of Hageman factor in prekallikrein-deficient plasma may occur by the Factor XIa-HMW kininogen complex and/or plasmin or by Hageman factor autoactivation.

III. PREKALLIKREIN

A. Purification and Properties of Human Prekallikrein

Human prekallikrein has been partially purified from plasma by fractionation on anion exchangers, such as DEAE-cellulose (or Sephadex) or QAE-Sephadex.[54-56,58,59,78] Under conditions of alkaline pH (8.0 to 8.5) at a conductivity of less than 1 mS, prekallikrein did not bind to these exchangers and was found in the effluent with the bulk of IgG. At this point, prekallikrein was effectively separated from Hageman factor and HMW-kininogen, as well as plasma protease inhibitors. It is interesting to note that the prekallikrein-HMW-kininogen complex was readily dissociated by a single passage over the ion exchanger. The other contaminating proteins identified after this first column step were β_2 glycoprotein I[22], Factor XI, and the complement components $C1_q$ and properdin. Further purification of human prekallikrein utilized fractionation on SP Sephadex and Sephadex G 150 to yield a product that was contaminated with IgG and variable quantities of β_2 glycoprotein I.[79] However, fractionation in the absence of inhibitors led to conversion of 25 to 35% of the material to kallikrein. Prekallikrein has been purified by Mandle and Kaplan,[80] utilizing each of the above steps followed by passage over a combined immunoadsorbent to IgG and β_2 glycoprotein I. Precautions taken to minimize conversion of prekallikrein to kallikrein included the addition of hexadimethrine bromide (360 mg/mℓ of the starting plasma), the addition of either 10 m*M* benzamidine or 10^{-4} *M* diisopropylfluorophosphate to all buffer systems, and use of plastic columns and test tubes. Estimates of the plasma concentration of prekallikrein range from 15 to 45 μg/mℓ, and the final yield based upon these estimates was approximately 5 to 10%.

The molecular weights reported for human prekallikrein as assessed by gel filtration have ranged from 100,000 to 127,000. However, when purified prekallikrein was examined by SDS gel electrophoresis, two molecular variants were identified at 88,000 and 85,000 daltons, respectively, (Figure 9) which have been designated prekallikrein I and II. Upon immunoelectrophoresis, in 1% agar at pH 8.3, prekallikrein migrated as a fast γ globulin, and its isoelectric point was determined to be between 8.5 and 9.0 (peak value at 8.7),[79] utilizing ampholytes of pH 7 to 10.

B. The Mechanism of Activation of Human Prekallikrein

Activation of human prekallikrein by either activated Hageman factor or Hageman factor fragments proceeds by limited proteolytic digestion. Each of the molecular forms of prekallikrein seen at 88,000 and 85,000 daltons is cleaved, and upon reduction a two-chain disulfide-linked enzyme results. A heavy chain of 52,000 daltons is linked to a light chain of either 36,000 or 33,000 daltons, corresponding to the two forms of the starting material. Figure 10 shows a preparation of ^{125}I prekallikrein which was partially activated so that approximately 50% was converted to kallikrein. The mixture was then reduced, subjected to SDS gel electrophoresis, and an autoradiogram of the gel was made. One can readily visualize the undigested prekallikrein, the kallikrein heavy chain, and two kallikrein light chains. On the same figure is an identical experiment in which nonradiolabeled prekallikrein was activated, incubated with ^3H-DFP, reduced, and subjected to SDS gel electrophoresis and autoradiography. All of the ^3H-DFP was seen in the light chains, indicating that this portion of the molecule contains the active site of kallikrein.[80] A time course of cleavage of 15 μg prekallikrein with 0.5 μg Hageman factor fragments as assessed after reduction and SDS gel electrophoresis is in Figure 11. As the two forms of prekallikrein were cleaved, there was a gradual formation of the kallikrein heavy chain and the two light chains. The evolution of functional activity has been shown to parallel the percent conversion to the cleaved form. In the absence of reducing agents, the molecular weight of prekallikrein and kallikrein were the same; thus, there was no evidence of release of any peptide during activation, and activation occurred by cleavage within a disulfide bridge. The difference in molecular weight of prekallikreins I and II (Figure 11) was reflected in the light chains. The evidence that both bands represent prekallikrein included:

1. Both were cleaved by Hageman factor fragments and yielded similar activation patterns.
2. They were not interconvertible upon activation by Hageman factor or incubation of prekallikrein with kallikrein.
3. They contained the same antigenic determinants.
4. DFP was incorporated into the light chains of each molecular form of the active enzymes.
5. Neither band was seen when prekallikrein-deficient plasma was fractionated.[80]

FIGURE 9. SDS gel electrophoresis of 20 μg of reduced, purified, human prekallikrein.

Prekallikrein has been purified in other species, and its mechanism of activation has been examined. Bovine prekallikrein[81,82] was shown to be a single chain proenzyme that was digested by bovine Hageman factor to yield a two-chain disulfide-linked enzyme in a fashion analagous to that seen in the human. Rabbit prekallikrein was found to be a β globulin with a molecular weight of 90,000 daltons and an isoelectric point of 5.9.[83] Upon conversion to kallikrein, not only was a kinin-generating enzyme

FIGURE 10. Autoradiogram of a mixture of ^{125}I-labeled kallikrein and prekallikrein, showing the prekallikrein, the kallikrein heavy chain, and the two kallikrein light chains (right gel). The left gel is an autoradiogram of a reduced SDS-polyacrylamide gel electrophoresis of ^{3}H-DFP-treated kallikrein, showing incorporation of ^{3}H-DFP into both kallikrein light chains.

formed, but the kallikrein was found to shorten the PTT of rabbit plasma; human kallikrein behaved similarly.[84] Thus, the function of kallikrein as a coagulation factor could be detected in rabbit plasma. Addition of kallikrein to human plasma or to congenitally deficient plasmas (other than Fletcher trait) has no significant effect. When the mechanism of conversion of rabbit prekallikrein to kallikrein was examined, activation was associated with the loss of an 8000-dalton peptide.[83] However, when

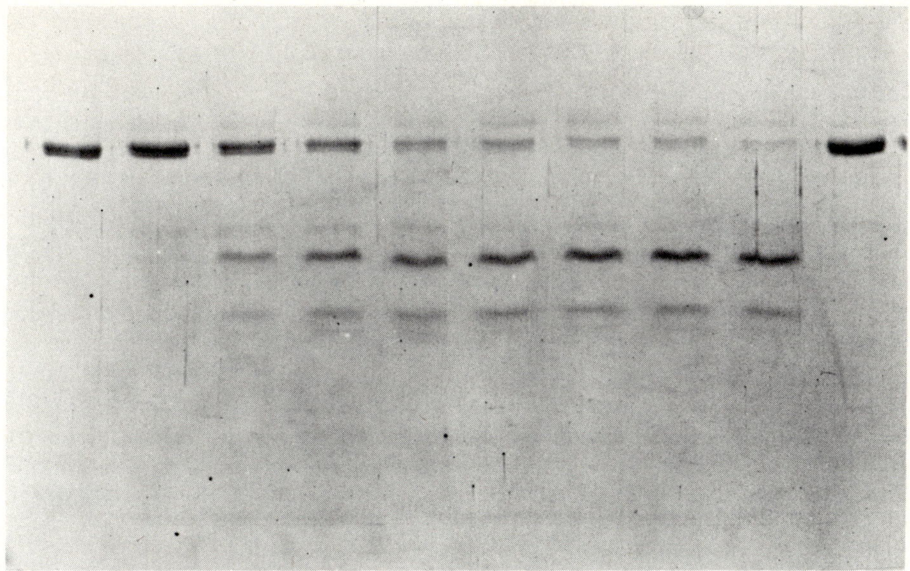

FIGURE 11. Kinetics of prekallikrein activation by Hageman factor fragments. From left to right the gel contains the starting material followed by time 0-, 2-, 5-, 10-, 15-, 25-, 40-, and 60-min time points after addition of Hageman factor. The final sample is a premixed control of SDS-buffer plus starting material and Hageman factor fragments incubated at 37°C for 60 min.

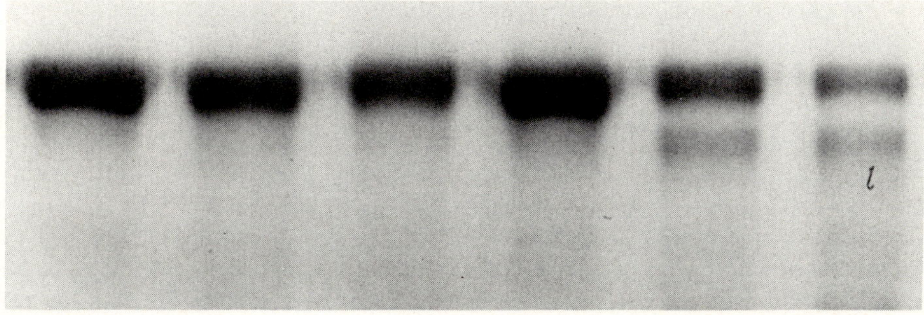

FIGURE 12. Autoradiograms of ^{125}I-labeled prekallikreon plus nonlabeled kallikrein. The samples from left to right are prekallikrein plus kallikrein plus 2000 units/mℓ Trasylol® incubated for 0, 30, and 60 min followed by prekallikrein plus kallikrein incubated for 60 min without any Trasylol®.

the mechanism was examined in greater detail, activation in the presence of Trasylol® yielded conversion to a two-chain disulfide-linked enzyme without any change in molecular weight.[85] Since Trasylol® inactivates kallikrein, but not Hageman factor,[59] it appeared that the peptide released was secondary to digestion of prekallikrein (or kallikrein) by the kallikrein produced. This phenomenon has been observed for human prekallikrein as in Figure 12. Digestion of ^{125}I prekallikrein with 5% nonradiolabeled kallikrein followed by SDS gel electrophoresis, and autoradiography resulted in the formation of a prekallikrein which was diminished in size by approximately 10,000 daltons.[80] The molecule remained as a single chain, and no conversion to kallikrein was detected.

IV. FACTOR XI

A. Purification and Properties

Factor XI[86] is a γ globulin of mol wt 158,000,[21,50] as assessed by SDS gel electrophoresis, and has an isoelectric point of 9.1.[87] It was first separated from Hageman factor by Schiffman et al.,[88] who showed that it would not adhere to DEAE cellulose under dilute, alkaline conditions, while Hageman factor was completely bound. This initial step has been utilized in most purification procedures. Factor XI is thereby found in a fraction containing other γ globulins, but it is free of virtually all the other plasma proteins. This is, however, the same fraction that contains prekallikrein, and complete separation of these two proteins is difficult. The first direct demonstration that these two factors could be separated was reported by Harpel,[89] who incubated a mixture of both active enzymes with α_2 macroglobulin and fractionated the mixture by gel filtration. Kallikrein binds to this inhibitor, while Factor XIa does not; thus, Sephadex® G-200 gel filtration of the mixture separated the kallikrein-α_2 macroglobulin complex from the Factor XIa. The first chromatographic separation of kallikrein from Factor XIa[16] and prekallikrein from Factor XI utilized a salt gradient on SP Sephadex;[79] prekallikrein was eluted first along the descending portion of the IgG peak at approximately 10 to 12 mS, and Factor XI eluted later at 18 to 20 mS. The Factor XI preparation at this stage was still contaminated with prekallikrein; however, over 90% of the IgG was removed. Fractionation on Sephadex G-200 yielded Factor XI essentially free of prekallikrein, since the Factor XI was eluted first at mol wt 175,000, and prekallikrein eluted later at 100,000. This combination of three steps was also utilized by other investigators[52,90] to prepare highly purified Factor XI. However, contamination with IgG and (at times) trace quantities of prekallikrein remained.

Schiffman utilized a five-step procedure to prepare human Factor XI of very high purity.[26] Assessment by gel analysis, however, was not reported, and the percent contamination with residual IgG was not given. Wuepper utilized a separation by Pevikon block electrophoresis in which Factor XI could be isolated such that it represented the major band seen upon SDS gel electrophoresis,[21] and Heck and Kaplan[87] removed residual IgG by passage over an antiIgG immunoadsorbant. The yield of Factor XI obtained was approximately 6%. Recently Koide et al.[91] have reported an isolation procedure for bovine Factor XI which utilized the ability of bovine Factor XI to bind to heparin Sepharose and benzamidine Sepharose. These methods have not yet been applied to human Factor XI, but if either one is applicable, an increase in yield and purity may result. In particular, the Sephadex G-200 gel filtration step causes the greatest loss, since only the first one half to two thirds of the peak is pooled in order to minimize contamination with prekallikrein.

B. Activation of Human Factor XI

Purified preparations of human Factor XI have a molecular weight of 155,000 to 160,000 upon SDS gel electrophoresis; however, upon reduction, the molecular weight is 80,000 to 82,000,[21,50,70] and only a single band is seen. Thus, it appears that Factor XI is a two-chain molecule, and the two constituent chains are virtually the same size. A similar observation has been made when highly purified bovine Factor XI was examined, and thus far incorporation of high concentrations of benzamidine and DFP into the isolation procedure has not resulted in the identification of a single-chain form of Factor XI.

Cleavage of human Factor XI by trypsin,[21,90] Hageman factor fragments,[50,70,87] or surface-bound activated Hageman factor[93] resulted in cleavage of the 80,000-dalton chains within a disulfide bridge. Thus, in the absence of reduction, the molecular weight of Factor XI and Factor XIa were essentially the same.[46,90,94,95] However, upon reduction, the two 80,000 chains of the starting material appeared to be cleaved to chains of 50,000 and 30,000. Factor XIa has been shown to be a serum protease[96] that can be inhibited by DFP. When Factor XI was activated by Hageman factor, inactivated by ^{3}H-DFP, and reduced, ^{3}H-DFP was incorporated into the 30,000-dalton light chain.[93] Since two 30,000-dalton fragments are formed (one from each 80,000-dalton chain), when the number of active sites per molecule was determined, two were found.[97] This suggests that Factor XI may contain two identical chains that are disulphide-linked.

Factor XI circulates as a complex with HMW-kininogen;[43] the rate of conversion of Factor XI to Factor XIa is augmented by HMW-kininogen,[38,66-73] and the rate of formation of activated Hageman factor (and Factor XIa) are dependent upon prekallikrein.[22-24,68-71,73] Yet prekallikrein circulates bound to HMW-kininogen as a separate complex from the Factor XI HMW-kininogen complex;[43] thus, a mechanism must exist in which Hageman factor that is activated by kallikrein can interact with the Factor XI HMW-kininogen complex. This may require movement of either kallikrein or activated Hageman factor along the surface or release and readsorption of activated molecules at the surface-fluid phase interface.

V. ISOLATION AND CHARACTERIZATION OF PLASMINOGEN PROACTIVATORS/ACTIVATORS OF HUMAN PLASMA

A. Conversion of Plasminogen to Plasmin: Identification of Prekallikrein and Factor XI as Plasminogen Proactivators

Hageman factor-dependent conversion of plasminogen to plasmin is readily demonstrable in whole plasma.[12,13,98] Since prekallikrein and HMW-kininogen are required for optimal activation and function of Hageman factor, they are also required for activation of the Hageman factor-dependent fibrinolytic pathway. However, identification of the molecule or molecules that directly convert plasminogen to plasmin has been the subject of numerous investigations, and the results have not been clear. Colman[99] first reported that incubation of kallikrein with plasminogen led to the generation of plasmin, and, utilizing caseinolysis as the assay for plasmin, the kinetics of the reaction appeared to be stoichiometric. Ogston et al.[100] demonstrated a cofactor requirement for Hageman factor-dependent fibrinolysis that appeared to be distinguishable from kallikrein and Factor XIa. However, the cofactor was clearly present in plasma fractions containing these factors. The assay for this protein was dependent upon reconstitution of glass-adsorbed plasma from which the fibrinolytic factor had been depleted. This "Hageman factor cofactor" had a molecular weight of 160,000, and it migrated with the γ globulins.[100] Kaplan and Austen subsequently demonstrated a Hageman factor-activatable plasma factor (called plasminogen proactivator) which upon activation was able to directly convert purified plasminogen to plasmin.[101] These authors proposed that the plasminogen activator derived was responsible for the plasminogen-converting activity in kallikrein preparations. The demonstration of plasminogen proactivator activity in the γ globulin fraction of prekallikrein-deficient plasma appeared to confirm their interpretation.[102] This postulate was challenged by Laake and Vennerod based upon their inability to separate prekallikrein from plasminogen proactivator, and they concluded that kallikrein and plasminogen-activating activities are functions of the same molecule.[103] When these authors examined the γ globulin effluent obtained from prekallikrein-deficient plasma, no plasminogen activator or proactivator activity was observed.[104]

The successful purification of human prekallikrein has shed further light upon this question. First, when human prekallikrein was isolated in the presence of proteolytic inhibitors, the prekallikrein and plasminogen proactivator activities coincided and the

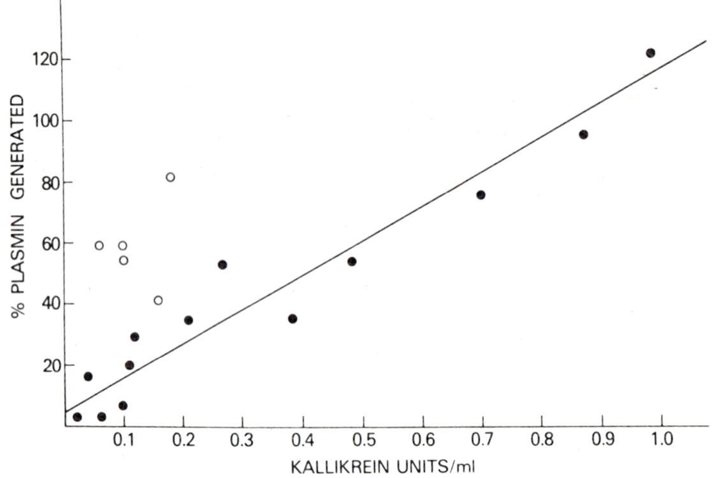

FIGURE 13. The relationship of plasmin generation to amidolytic activity of kallikrein preparations at the initial stage of purification (QAE-Sephadex® effluent, open circles) and later stages of purification (closed circles). The QAE-Sephadex® effluent had a significantly greater ratio of plasmin generation to amidolytic activity.

gel pattern which contained two bands was later shown to represent prekallikrein heterogeneity rather than two separate Hageman factor substrates.[80] Second, kallikrein was shown to cleave prekallikrein and decrease its molecular weight by 10,000 daltons (Figure 4); this difference in size corresponded to the previously reported difference in size between prekallikrein and plasminogen proactivator.[101] Finally, fractionation of prekallikrein-deficient plasma demonstrated that the plasminogen proactivator activity seen associated with prekallikrein was absent.[80] Hence, the conclusion was reached that prekallikrein is a plasminogen proactivator and that the previously reported activity was a property of prekallikrein and/or the prekallikrein degradation product. However, plasminogen activating activity was also found in the γ globulin fraction of normal plasma[105] which was not attributable to prekallikrein (Figure 13), and this same activity was found in prekallikrein-deficient plasma. Further fractionation of this material demonstrated that the activity was superimposed upon the elution profile of Factor XI.[80] In addition, two plasminogen proactivator peaks have been reported upon subsequent chromatography of the γ globulin fraction obtained from normal plasma,[70] suggesting that Factor XI may be a second proactivator. The observation that plasminogen activating activity does indeed reside in the γ globulin effluent of prekallikrein-deficient plasma has been confirmed;[106] however, these authors did not demonstrate that the activity was Hageman factor activatable and considered prekallikrein to be the only plasminogen proactivator. Clearly, the gradual conversion of plasminogen to plasmin observed in prekallikrein-deficient plasma is due to a Hageman factor-dependent enzyme that is not kallikrein. It has been suggested by one laboratory that activated Hageman factor itself can function as a plasminogen activator.[107] When the fibrinolytic capacity of prekallikrein is assessed, a necessary control is included, i.e., Hageman factor fragments plus plasminogen, and under these conditions less than 5% of the activity seen with kallikrein is observed. Figure 14 illustrates the detection of the plasminogen-activating potential of prekallikrein as it is eluted from the second (SP-Sephadex) step utilized by us in its purification. No fibrinolytic activity is detected in the absence of activated Hageman factor, while the mixture of activated Hageman factor and plasminogen alone did not yield significant fibrino-

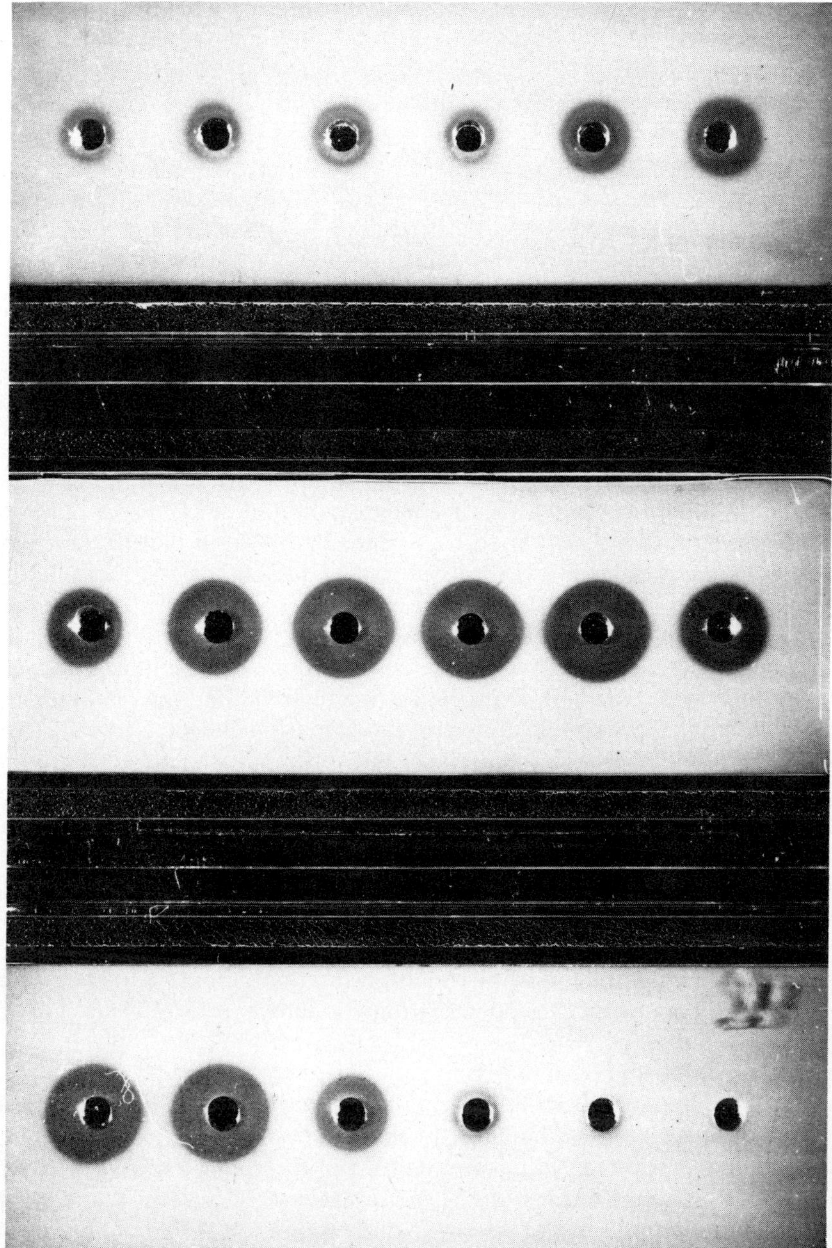

FIGURE 14. Fibrin plate assay of the generation of the plasminogen-activating capacity of Hageman factor-activated prekallikrein as it is eluted from the SP Sephadex® step utilized in its purification. All fractions were incubated with equal volumes of Hageman factor fragment (25 μg/mℓ) for 10 min at 37°C and then incubated with equal volumes of plasminogen (200 μg/mℓ) for 1 hr at 37°C.

lytic activity. Thus, large quantities of activated Hageman factor may be required for its ability to directly convert plasminogen to plasmin to reach significant levels. It appears clear that prekallikrein is a plasminogen proactivator, however, further work is needed to distinguish whether Factor XI can function as a second proactivator or if the activity observed in Factor XI preparations is due to a contaminant. Figure 15

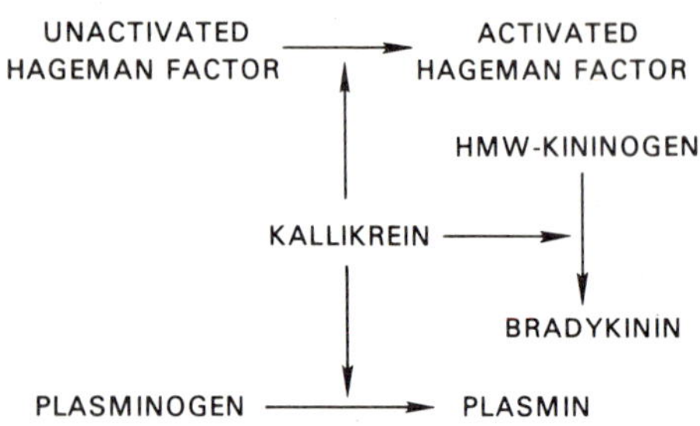

FIGURE 15. Schematic diagram depicting the enzymatic functions of kallikrein in coagulation and fibrinolysis.

shows the three proteolytic activities of kallikrein described herein; namely, the ability to activate Hageman factor (in the presence of HMW-kininogen), digest HMW-kininogen and liberate bradykinin, and to convert plasminogen to plasmin.

The identity of the Hageman factor cofactor is not clear. However, the necessity for this material does not appear to be distinguishable from that of already-known Hageman factor substrates. Glass adsorbed plasma, used in the assay for the Hageman factor cofactor, has been shown to be depleted of prekallikrein;[108] thus, the kallikrein present in Hageman factor cofactor preparations may contribute to the fibrinolysis observed by its effect upon Hageman factor activation. Yet the molecular weight reported for this factor was quite different from kallikrein, and the factor appeared to be separable from the bulk of kallikrein, but not from Factor XI.[100,109] The active factor was also inhibited by α_1 antitrypsin, a property it shares with Factor XIa.[109] The molecular properties of this cofactor most closely resemble the activity we have observed with our Factor XI preparation; thus, it is possible that the activity being measured was a function of more than one protein.

Further studies in whole plasma are needed to distinguish the effect of kallikrein upon fibrinolysis via its ability to activate Hageman factor from its ability to convert plasminogen to plasmin. It is of interest that one estimate of the direct contribution of kallikrein to the conversion of plasminogen to plasmin was approximately 50%[110] of the total Hageman factor-dependent fibrinolytic activity present in plasma.

B. Conversion of Plasminogen to Plasmin

We have now begun to examine in detail the interaction of kallikrein with plasminogen at a molecular level. No binding of kallikrein to plasminogen was detected when ^{125}I kallikrein was incubated with plasminogen and the mixture subjected to Sephadex G-200 gel filtration.[111] Thus, an initial binding step as is seen in the streptokinase-plasminogen interaction was not observed; furthermore, the active site for the reaction is known to reside in the kallikrein, since DFP-kallikrein has no ability to generate fibrinolytic activity.[101] When ^{125}I plasminogen was interacted with kallikrein with plasminogen at a tenfold molar excess, the formation of plasmin heavy and light chains were observed as fibrinolytic activity evolved.[111] Over 90% of the plasminogen was converted to plasmin during a 2-hr incubation, suggesting that there is no stoichiometry involved in the conversion of plasminogen to plasmin; however, a true catalytic mechanism as is seen with urokinase or the plasminogen activator formed upon interaction of streptokinase with plasminogen has not yet been demonstrated. These studies are impeded by the lack of a selective inhibitor which rapidly destroys plasmin, but not kallikrein; thus, any bond cleavage observed has not been shown to be due specifically to kallikrein rather than to the plasmin that is generated. Conversely, a kallikrein inhibitor that spares plasmin is also not available, and direct contributions of kallikrein to caseinolysis or cleavage of other synthetic substrates limit the molar ratio of kallikrein/plasminogen that can be used. At ratios of 1:100 or less, plasmin is generated slowly, lengthy incubations are required, and it is difficult to distinguish a stoichiometric reaction (which is not instantaneous) from a catalytic mechanism that is slow, given the above constraints. We are presently utilizing active site titrants to determine the rate of formation of plasmin active sites for fixed inputs of kallikrein sites in an attempt to further delineate the kinetic mechanism.

REFERENCES

1. **Denys, J. and de Marbaix, H.**, Les peptonisations provoquees par le chloroforme, *La Cellule,* 5, 197, 1889.
2. **Dastre, A.**, Action proteolytique du serum sanguin prealablement thaite par le chloroforme, *Arch. Physiol. Norm. Pathol.,* 5, 661, 1893.
3. **Delezenne, C. and Pozerski, E.**, Fibrinolyse dans le sang, *C. R. Soc. Biol.,* 55, 690, 1903.
4. **Hedin, S. G.**, On the presence of a proteolytic enzyme in the normal serum of the ox, *J. Physiol. (London),* 30, 195, 1904.
5. **Christensen, L. R. and MacLeod, C. M.**, A proteolytic enzyme of serum: characterization, activation, and reaction with inhibitors, *J. Gen. Physiol.,* 28, 559, 1945.
6. **Loomis, E. C., George, C., Jr., and Ryder, A.**, Fibrinolysin: nomenclature, unit, assay, preparation and properties, *Arch. Biochem.,* 12, 1, 1947.
7. **Lewis, J. H. and Ferguson, J. H.**, Studies on a proteolytic enzyme system of blood. IV. Activation of profibrinolysin by serum fibrinolysokinase, *Proc. Soc. Exp. Biol. (N.Y.),* 78, 184, 1951.
8. **Ratnoff, O. D. and Colopy, J. E.**, A familial hemorrhagic trait associated with a deficiency of clot-promoting fraction of plasma, *J. Clin. Invest.,* 34, 602, 1955.
9. **Ratnoff, O. D. and Rosenblum, J. M.**, Role of Hageman factor in the initiation of clotting by glass: evidence that glass frees Hageman factor from inhibition, *Am. J. Med.,* 25, 160, 1958.
10. **Iatridis, S. G.**, The effects of surface on plasminogen activation, *Fed. Proc. Fed. Am. Soc. Exp. Biol.,* 20, 58, 1961.
11. **Iatridis, S. G. and Ferguson, J. H.**, Effects of surface on Hageman factor on the endogenous or spontaneous activation of the fibrinolytic system, *Thromb. Diath. Haemorrh.,* 6, 411, 1961.
12. **Niewierowski, S. and Prow-Wartelle, O.**, Role du facteur contact (Facteur Hageman) dans la fibrinolyse, *Thromb. Diath. Haemorrh.,* 3, 593, 1959.
13. **Iatridis, S. G. and Ferguson, J. H.**, Active Hageman factor. A plasma lysokinase of the human fibrinolytic system, *J. Clin. Invest.,* 41, 1277, 1962.
14. **McDonagh, K. S. and Ferguson, J. H.**, Studies on the participation of Hageman factor in fibrinolysis, *Thromb. Diath. Haemorrh.,* 24, 1, 1970.
15. **Margolis, J.**, Plasma pain-producing substance and blood clotting, *Nature (London),* 180, 1464, 1957.
16. **Margolis, J.**, Activation of plasma by contact with glass. Evidence for a common reaction which releases plasma kinin and initiates coagulation, *J. Physiol. (London),* 144, 1, 1959.
17. **Margolis, J.**, The interrelationship of coagulation of plasma and release of peptides, *Ann. N. Y. Acad. Sci.,* 104, 133, 1963.
18. **Hathaway, W. E., Belhausen, L. P., and Hathaway, H. S.**, Evidence of a new plasma coagulation factor. I. Case report, coagulation studies, and physicochemical properties, *Br. J. Haematol.,* 26, 521, 1965.
19. **Hathaway, W. E. and Hayse, D.**, Fletcher factor deficiency. A report of three unrelated cases, *Br. J. Haematol.,* 18, 411, 1970.
20. **Hathaway, W. E. and Alsever, J.**, The relation of "Fletcher factor" to factors XI and XII, *Br. J. Haematol.,* 18, 161, 1970.
21. **Wuepper, K. D.**, Biochemistry and biology of components of the plasma kinin-forming system, in *Inflammation: Mechanisms and Control,* Lepow, I. H. and Ward, P. A., Eds., Academic Press, New York, 1972, 93.
22. **Wuepper, K. D.**, Prekallikrein deficiency in man, *J. Exp. Med.,* 138, 1345, 1973.
23. **Weiss, A. S., Gallin, J. I., and Kaplan, A. P.**, Fletcher factor deficiency. Abnormalities of coagulation, fibrinolysis, chemotactic activity, and kinin generation attributable to absence of prekallikrein, *J. Clin. Invest.,* 53, 622, 1974.

24. **Saito, H., Ratnoff, O. D., and Donaldson, V. H.,** Defective activation of clotting, fibrinolytic, and permeability enhancing systems in human Fletcher trait plasma, *Circ. Res.,* 34, 641, 1974.
25. **Webster, M. E. and Pierce, J. V.,** Activators of Hageman factor (Factor XII): identification and relationship to kallikrein-kinin system, *Fed. Proc. Fed. Am. Soc. Exp. Biol.,* 32, 845, 1973.
26. **Schiffman, S. and Lee, P.,** Preparation, characterization, activation of a highly purified factor XI. Evidence that a hitherto unrecognized plasma activity participates in the interaction of factors XI and XII, *Br. J. Haematol.,* 27, 101, 1974.
27. **Colman, R. W., Bagdasarian, A., Talamo, R. C., and Kaplan, A. P.,** Williams trait: a new deficiency with abnormal levels of prekallikrein, plasminogen proactivator, and kininogen, in The Chemistry and Biology of the Kallikrein-Kinin System in Health and Disease, Pisano, J. J. and Austen, K. F., Eds., Fogarty Int. Proc. No. 27, U.S. Government Printing Office, Washington, D.C., 1974, 65.
28. **Saito, H. and Ratnoff, O. D.,** Fitzgerald trait: an assymptomatic disorder with impaired blood coagulation, fibrinolysis, kinin generation, and generation of permeability factor of dilution, in The Chemistry and Biology of the Kallikrein-Kinin System in Health and Disease, Pisano, J. J. and Austen, K. F., Eds., Fogarty Int. Proc. No. 27, U.S. Government Printing Office, Washington, D.C., 1974, 73.
29. **LaCombe, M. J.,** Deficit constitutionnel en un nouveau facteur de la coagulation intervenant au niveau de contact: Le facteur "Flaujeac", *C. R. Acad. Sci. Ser. D.,* 280, 1039, 1975.
30. **Waldman, R. and Abraham, J.,** Fitzgerald factor: a heretofore unrecognized coagulation factor, *Blood,* 46, 761, 1975.
31. **Saito, H., Ratnoff, O. D., Waldmann, R., and Abraham, J. P.,** Fitzgerald trait. Deficiency of a hitherto unrecognized agent, Fitzgerald factor, participating in surface-mediated reactions of clotting, fibrinolysis, generation of kinins, and the property of diluted plasma enhancing vascular permeability (PF-dil), *J. Clin. Invest.,* 55, 1082, 1975.
32. **Wuepper, K. D., Miller, D. R., and LaCombe, M. J.,** Flaujeac trait: deficiency of kininogen in man, *Fed. Proc. Fed. Am. Soc. Exp. Biol.,* 34, 859, 1975.
33. **Wuepper, K. D., Miller, D. R., and LaCombe, M. J.,** Flaujeac trait. Deficiency of human plasma kininogen, *J. Clin. Invest.,* 56, 1663, 1975.
34. **Colman, R. W., Bagdasarian, A., Talamo, R. C., Seavey, M., Scott, C. F., and Kaplan, A. P.,** Williams trait: combined deficiency of plasma plasminogen proactivator, kininogen, and a new procoagulant factor, *Fed. Proc. Fed. Am. Soc. Exp. Biol.,* 34, 859, 1975.
35. **Colman, R. W., Bagdasarian, A., Talamo, R. C., Scott, C. F., Seavey, M., Guimaraes, J. A., Pierce, J. V., and Kaplan, A. P.,** Williams trait. Human kininogen deficiency with diminished levels of plasminogen proactivator and prekallikrein associated with abnormalities of the Hageman factor-dependent pathways, *J. Clin. Invest.,* 56, 1650, 1975.
36. **Donaldson, V. H., Glueck, H. I., Miller, M. A., Movat, H. Z., and Habal, F.,** Kininogen deficiency in Fitzgerald trait: role of high molecular weight kininogen in clotting and fibrinolysis, *J. Lab. Clin. Med.,* 87, 327, 1976.
37. **Schiffman, S., Lee, P., and Waldmann, R.,** Identity of contact activation cofactor and Fitzgerald factor, *Thromb. Res.,* 6, 451, 1975.
38. **Schiffman, S., Lee, P., Feinstein, D. I., and Pecci, R.,** Relationship of contact activation cofactor (CAC) procoagulant activity to kininogen, *Blood,* 49, 935, 1977.
39. **Ratnoff, O. D., Davie, E. W., and Mallet, D. L.,** Studies on the action of Hageman factor: evidence that activated Hagemen factor in turn activated plasma thromboplastin antecedent, *J. Clin. Invest.,* 40, 803, 1961.
40. **Wendel, U., Vogt, W., and Seidel, G.,** Purification and some properties of a kininogenase from human plasma activated by surface contact, *Hoppe-Seylers Z. Physiol. Chem.,* 353, 1591, 1972.
41. **Nagasawa, S. and Nakayasu, T.,** Human plasma prekallikrein as a protein complex, *J. Biochem. (Tokyo),* 74, 401, 1973.
42. **Mandle, R., Jr., Colman, R. W., and Kaplan, A. P.,** Identification of prekallikrein and HMW-kininogen as a circulating complex in human plasma, *Proc. Natl. Acad. Sci. U.S.A.,* 73, 4179, 1976.
43. **Thompson, R., Mandle, R., Jr., and Kaplan, A. P.,** Association of factor XI and high molecular weight kininogen in human plasma, *J. Clin. Invest.,* 59, 1376, 1977.
44. **Ratnoff, O. D. and Davie, E. W.,** The purification of activated Hageman factor (Activated XII), *Biochemistry,* 1, 967, 1962.
45. **Speer, R. J., Ridgway, H., and Hill, J. M.,** Activation of human Hageman factor (XII), *Thromb. Diath. Haemorrh.,* 14, 1, 1965.
46. **Kaplan, A. P., Spragg, J., and Austen, K. F.,** The bradykinin-forming system in man, in *Biochemistry of the Acute Allergic Reaction,* Austen, K. F. and Becker, E. L., Eds., Blackwell Scientific, Oxford, 1971, 279.
47. **Cochrane, C. G. and Wuepper, K. D.,** The first component of the kinin-forming system in human and rabbit plasma. Its relationship to clotting factor XII (Hageman factor), *J. Exp. Med.,* 134, 986, 1971.

48. **Revak, S. D., Cochrane, C. G., Johnston, A., and Hugli, T.**, Structural changes accompanying enzymatic activation of Hageman factor, *J. Clin. Invest.*, 54, 619, 1974.
49. **Meier, H. L. and Kaplan, A. P.**, A new method for the rapid purification of human unactivated Hageman factor, *Fed. Proc. Fed. Am. Soc. Exp. Biol.*, 34, 860, 1975.
50. **Kaplan, A. P., Meier, H. L., Yecies, L. D., and Heck, L. W.**, Hageman factor and its substrates: the role of factor XI (PTA), prekallikrein, and plasminogen proactivator in coagulation, fibrinolysis, and kinin-generation, in Chemistry and Biology of the Kallikrein-Kinin System in Health and Disease, Pisano, J. J. and Austen, K. F., Eds., Fogarty Int. Center Proc. No. 27, U.S. Government Printing Office, Washington, D.C., 1974, 237.
51. **Chan, J. Y. C. and Movat, H. Z.**, Purification of factor XII (Hageman factor) from human plasma, *Thromb. Res.*, 8, 337, 1976.
52. **Movat, H. Z. and Ozge-Anwar, A. H.**, The contact phase of blood coagulation: clotting factors XI and XII, their isolation and interaction, *J. Lab. Clin. Med.*, 84, 861, 1974.
53. **Griffin, J. H. and Cochrane, C. G.**, Human factor XII, in *Methods in Enzymology*, Vol. 45 (Part B), Lorand, L., Ed., Academic Press, New York, 1976, 56.
54. **Kaplan, A. P. and Austen, K. F.**, A prealbumin activator of prekallikrein, *J. Immunol.*, 105, 802, 1970.
55. **Kaplan, A. P. and Austen, K. F.**, A prealbumin activator of prekallikrein. II. Derivation of activators of prekallikrein from active Hageman factor by digestion with plasmin, *J. Exp. Med.*, 133, 672, 1971.
56. **Wuepper, K. D., Tucker III, E. S., and Cochrane, C. G.**, Plasma kinin system: proenzyme components, *J. Immunol.*, 105, 1307, 1970.
57. **Treloar, M. P. and Movat, H. Z.**, Isolation of two small molecular activators of the plasma kinin system in the guinea pig, *Fed. Proc. Fed. Am. Soc. Exp. Biol.*, 59, 576, 1970.
58. **Movat, H. Z., Poon, M. C., and Tukeuchi, Y.**, The kinin system of human plasma. I. Isolation of a low molecular weight activator of prekallikrein, *Int. Arch. Allergy Appl. Immunol.*, 40, 89, 1971.
59. **Wuepper, K. D. and Cochrane, C. G.**, Isolation and mechanism of activation of components of the plasma kinin-forming system, in *The Biochemistry of the Acute Allergic Reactions — Second International Symposium*, Austen, K. F. and Becker, E. L., Eds., Blackwell Scientific, Oxford, 1971, 299.
60. **Soltay, M. J., Movat, H. Z., and Ozge-Anwar, A. H.**, The kinin system of human plasma. V. The probable derivative of prekallikrein activator from activated Hageman factor, *Proc. Soc. Exp. Biol. Med.*, 138, 952, 1972.
61. **Burrowes, C. E., Movat, H. Z., and Soltay, M. J.**, The kinin system of human plasma. VI. The action of plasmin, *Proc. Soc. Exp. Biol. Med.*, 135, 959, 1975.
62. **Cochrane, C. G., Revak, S. D., and Wuepper, K. D.**, Activation of Hageman factor in solid and fluid phases, *J. Exp. Med.*, 138, 1564, 1973.
63. **Revak, S. D. and Cochrane, C. G.**, The relationship of structure and function in human Hageman factor. The association of enzymatic and binding activities with separate regions of the molecule, *J. Clin. Invest.*, 57, 852, 1976.
64. **Bagdasarian, A., Lahiri, B., and Colman, R. W.**, Origin of the high molecular weight activator of prekallikrein, *J. Biol. Chem.*, 248, 7742, 1973.
65. **Bagdasarian, A., Talamo, R. C., and Colman, R. W.**, Isolation of high molecular weight activators of plasma prekallikrein, *J. Biol. Chem.*, 248, 3456, 1972.
66. **Meier, H. L., Webster, M., Liu, C. Y., Colman, R. W., and Kaplan, A. P.**, Enhancement of surface dependent Hageman factor activation by high molecular weight kininogen, *Fed. Proc. Fed. Am. Soc. Exp. Biol.*, 35, 692, 1976.
67. **Liu, C. Y., Bagdasarian, A., Meier, H., Scott, C. F., Pierce, J., Kaplan, A. P., and Colman, R. W.**, Potentiation of the action of Hageman factor fragments (HF_f) by high molecular weight kininogen (HMW kng), *Fed. Proc. Fed. Am. Soc. Exp. Biol.*, 35, 692, 1976.
68. **Griffin, J. H. and Cochrane, C. G.**, Involvement of high M. W. kininogen (HK) in surface dependent reactions of Hageman factor, *Fed. Proc. Fed. Am. Soc. Exp. Biol.*, 35, 692, 1976.
69. **Griffin, J. H. and Cochrane, C. G.**, Mechanism for the involvement of high molecular weight kininogen in surface-dependent reactions of Hageman factor, *Proc. Natl. Acad. Sci. U.S.A.*, 73, 2559, 1976.
70. **Kaplan, A. P., Meier, H. L., and Mandle, R., Jr.**, The Hageman factor dependent pathways of coagulation, fibrinolysis, and kinin-generation, *Semin. Thromb. Haemostas.*, 3, 1, 1976.
71. **Meier, H. L., Scott, C. F., Mandle, R., Jr., Webster, M. E., Pierce, J. V., Colman, R. W., and Kaplan, A. P.**, Requirements for contact activation of human Hageman factor, *Ann. N. Y. Acad. Sci.*, 283, 93, 1977.
72. **Liu, C. Y., Scott, C. F., Bagdasarian, A., Pierce, J. V., Kaplan, A. P., and Colman, R. W.**, Potentiation of the function of Hageman factor fragments by high molecular weight kininogen, *J. Clin. Invest.*, 60, 7, 1977.

73. **Meier, H. L., Pierce, J. V., Colman, R. W., and Kaplan, A. P.**, Activation and function of human Hageman factor. The role of high molecular weight kininogen and prekallikrein, *J. Clin. Invest.*, 60, 18, 1977.
74. **Revak, S. D., Cochrane, C. G., and Griffin, J. H.**, The binding and cleavage characteristics of human Hageman factor during contact activation. A comparison of normal plasma with plasmas deficient in factor XI, prekallikrein, or high molecular weight kininogen, *J. Clin. Invest.*, 59, 1167, 1977.
75. **Griffin, J. H.**, New hypothesis for the molecular mechanism of surface-dependent activation of Hageman factor, *Thromb. Haemostas.*, 38, 50, 1977.
76. **McMillin, C. R., Saito, H., Ratnoff, O. D., and Walton, A. G.**, The secondary structure of human Hageman factor (Factor XII) and its alteration by activating agents, *J. Clin. Invest.*, 54, 1312, 1974.
77. **Meier, H. L., Thompson, R. E., and Kaplan, A. P.**, Activation of Hageman factor by factor XIa-HMW-kininogen, *Thromb. Haemostas.*, 38, 14, 1977.
78. **McConnell, D. J. and Mason, B.**, The isolation of human plasma prekallikrein, *Br. J. Pharm.*, 38, 490, 1970.
79. **Kaplan, A. P., Kay, A. B., and Austen, K. F.**, A prealbumin activator of prekallikrein III. Appearance of chemotactic activity in human neutrophils by the conversion of human prekallikrein to kallikrein, *J. Exp. Med.*, 135, 81, 1972.
80. **Mandle, R., Jr. and Kaplan, A. P.**, Hageman factor substrates. Human plasma prekallikrein: mechanism of activation by Hageman factor and participation in Hageman factor-dependent fibrinolysis, *J. Biol. Chem.*, 252, 6097, 1977.
81. **Nagasawa, S., Takahashi, H., Koida, M., and Suzuki, T.**, Partial purification of bovine plasma kallikreinogen, its activation by the Hageman factor, *Biochem. Biophys. Res. Commun.*, 32, 644, 1968.
82. **Takahashi, H., Nagasawa, S., and Suzuki, T.**, Studies on prekallikrein of bovine plasma I. Purification and properties, *J. Biochem. (Tokyo)*, 71, 471, 1972.
83. **Wuepper, K. D. and Cochrane, C. G.**, Plasma prekallikrein: isolation, characterization and mechanism of activation, *J. Exp. Med.*, 135, 1, 1972.
84. **Wuepper, K. D. and Cochrane, C. G.**, Effect of plasma kallikrein on coagulation in vitro, *Proc. Soc. Exp. Biol. Med.*, 141, 271, 1972.
85. **Johnson, A. R., Ulevitch, R. J., and Ryan, K.**, Biochemical and biological properties of rabbit prekallikrein, *Fed. Proc. Fed. Am. Soc. Exp. Biol.*, 35, 693, 1976.
86. **Rosenthal, R. L., Dreskin, O. H., and Rosenthal, N.**, New hemophilia-like disease caused by deficiency of a third plasma thromboplastin factor, *Proc. Soc. Exp. Biol. Med.*, 82, 171, 1953.
87. **Heck, L. W. and Kaplan, A. P.**, Substrates of human Hageman factor I. Isolation and characterization of PTA (Factor XI) and its inhibition by α_1 antitrypsin, *J. Exp. Med.*, 140, 1615, 1974.
88. **Schiffman, S., Rapaport, S. I., Ware, A. O., and Mehl, J. W.**, Separation of plasma thromboplastin antecedent (PTA) and Hageman factor (HF) from human plasma, *Proc. Soc. Exp. Biol. Med.*, 105, 453, 1960.
89. **Harpel, P. C.**, Separation of plasma thromboplastin antecedent from kallikrein by the plasma α_2 macroglobulin, kallikrein inhibitor, *J. Clin. Invest.*, 50, 2084, 1971.
90. **Saito, H., Ratnoff, O. D., Marshall, J. S., and Pensky, J.**, Partial purification of plasma thromboplastin antecedent (factor XI) and its activation by trypsin, *J. Clin. Invest.*, 52, 850, 1973.
91. **Koide, T., Kato, H., and Davie, E. W.**, Bovine factor XI (plasma thromboplastin antecedent), in *Methods in Enzymology*, Vol. 45 (Part B), Lorand, L., Ed., Academic Press, New York, 1976, 65.
92. **Kaode, T., Hermodson, M. A., and Davie, E. W.**, Active site of bovine Hageman factor XI (plasma thromboplastin antecedent), *Nature (London)*, 266, 729, 1977.
93. **Bouma, B. N. and Griffin, J. H.**, Human blood coagulation Factor XI: purification, properties, and mechanism of activation by activated Factor XII, *J. Biol. Chem.*, 252, 6432, 1977.
94. **Forbes, C. D. and Ratnoff, O. D.**, Studies on plasma thromboplastin antecedent (factor XI), PTA deficiency, and inhibition of PTA by plasma, pharmacologic inhibitors, and specific antiserum, *J. Lab. Clin. Med.*, 79, 113, 1972.
95. **Ratnoff, O. D.**, Studies on the product of the reaction between activated Hageman factor (factor XII) and plasma thromboplastin antecedent, *J. Lab. Clin. Med.*, 80, 704, 1972.
96. **Kingdon, H. S., Davie, E. W., and Ratnoff, O. D.**, The reaction between activated plasma thromboplastin antecedent and diisopropylphosphofluoridate, *Biochemistry*, 3, 166, 1964.
97. **Kurachi, K. and Davie, E. W.**, Activation of human Factor XI (plasma thromboplastin antecedent) by Factor XIIa (activated Hageman factor), *Biochemistry*, 16, 5831, 1977.
98. **McDonagh, K. S. and Ferguson, J. H.**, Studies on the participation of Hageman factor in fibrinolysis, *Thromb. Diath. Haemorrh.*, 24, 1, 1970.
99. **Colman, R. W.**, Activation of plasminogen by human plasma kallikrein, *Biochem. Biophys. Res. Commun.*, 351, 273, 1969.

100. **Ogston, D., Ogston, C. M., Ratnoff, O. D., and Forbes, C. O.,** Studies on a complex mechanism for the activation of plasminogen by kaolin and by chloroform: the participation of Hageman factor and additional cofactors, *J. Clin. Invest.,* 48, 1786, 1969.
101. **Kaplan, A. P. and Austen, K. F.,** The fibrinolytic pathway of human plasma. Isolation and characterization of the plasminogen proactivator, *J. Exp. Med.,* 136, 1378, 1972.
102. **Kaplan, A. P., Goetzl, E. J., and Austen, K. F.,** The fibrinolytic pathway of human plasma II. Generation of chemotactic activity by activation of plasminogen proactivator, *J. Clin. Invest.,* 52, 2591, 1973.
103. **Laake, K. and Vennerod, A. M.,** Factor XII-induced fibrinolysis. Studies on the separation of prekallikrein, plasminogen proactivator, and factor XI in human plasma, *Thromb. Res.,* 4, 285, 1974.
104. **Vennerod, A. M. and Laake, K.,** Prekallikrein and plasminogen proactivator: absence of plasminogen proactivator in Fletcher factor deficient plasma, *Thromb. Res.,* 8, 519, 1976.
105. **Mandle, R., Jr. and Kaplan, A. P.,** Plasminogen proactivators of human plasma: relationship to prekallikrein and factor XI, *Fed. Proc. Fed. Am. Soc. Exp. Biol.,* 36, 329, 1977.
106. **Bouma, B. N. and Griffin, J. H.,** Human prekallikrein (plasminogen proactivator): purification, characterization and activation by activated factor XII, *Thromb. Haemostas.,* 38, 136, 1977.
107. **Goldsmith, G., Saito, H., and Ratnoff, O. D.,** The activation of plasminogen by Hageman factor and Hageman factor fragments, *Clin. Res.,* 25, 340, 1977.
108. **Wuepper, K. D.,** Prekallikrein-Hageman factor cofactor — Fletcher factor: are they identical?, *Clin. Res.,* 21, 484, 1973.
109. **Robyn, J. C., Ogston, D., and Douglas, A. T.,** Further purification and properties of Hageman factor cofactor, *Biochem. Biophys. Acta,* 271, 371, 1972.
110. **Kluft, C.,** An inventory of plasminogen activators in human plasma, *Thromb. Haemostas.,* 38, 134, 1977.
111. **Yecies, L. D. and Kaplan, A. P.,** Studies of human plasminogen and its activation with plasminogen activator, *Fed. Proc. Fed. Am. Soc. Exp. Biol.,* 34 (Abstr.), 874, 1975.

Chapter 4

MECHANISM OF ACTIVATION OF HUMAN PLASMINOGEN BY STREPTOKINASE

K. N. N. Reddy*

TABLE OF CONTENTS

* Supported by National Institute of Health Grants 1-K04-HL 00420-01 (RCDA) and 2-RO1-HL 11172-12.

I. INTRODUCTION

The subject of this chapter* has a short history, beginning with the discovery of streptokinase by Tillett in 1933. Streptokinase is an extracellular bacterial protein isolated from the growth medium of hemolytic streptococcal cultures and is one of the most potent inducers of fibrinolysis so far known. Hence, it holds promise as a therapeutic agent for dissolving human blood clots. How the bacterial product is able to bring about the dissolution of human blood clots has occupied the attention of many scientists and lasted a lifetime for some of them. Studies on the properties of streptokinase were responsible for the identification of plasmin as the proteolytic enzyme-possessing fibrinolytic activity in human blood. The enzyme plasmin is normally present in blood as an inactive precursor, plasminogen, which is converted to the active form by streptokinase. This conversion of plasminogen to plasmin involves an enzymatic process, and yet streptokinase, the agent responsible for this process, is inappropriately named, since it is not an enzyme. In the following pages, I have described the search for an answer to this apparent paradox and the considerable effort made by many workers which led to our present understanding of the mechanism of activation of plasminogen by streptokinase. In the words of Beaumont, "I submit a body of facts which cannot be invalidated. My opinions may be doubted, denied, or approved, according as they conflict or agree with the opinions of each individual who may read them; but their worth will be best determined by the foundation on which they rest — the incontrovertible facts" (William Beaumont, M.D., 1833).

The presence of a substance in culture filtrates of certain β-hemolytic streptococci which caused rapid lysis of clotted human plasma was first reported by Tillett and Garner in 1933. The pioneering studies of Tillett and co-workers[1-3] established the following facts:

1. The streptococcal fibrinolysin did not have the capacity to hydrolyze proteins, such as casein, gelatin, and peptone. Thus, it differed significantly from other known proteolytic enzymes.
2. Clot dissolution occurred much more rapidly when the streptococcal fibrinolysin was added to plasma before inducing clot formation than when it was added to a preformed clot. They therefore recognized the important point that diffusion of the active bacterial agent within the body of the clot as it forms promoted rapid clot lysis.
3. Plasma of patients recovering from acute streptococcal infections was found to contain a specific antisubstance for the streptococcal fibrinolysin.
4. Clots made with rabbit plasma were resistant to the lytic action of the streptococcal fibrinolysin. However, when human thrombin was used for the coagulation of rabbit plasma, the clots were lysed rapidly by the bacterial agent, indicating that resistance to lysis was not the property of the fibrin itself, but involved species specificity.

The first important clue to our understanding of the mechanism by which the bacterial agent causes fibrinolysis came from the work of Milstone in 1941.[4] He found that with progressive purification of human fibrinogen and thrombin preparations, the clots became less susceptible to the streptococcal fibrinolysin. However, the addition of a euglobulin fraction prepared from human serum (along with the fibrinolysin) to the resistant clots resulted in rapid liquefaction, while the euglobulin fraction alone

* This chapter is dedicated to my teacher, Dr. Paul J. Vithayathil, whose studies on protein structure and function were a source of inspiration and guidance for my own work.

ogen was not activated by SK alone, it reacted if a small amount of normal human plasma euglobulin was added to the reaction mixture. The reaction consisted of two fraction. Since neither the euglobulin preparation nor the streptococcal fibrinolysin alone were active, but together caused clot lysis, it was clear that the euglobulin fraction from human plasma contained a factor important in the lytic process.

II. NATURE OF HUMAN FIBRINOLYTIC FACTOR

That serum contains a fibrinolytic enzyme whose activity becomes apparent after treatment of serum with chloroform or ether was known as early as 1889.[5] Kaplan[6] and Christensen[7] independently discovered that the "lytic factor" in human euglobulin preparation described by Milstone could be activated not only by the streptococcal fibrinolysin, but also by chloroform. Thus, it became clear that fibrinolysis was the result of the action of a proteolytic enzyme present in precursor form in the euglobulin fraction.

Christensen[7] and Christensen and McLeod[8] in a detailed study of the interaction of the streptococcal fibrinolysin with human euglobulin preparations made the following important observations:

1. Samples of lysin factor prepared from human plasma which have been stored in the cold developed proteolytic activity spontaneously.
2. In the presence of excess bacterial fibrinolysin, the proteolytic activity developed was directly proportional to the concentration of the human lysin factor in the system.
3. The rate of activation of the human lysin factor was proportional to the fibrinolysin concentration.
4. A comparison of the chloroform-activated serum protease and fibrinolysin-activated lysin factor with respect to their pH of optimum activity, pH of maximum stability, and temperature-activity relationships indicated that these proteolytic enzyme preparations were identical. Moreover, both the enzyme preparations were found to be inhibited in an identical manner when reacted with pancreatic trypsin inhibitor and with serum inhibitor.

Based on these results, Christensen and McCleod concluded that human plasma contains a proteolytic enzyme in a precursor or "zymogen" form which is activatable by streptococcal fibrinolysin or by chloroform treatment. In view of the similarities between the serum proteolytic enzyme and the proteolytic enzymes of the pancreas, chymotrypsinogen and trypsinogen, they suggested a new nomenclature for the fibrinolytic system which was universally accepted. The inactive enzyme in human plasma was called "plasminogen" and the activated enzyme, "plasmin". The streptococcal fibrinolysin was renamed "streptokinase" (SK) in view of its apparent catalytic role in the activation process. Christensen suggested that the activation of plasminogen which occurs when serum is shaken with chloroform is due to the removal of a serum inhibitor which prevents the spontaneous activation of plasminogen to plasmin. Thus, studies aimed at an understanding of the action of a bacterial protein led to the identification of a major proteolytic enzyme in human plasma.

III. PROACTIVATOR THEORY

Geiger[9] in 1952 found that a substance in human plasma was required for SK to act as a catalyst in the activation of plasminogen in the guinea pig, rabbit, chicken, and duck. Müllertz and Lassen and Troll and Sherry showed that although bovine plasmin-had no effect. Also, clots made with rabbit plasma which were known to be resistant to the action of the fibrinolysin promptly lysed in the presence of the human euglobulin steps; in Step 1, SK reacted stoichiometrically with a component in human euglobulin to produce an activator which in Step 2 catalytically activated plasminogen.[10,11]

Thus, human globulin fraction was found to contain a factor called "proactivator" which participated in the activation of plasminogen by SK. According to the proactivator theory, animal plasmas were assumed to be resistant to the action of SK by virtue of their lack of proactivator. SK was therefore no longer assumed to function as a catalytic enzyme, but assigned a role as a cofactor for proactivator activation.

The introduction of a simple method by Kline[12] for the purification of human plasminogen led Sherry[13] to test highly purified preparations of human plasminogen for proactivator activity, and indeed, he found that small amounts of human plasminogen or plasmin when mixed with SK, activated bovine, dog, and rabbit plasminogens equally well. Since human plasminogen preparations upon treatment with SK were found to give rise to two enzymatic activities, activator activity, i.e., the ability to activate plasminogen from different species, and plasmin activity, the question naturally arose whether human plasminogen preparations contained two different enzyme precursors (proactivator and plasminogen) or whether plasminogen itself gave rise to the two enzyme activities.

Sherry[13] found that acid treatment of a mixture of SK and human plasmin resulted in the loss of activator activity which could be restored by the addition of fresh SK to the reaction mixture. When SK was added to human plasminogen preparations of varying purity, the amount of plasmin formed and the amount of activator activity generated maintained a constant ratio.[14-16]

These results argued against a proactivator that is distinct from plasminogen and strongly suggested the possibility that human plasminogen itself might be the proactivator. Since the addition of SK to human plasminogen results in the rapid generation of plasmin, the active proactivator molecule could possibly be human plasmin. Ablondi and Hagan[15] did not believe that plasmin could be the proactivator, since in their studies, when human plasmin was prepared by the autocatalytic activation of plasminogen in the absence of added SK, such preparations did not exhibit proactivator activity. When human plasmin was prepared by activation of plasminogen with trypsin, once again these preparations lacked proactivator activity.[17] Therefore, these workers believed that activator activity arises when SK reacts with human plasminogen and not with plasmin.

Zylber et al.[18] found that contrary to the report of Ablondi and Hagan, human plasmin had proactivator activity. By treating their human plasmin preparations with SK, they obtained bovine plasminogen activator activity. When a mixture of SK and human plasmin was adjusted to pH 2.0, there was a striking loss of activator activity. Upon neutralization of the reaction mixture, addition of fresh SK restored the activator activity to pretreatment levels. In another experiment, when they treated their plasmin preparation with pancreatic trypsin inhibitor prior to the addition of SK, they found that the bovine plasminogen activator activity was significantly reduced. Based on these studies, they proposed that human plasmin combines with SK to form a complex which activates bovine plasminogen.

The studies of Kline and Fishman[19] provided strong evidence that human plasmin is the proactivator with which SK reacts to form the plasminogen activator. They discovered that the effect of soybean trypsin inhibitor on plasmin and on the activator (mixture of SK and plasmin) was quite different: while the lysine methyl esterase activity

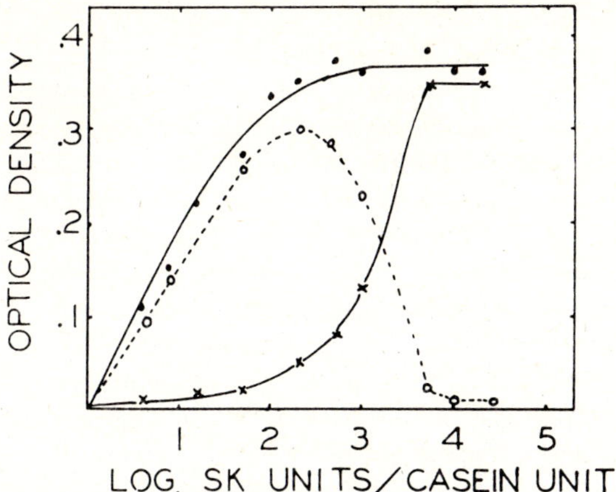

FIGURE 1. The effect upon LME hydrolysis of adding increasing amounts of streptokinase, SK, to a fixed quantity of plasminogen. Total LME hydrolysis (•-•) represents plasmin plus activator activity. LME hydrolysis in the presence of soybean trypsin inhibitor (X-X) measures activator activity, and the calculated difference between these curves (O—-O) is plasmin activity. Note the appearance of activator activity instead of plasmin at high streptokinase levels.

of plasmin was completely inhibited, the esterase activity of the activator was not affected by the presence of the inhibitor. This enabled them to investigate on a quantitative basis the formation of plasmin and activator in reaction mixtures containing human plasminogen and SK. To a fixed amount of human plasminogen, increasing amounts of SK were added to obtain increasing ratios from 40 to 20,000 streptokinase units per casein unit, and the amounts of plasmin and activator formed were determined. Their results are in Figure 1. With increasing concentrations of SK in the reaction mixture, it can be seen that the amount of plasmin plus activator increased and reached a plateau at 750 units of SK. Activator activity was initially low and then rapidly rose until a maximum was reached at 8000 units. Plasmin activity, however, steadily increased at low levels of SK, reached a plateau between 75 and 1000 units of SK, and then fell to zero with higher concentrations of SK. If human plasminogen preparations contained a separate proactivator with which SK reacted to form an activator, then addition of 100 units of SK to the reaction mixture (Figure 1) should have resulted in maximum activator formation, since at this level of SK, complete activation of plasminogen to plasmin had occurred. However, it can be seen that the activator activity continued to rise beyond 100 units of SK and reached a plateau only after 8000 units of SK. Earlier, Alkjaersig et al.[20] had also found that at low SK levels, proteolytic activity appears in the reaction mixture, while increasing the amounts of SK results in increasing activator activity. It can be seen from Figure 1 that the rise in activator activity at high SK levels was accompanied by a mirror-image fall in plasmin, indicating that the activator activity appeared at the expense of plasmin activity. These studies provided strong experimental support to the suggestion of earlier workers that the plasminogen activator is a complex of SK and human plasmin.

IV. THE STREPTOKINASE-HUMAN PLASMIN COMPLEX

The finding that a complex of SK and human plasmin possesses the ability to activate plasminogen to plasmin was followed by studies on the physicochemical properties of the complex. Physical evidence for the formation of a complex between SK and plasmin was independently obtained by Baumgarten,[21] DeRenzo,[22] and by Heimburger and Schwick.[23] Ultracentrifugal analysis of a reaction mixture prepared by mixing SK and human plasminogen in a 1:1 molar ratio showed a single boundary with a sedimentation coefficient of 5.2 S for the complex. The calculated molecular weight of approximately 130,000 for the complex corresponded very well with the sum of the molecular weights of the individual proteins, 47,000 for SK and 84,000 for plasminogen.[24,25] Based on the decrease in caseinolytic activity which occurred when SK was bound to plasmin, Blatt et al.[26] were able to calculate that complex formation occurred at 1:1 molar ratio of SK and plasmin. Complex formation between SK and plasmin was also demonstrated by starch gel electrophoresis,[25,27,28] column chromatography on Sephadex® G-200,[28] and by polyacrylamide-gel discontinuous electrophoresis.[29] When electrophoresis of the complex was carried out under dissociating conditions, the components separated and migrated individually. However, the mobility of the SK was different from that of the native SK, indicating that the SK molecule in the complex was present in an altered form.[25,28]

Chemical studies of the SK-plasmin complex revealed the following: treatment of the complex with di-isopropylflourophosphate (DFP) led to the incorporation of 1 mol of DFP into the active site of the complex and resulted in a loss of activator activity. Plasmin alone also incorporated 1 mol of DFP and lost its proteolytic activity, while treatment of SK with DFP did not impair its ability to activate plasminogen.[30,31] Starch-gel electrophoretic analysis of the DFP-treated SK-plasmin complex after dissociation in 8 *M* urea showed that the DFP-sensitive active site was present in the plasmin moiety of the complex.[30] Peptide mapping of tryptic digests of the SK-plasmin complex treated with radiolabeled DFP also showed that the active site was located on the plasmin moiety of the complex.[31,32] The activator activity of the complex was inhibited by treatment with tosyllysinechloromethyl ketone (TLCK).[31] These studies showed that the plasmin molecule contains a single active site serine residue and a histidine residue responsible for its proteolytic activity and that it is this same active site that is required for activator activity when plasmin forms a complex with SK. Further, that the active site region of the plasmin molecule may have undergone a conformational change as a result of binding to SK was indicated by the observations of Markus and Werkheiser.[33] They found that with azocasein as the substrate, the V_{max} for the proteolytic activity of the SK-plasmin complex was much less than for free plasmin, while the K_m was greatly increased. The esterase activity of plasmin towards tosyl arginine methyl ester, however, was not affected by the formation of a complex with SK. Sherry et al. in a detailed study compared the esterase activities of plasmin with the SK-plasmin complex.[34] When a variety of substituted arginine and lysine esters were used as substrates, more hydrolysis was observed with the SK-plasmin complex than with plasmin alone. While plasmin hydrolyzed benzoyl arginine methyl ester and tosyl arginine methyl ester equally well, the SK-plasmin complex hydrolyzed benzoyl arginine methyl ester three times more rapidly.

The above studies provide evidence to suggest that human plasmin is the "proactivator" with which SK reacts to form the activator of bovine plasminogen. It may be recalled that the proactivator concept was introduced by Mullertz and Lassen[10] to explain the ability of SK to activate human, but not bovine plasminogen. They assumed that human plasminogen preparations contained proactivator with which SK reacted to form the activator. The proactivator was thought to be lacking in bovine plasminogen preparations. The finding that human plasmin functions as a proactivator implies that the activation of human plasminogen by SK might also proceed by a prior interaction of SK with human plasmin to form the activator complex.

V. ACTIVATION OF HUMAN PLASMINOGEN BY STREPTOKINASE

A mechanism for the activation of human plasminogen by SK, in line with the proactivator concept, can be proposed as follows: if human plasminogen preparations were to contain some preformed plasmin, then the added SK can react with the latter to form a complex and initiate activation. The newly formed plasmin can then combine with any free SK present in the reaction mixture and form more activator. A simple requirement for such a mechanism is the presence of some "spontaneous plasmin" in human plasminogen preparations. Many workers have indeed found that plasminogen preparations were contaminated with varying amounts of plasmin, ranging as high as 30% of the total protein content. Particularly interesting in this context was the observation of Summaria et al.[30] that the plasmin contaminant in their plasminogen preparation existed as caseinolytically active and inactive forms. The caseinolytically inactive form was found to be capable of reacting with DFP and of forming a complex with SK. Thus, it was tempting to ascribe a proactivator function to the plasmin molecule.

However, detailed studies on the role of "spontaneous" plasmin in the activation of human plasminogen by SK showed that the activation of plasminogen did not depend on the presence of preformed plasmin. Treatment of plasminogen with DFP, under conditions which completely inactivated the plasmin present in the preparation, nevertheless was activated by the addition of SK. Similarly, inactivation of the plasmin contaminant by treatment with soybean trypsin inhibitor and by TLCK did not prevent the activation of plasminogen by SK. The strongest evidence came from experiments in which human plasminogen was found to be activated by SK when 10^{-2} *M* DFP was present throughout the period of incubation of the reaction mixture.[35] Since the presence of DFP was expected to inhibit any SK-plasmin complex that might be formed in the activation mixture, the fact that activation did occur led Summaria et al.[36] to propose that SK activates human plasminogen directly. Similar results were also obtained by Kline and Tsao.[35] They found that SK activated human plasminogen even in the presence of pancreatic trypsin inhibitor (PTI) added at a level 100 times more than was necessary to inhibit its content of preformed plasmin. Since control experiments showed that SK was not displacing the PTI from PTI-plasmin complex, the observed activation could not have been due to the participation of spontaneous plasmin. Kline and Tsao[36] concluded that SK could be capable of playing two roles in the activation of plasminogen: (1) as an enzyme in the direct conversion of human plasminogen to plasmin and (2) as a cofactor in the formation of a plasmin-SK complex which is a nonspecies specific activator. However, although the experimental results establish beyond doubt that activation of human plasminogen by SK does take place in the absence of spontaneous plasmin, the conclusion that SK acts as an enzyme is difficult to accept, since SK does not exhibit any other substrate specificity.

During the course of studies on the nature of the proactivator as evidence began to accumulate that human plasminogen preparations may not contain a separate proactivator molecule, several workers proposed that interaction of SK with human plasminogen itself results in activator activity. Werkheiser and Markus,[37] while studying the kinetics of activation of human plasminogen by SK, made the following observation: when they mixed human plasminogen with SK and analyzed the reaction mixture for its ability to activate bovine plasminogen, they found that maximum activator activity was formed within 1 min after the addition of SK to the human plasminogen solution, whereas the appearance of maximum amounts of human plasmin required more than 5 min. They interpreted this result to indicate that SK must have reacted with human plasminogen to give rise to bovine plasminogen activator activity. However, Ling et al.[38] questioned the above conclusion, since under the assay conditions used by Werkheiser and Markus (the time required to lyse a bovine clot), the SK-plasminogen could have been rapidly converted to the SK-plasmin complexes. Buck et al.[31] also proposed that the SK interacts with human plasminogen to give rise to an SK-plasminogen complex possessing activator activity, based on their results which were similar to those of Werkheiser and Markus.[37] They reported that while maximum plasmin formation required more than 10 min in a reaction mixture containing equimolar amounts of SK and human plasminogen, maximum activator activity was detectable in 3 min, indicating that the latter activity was due to the SK-plasminogen complex. However, a critical examination of their data shows that in order to detect the enzymatic activity of the SK-plasminogen complex, the assay conditions employed required a further incubation period, during which time the SK-plasminogen would be converted to the SK-plasmin complex. The authors' contention that the presence of 0.025 *M* ε-aminocaproic acid in the assay medium would have been sufficient to prevent any conversion of SK-plasminogen to SK-plasmin was not valid, since Gajewski and Markus[39] have found that for complete and practically instantaneous arrest of activation, the assay conditions required were quite different from those used by Buck et al.[31]

Although the hypothesis that the interaction of SK with human plasminogen results in the formation of a SK-plasminogen complex with enzymatic activity is very attractive, to establish it as a fact requires the unequivocal demonstration that (1) a complex indeed exists between SK and human plasminogen and (2) that such a complex possesses the enzymatic properties of an activator. Studies on the interaction of SK with plasminogen in ultracentrifuge and starch-gel electrophoresis experiments to demonstrate formation of a SK-plasminogen complex were not conclusive, since it was not clearly established that the observed complex was indeed SK-plasminogen and not SK-plasmin. This was due to the fact that these experimental methods were not capable of satisfactorily distinguishing between plasminogen and plasmin. Thus, when human plasmin was reacted with SK, the product formed was identical to that derived from the interaction of SK with human plasminogen.[28,30] By mixing SK with human plasminogen at 0°C and isolating the resultant product by a specific precipitation procedure, Summaria et al.[30] were able to show that the isolated product contained at least 50% of the SK-plasminogen. However, the possibility that the observed complex of SK-plasminogen could have enzyme properties was not explored by these workers.

Rimon and co-workers[40,41] have also presented experimental results, suggesting that a complex of SK-plasminogen exhibits activator activity. They prepared an insoluble derivative of human plasminogen by coupling it to a diazotized copolymer of *p*-amino-DL-phenylalanine and α-leucine. When SK was added to the product, activator activity appeared, but not plasmin activity. They concluded that the coupling of human plasminogen to the copolymer occurred in such a way as to prevent plasmin formation, while allowing the formation of the activator. Unfortunately, they did not report on whether their plasminogen preparation contained any preformed plasmin. If some plasmin were present in the plasminogen preparation, then that plasmin could also have become coupled to the copolymer, and therefore the observed activator activity could have been due to the SK-plasmin complex. Moreover, the observation that no caseinolytic activity could be detected upon addition of SK to the insoluble plasminogen preparation can be interpreted in a different way. If plasmin were to have been formed upon the addition of SK to the insoluble plasminogen preparation, it is possible that it was unable to react with casein due to steric hindrance. It may be pointed out that it remains to be established whether Rimon's insoluble plasminogen preparation is capable of forming an activator with SK without itself being converted to plasmin.

While the above-mentioned theories for the mechanism of activation of human plasminogen by SK depend on the interaction of SK with human plasmin or plasminogen to form the activator, Takada et al.[42] suggest the participation of a proactivator distinct from plasmin or plasminogen. They reported the isolation of a proactivator from human plasma with properties different from those of human plasminogen. Euglobulin fractions from human plasma were subjected to various column chromatographic procedures to yield a protein preparation which with SK activated human and bovine plasminogens. Whether or not this newly discovered proactivator had any role in the mechanism of activation of human plasminogen by SK remained doubtful in view of the fact that while small amounts of SK (one unit) required the presence of their proactivator to activate human plasminogen, large amounts of SK (500 units) were able to activate human plasminogen in the absence of the proactivator.

An interesting hypothesis for the mechanism of activation of plasminogen by SK was presented by Kline and Bowlds[43] and by Taylor and Beisswenger.[44] They proposed that the interaction of SK with human plasminogen results in the formation of a modified derivative of SK which is capable of activating human and bovine plasminogens directly. The modification of SK was believed to be brought about by the preformed plasmin normally present as a contaminant in human plasminogen preparations.

When we began our investigations into the mechanism of activation of human plasminogen by SK in 1968, we ruled out the possibility of SK acting as an enzyme based on the following reasoning: the activation of plasminogen to plasmin involves the cleavage of an arginyl-valyl peptide bond in the plasminogen molecule.[45] If SK were an enzyme, then it must be a proteolytic enzyme with a specificity towards basic amino acid residues. Since the pioneering studies of Bergmann and co-workers, it had been established that proteolytic enzymes in general catalyze the hydrolysis of ester and amide bonds in synthetic substrates comprising the same amino acid residues that were found to be susceptible to hydrolysis in the natural substrates. Since SK was found to be inactive towards arginine or lysine derivatives, it appeared highly unlikely that it would act as a proteolytic enzyme. A critical evaluation of all the information available in the literature on the interaction of SK with plasminogen gave the following incontrovertible facts:

1. SK reacts with human plasmin to form a stoichiometric complex.
2. This complex activates plasminogen from different species.
3. This complex possesses an active site serine residue.
4. The SK-plasmin complex is active against synthetic substrates of arginine and lysine.

Thus, it can be seen that the SK-human plasmin complex ideally fulfills the requirements of an activator enzyme. The formation of such an activator can occur readily when SK is added to plasminogen, since the latter is invariably contaminated with some preformed plasmin. However, the main objection to this mechanism of activation was the fact that Kline and Ts'ao[35] and Summaria et al.[36] have reported that inhibition of the spontaneous plasmin in human plasminogen preparation did not result in a loss of activatability of plasminogen by SK. It appeared to us that the problem could be resolved if it could be demonstrated that some plasmin molecules escape reaction with the inhibitors. Then, even these trace amounts of plasmin would be sufficient for activation, since once activation was initiated, the newly formed plasmin would combine with SK to form more activator. Therefore, we reinvestigated the role of spontaneous plasmin in the activation mechanism.

The inhibitor, *p*-nitrophenyl-*p*-guanidinobenzoate (NPGB) reacts with plasmin as an active center-specific reagent,[46] giving a burst of *p*-nitrophenol and inactive, acylated enzyme. The ease and rapidity with which this reagent reacts with plasmin and the mild conditions necessary to destroy excess reagent prompted us to use NPGB to inhibit the spontaneous plasmin present in our plasminogen in order to see whether SK could still activate plasminogen. The plasminogen preparation was treated with

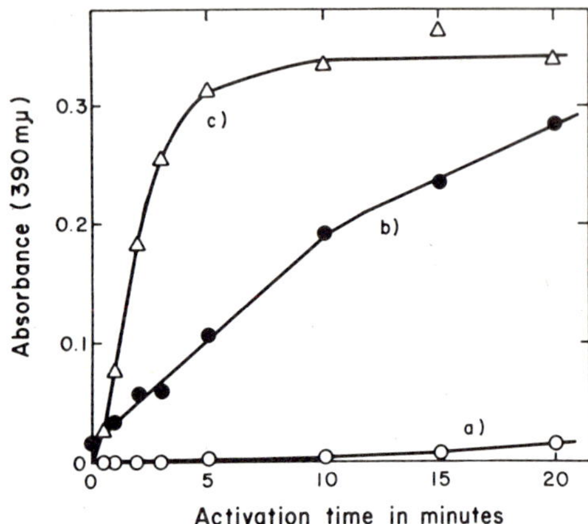

FIGURE 2. Effect of NPGB-inhibition of the spontaneous plasmin content of plasminogen on activation rates of streptokinase at two levels. (a) Spontaneous plasmin inhibited, activation with "low streptokinase"; (b) spontaneous plasmin not inhibited, activation as in (a); and (c) spontaneous plasmin inhibited, activation with "high streptokinase". Plasmin, formed by the activation of plasminogen, was determined by its hydrolysis of azocasein. (From Reddy, K. N. N. and Markus, G., *J. Biol. Chem.*, 247, 1683, 1972. American Society of Biological Chemists, Inc., Bethesda, Md. With permission.)

NPGB to inactivate the spontaneous plasmin, and the excess reagent destroyed by nonspecific hydrolysis. Curve A in Figure 2 shows the rate of activation of this plasminogen preparation when activated with 490 units of SK, an amount less than equimolar (4500 units) to the spontaneous plasmin content. Curve B shows the rate of activation of the uninhibited, control preparation by the same amount of SK. Curve C illustrates the rate of activation of the inhibited preparation by 5900 units of SK, an amount in excess of equivalence with the blocked spontaneous plasmin content.

It can be seen that the low amount of SK poorly activated the inhibited sample after a long lag period, yielding only 5% of the uninhibited control value in 20 min, indicating that the SK had indeed reacted with the spontaneous plasmin forming an inactive complex. When the larger amount of SK was used, vary fast activation of the inhibited sample occurred. Curve A shows that very little plasmin had formed in 10 min, and yet activation had reached completion in Curve C in the same interval. Therefore, activation in this system could not have been due to the formation of an SK-plasmin complex involving any newly formed plasmin. These results clearly showed that the activation of human plasminogen by SK can proceed by a mechanism not involving plasmin as the cofactor.

In seeking an explanation for the activation of human plasminogen by SK, it was essential to remember that the activation process involves the cleavage of an arginyl-valyl peptide bond in the plasminogen molecule. It was reasonable to expect that the activator, whatever it might be, possessed specificity towards basic amino acid residues. In analogy with other known proteolytic enzymes of similar specificity, the activator enzyme can also be expected to possess a serine residue in its active site. It can then be argued that if the activation of plasminogen by SK involves the formation of an intermediate activator species, the presence of a serine-active site-specific inactiva-

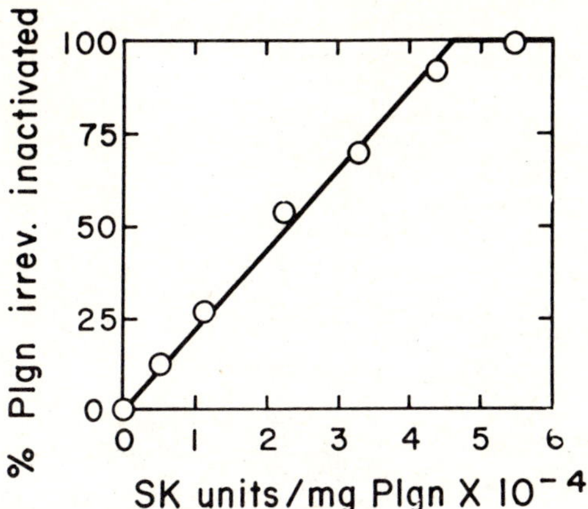

FIGURE 3. Irreversible inactivation of plasminogen by NPGB in the presence of increasing amounts of streptokinase. A 1:1 *M* ratio of streptokinase to plasminogen corresponds to 46,000 units of streptokinase per milligram of the plasminogen used in the experiment. (From Reddy, K. N. N. and Markus, G., *J. Biol. Chem.*, 247, 1683, 1972. American Society of Biological Chemists, Inc., Bethesda, Md. With permission.)

tor in the reaction mixture should prevent activation. To demonstrate this, one condition that must be fulfilled is that the rate with which the reagent reacts with the activator molecule must be faster than the rate with which the activator reacts with the plasminogen substrate. The serine-active site-specific reagent, NPGB, met this requirement.

When SK is added to plasminogen in the presence of NPGB, if NPGB were to inactivate the activator molecule, the plasminogen should remain unchanged. In the experiment to test this theory, increasing amounts of SK were added to plasminogen solutions containing excess NPGB, and the solutions were incubated for 1 hr at 25°C. Samples were then analyzed for activatable plasminogen. The results (Figure 3) show that instead of a constant amount of activatable plasminogen being present in the reaction mixtures, the amounts actually decreased. At an equimolar ratio of SK to plasminogen in the reaction mixture, practically no activatable plasminogen was present. Control experiments in which plasminogen alone was treated with NPGB showed that plasminogen did not lose its activatability. The linear correlation between the amount of SK added and the amount of plasminogen inactivated indicated that:

1. SK reacted with human plasminogen in a stoichiometric ratio.
2. As a result of complex formation, the plasminogen had acquired the ability to react with the active center specific reagent.
3. The inactivated SK-plasminogen existed as a complex.

If SK did not form a complex or was able to dissociate from the complex after reaction with NPGB, when a catalytic amount of SK was added in the above experiment, the SK would have been free to react further with all of the plasminogen molecules present in the reaction mixture making them susceptible to inactivation by NPGB. However, the results clearly showed that all of the plasminogen became inactivated only when an equimolar amount of SK was added. Similarly, if NPGB were to have reacted with

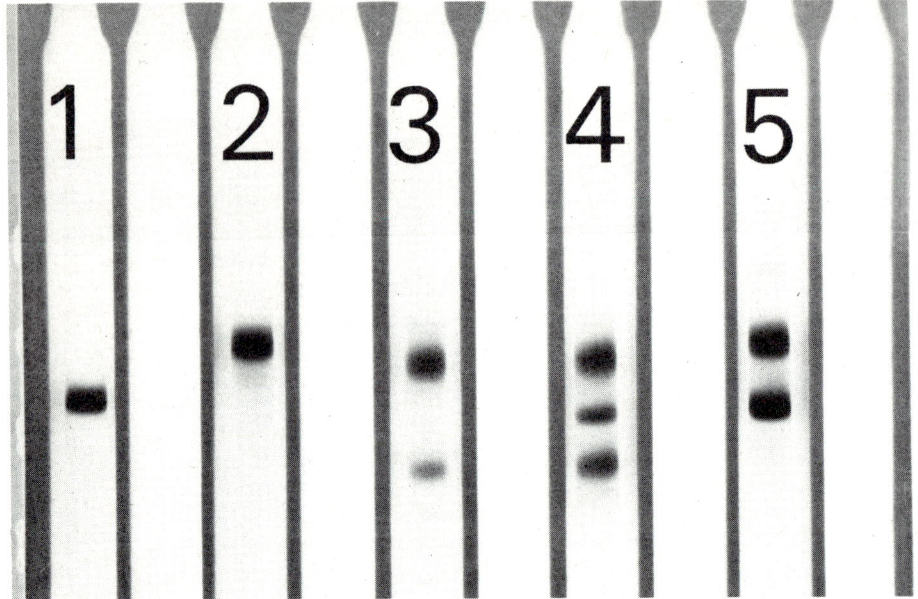

FIGURE 4. Acrylamide gel electrophoretic analysis of the reaction between streptokinase and plasminogen in the presence of NPGB. (1) Streptokinase alone; (2) plasminogen alone; (3) plasmin; (4) equimolar complex of streptokinase-plasmin treated with NPGB after complete activation; and (5) plasminogen incubated with equimolar amount of streptokinase in the presence of NPGB. (From Reddy, K. N. N. and Markus, G., *J. Biol. Chem.*, 247, 1683, 1972. With permission.)

an active site on the SK molecule, then all of the plasminogen would have been found to be activatable if it had not formed a complex with SK. Thus, it was clear that the interaction of SK with human plasminogen in the presence of NPGB resulted in the formation of an inactive SK-plasminogen complex.

However, one could argue that the activation of plasminogen to plasmin had proceeded normally, and the plasmin formed had been inactivated by the NPGB present in the reaction mixture. Thus, the inability to detect any activatable plasminogen in the above experiment could be due to the fact that the caseinolytic assay used was not capable of detecting the inhibited plasmin. It was, therefore, necessary to employ a method that would unambiguously distinguish between inactive plasmin and plasminogen.

Advantage was taken of the fact that plasminogen consists of a single polypeptide chain, whereas plasmin contains two chains held together by disulfide bonds. To plasminogen in the presence of excess NPGB was added an equimolar amount of SK, and the reaction mixture incubated for 30 min at room temperature. It was then reduced with β-mercaptoethanol in the presence of sodium dodecyl sulfate. As controls, plasmin was prepared by activation with catalytic and with equimolar amounts of SK, reacted with NPGB, and then reduced. The preparations were then subjected to polyacrylamide gel electrophoresis in the presence of sodium dodecyl sulfate, and the gel patterns obtained are in Figure 4. It can be seen that the SK and plasminogen controls migrated as single bands. Plasmin as expected gave two bands corresponding to the heavy and light chains. The equimolar complex of SK-plasmin gave a third band corresponding to a modified form of native SK. The NPGB-pretreated SK-plasminogen reaction mixture exhibited only two bands corresponding to native SK and plasminogen, indicating that this preparation did not contain detectable amounts of plasmin.

Since this preparation was incubated for 30 min in NPGB after the addition of SK, the absence of plasmin clearly shows that NPGB must have reacted with plasminogen. It is evident therefore that due to complex formation with SK, human plasminogen acquired the ability to react with NPGB, indicating that an active center on the plasminogen molecule had become available presumably as a result of a conformational change. Simultaneous with our report,[47] McClintock and Bell also reported their finding that NPGB reacts with the SK-plasminogen complex.[48]

Thus, when SK is added to human plasminogen, a stoichiometric complex of SK-plasminogen is formed. As a result of this complex formation, an active center becomes exposed in the plasminogen moiety of the complex by a conformational change. The obvious conclusion can be made that this active site is capable of activating plasminogen to plasmin. However, then the question can be asked, does catalysis by an enzyme depend on just the presence of a highly reactive catalytic group on the enzyme molecule? The SK-plasminogen complex could merely represent a first step leading to the formation of another true activator species. Moreover, Kline and Bowlds[43] and Taylor and Beisswenger[49] have also presented their views at the same session of the FASEB meetings in Chicago in 1971, where we presented our work on the SK-plasminogen complex that a modified derivative of SK might be the activator. Therefore, it appeared quite possible that the active site in the SK-plasminogen complex may be involved in the modification of the SK molecule and that the modified SK-plasminogen complex may be the true activator species. However, our results not only established the fact that the interaction of SK with human plasminogen results in the appearance of an active site before any proteolytic cleavage occurs, but also proved that this active site catalyzes the conversion of plasminogen to plasmin.[50] Later, Schick and Castellino[51] found that the activation of rabbit plasminogen by SK also proceeds by the intermediate formation of a SK-rabbit plasminogen complex as the activator species.

Based on the above studies, Reddy and Markus described the mechanism of activation of human plasminogen by SK as follows:[50]

1. SK reacts almost instantaneously with human plasminogen to form an equimolar complex of SK-plasminogen.
2. This complex then acquires the properties of an enzyme by exposing an active center in the plasminogen moiety of the complex without any peptide bonds cleaved in the process.
3. The enzyme (SK-plasminogen complex) generated thus in the reaction mixture catalyzes the conversion of plasminogen to plasmin by cleaving an arginyl-valyl peptide bond in the plasminogen molecule.
4. The SK-plasminogen also cleaves the same peptide bond in the plasminogen moiety of another SK-plasminogen molecule, and thus, it itself is converted within minutes to the SK-plasmin complex.

During this conversion the SK moiety of the complex also undergoes peptide bond hydrolysis, giving rise to a modified SK still attached to the plasmin molecule. Thus, when a catalytic amount of SK is used to activate human plasminogen, the products of activation will be plasmin and an amount of modified SK-plasmin complex equivalent to the amount of SK added. When plasminogen is activated with an equimolar amount of SK, modified SK-plasmin will be the only product formed. Since activation is initiated by the formation of a stoichiometric complex between SK and plasminogen, it can be seen that when a catalytic amount of SK is added to plasminogen, the SK-plasminogen complex formed acts on the free plasminogen as the substrate. When an equimolar amount of SK is used to activate plasminogen, the SK-plasminogen complex will act both as the substrate and as the activator enzyme. Therefore, the rate of activation of human plasminogen to plasmin can be expected to be influenced by the amount of SK added to the activation mixture. Indeed, Werkheiser and Markus[37] found that plasminogen was activated at a much faster rate with catalytic amounts of SK than with equimolar SK, indicating that the binding of SK to the plasminogen molecule caused steric hindrance for catalysis.

VI. THE STREPTOKINASE-PLASMINOGEN COMPLEX

As discussed in the preceding sections, the interaction of SK with human plasminogen results in the formation of a stoichiometric complex of SK-plasminogen. This complex is not stable in solution, being rapidly converted to the modified SK-plasmin complex. Formation of complexes by SK with human plasmin and plasminogen occurs by noncovalent bonds, since the components can be dissociated by lowering the pH and by treatment with urea and sodium dodecyl sulfate. The most striking feature of the SK-plasminogen complex is its enzyme activity, its ability to catalyze the conversion of plasminogen to plasmin being even higher than that of the SK-plasmin complex. We have investigated this newly discovered enzyme species for properties other than its ability to activate plasminogen or to react with the active center-specific reagent NPGB. We found that pancreatic trypsin inhibitor, an inhibitor known to react with plasmin and SK-plasmin complex, also reacts with the SK-plasminogen complex.[52] When stoichiometric amounts of SK and human plasminogen were mixed together in the presence of a twofold excess of PTI and the reaction mixture incubated for 20 min at room temperature, the plasminogen remained unactivated, indicating that PTI must have blocked the active site on the SK-plasminogen complex. The possibility that PTI might have prevented activation by displacing SK from the plasminogen was ruled out by the fact that upon gel filtration of the reaction mixture on a Sephadex G-200 column, the protein peak fraction was found to contain SK, plasminogen, and PTI as a triple complex. Moreover, NPGB which we know to be capable of reacting with the SK-plasminogen complex was unable to do so when PTI was present in the reaction mixture. This result was significant in that it demonstrated clearly that the NPGB-sensitive active site was located on the plasminogen moiety of the complex. Earlier workers have unequivocally demonstrated that a complex of SK-plasmin which is an activator of plasminogen contains one active site responsible for its esterase, protease, and activator activities. More importantly, it was established that this active site was located on the plasmin moiety of the complex. When plasmin reacts with PTI, a tight complex forms, and plasmin loses its esterase and protease activities. Similarly, when PTI reacts with the SK-plasmin complex, the complex loses its esterase, protease, and activator activities as well, showing that the PTI is blocking the only available catalytic site in the plasmin moiety of the complex.[52]

Since the activator activity of the SK-plasminogen complex involves the cleavage of an arginyl-valyl peptide bond in the plasminogen molecule, it was of interest to see whether the complex can also hydrolyze appropriate synthetic substrates. We chose lysine methyl ester, acetyl lysine methyl ester, and tosyl arginine methyl ester, since they have been shown earlier by Sherry et al.[34] to be excellent substrates for plasmin and for the SK-plasmin complex. When an equimolar amount of SK was mixed with plasminogen in the presence of 0.1 *M* acetyl lysine methyl ester, activation of plasminogen was found to be considerably delayed.[53] This delay in activation was directly related to the concentration of ester, suggesting that the ester may act either as competitive inhibitor or as a competitive substrate for the SK-plasminogen activator. If the ester acted as a competitive substrate, its hydrolysis should be observable immediately after mixing of the two proteins before any plasmin formation occurs. The experimental results indeed showed that hydrolysis of acetyl lysine methyl ester started

TABLE 1

Kinetic Constants for the Hydrolysis of Ac-Lys-OMe by Plasmin and Its Streptokinase Complexes

Enzyme	K_m (m*M*)	V_{max} (Asso)	Turnover number	Km/V_{max} (μmol substrate/nmol enzyme/hr
Plasmin	7.48 ± 2.3[a]	1.86 ± 0.52[a]	385	4.02
Streptokinase-plasmin	19.65 ± 7.6	5.34 ± 1.9	1105	3.68
Streptokinase-plasminogen	7.47 ± 2.3	1.58 ± 0.44	327	4.73

[a] SD calculated on the basis of two limiting visual estimates for the slopes.

From Reddy, K. N. N. and Markus, G., *J. Biol. Chem,* 249, 4851, 1974. American Society of Biological Chemists, Inc., Bethesda, Md., with permission.

as soon as the two components were mixed due to the catalytic activity of the SK-plasminogen complex. The kinetic constants for the hydrolysis of acetyl lysine methyl ester by SK-plasminogen complex are in Table 1, along with the constants for plasmin and SK-plasmin complex. The SK-plasminogen complex was also found to hydrolyze lysine methyl ester and tosyl arginine ester. Recently Wohl et al.[54] reported that the substrate *Nα*-CB2-L-lysine-*p*-nitrophenyl ester was also hydrolyzed by the SK-plasminogen complex.

The SK-plasminogen complex thus exhibits many of the characteristics of a proteolytic enzyme:

1. It reacts with active center-specific reagents (NPGB).
2. It possesses proteolytic specificity for a natural substrate (plasminogen).
3. It interacts with a naturally occurring inhibitor (PTI).
4. It exhibits esterase activity towards synthetic substrates.

It is of interest to note that the ability of the SK-plasminogen to hydrolyze acetyl lysine methyl ester is shared by another enzyme, urokinase, which is also an activator of plasminogen. The most striking feature of the SK-plasminogen enzyme is the fact that it is formed by an interaction of two inactive proteins, SK and plasminogen. Unlike other zymogens of serine proteases, such as chymotrypsinogen and trypsinogen,[55] human plasminogen does not appear to contain a preformed active site. The active site in the plasminogen molecule is formed when plasminogen is converted to plasmin by cleavage of a peptide bond. Yet this same active site becomes exposed without peptide bond cleavage when plasminogen forms a complex with SK. Esterase activity studies show that the catalytic site in the complex compares very well with that of the plasmin molecule. However, no caseinolytic activity has been demonstrable in the complex so far, although its proteolytic activity towards the physiological substrate plasminogen is expressed fully. It is possible that the plasminogen molecule is contributing a conformation specificity for the reaction with the activator enzyme or that some of the amino acid residues on the SK molecule may be participating in the activator activity as was suggested by Buck and Boggiano.[56] A comparison of some of the properties of SK-plasminogen complex with those of plasmin and the SK-plasmin complex is in Table 2.

TABLE 2

Comparison of Some Properties of Plasmin and Its Streptokinase Complexes

Relative activities[a]

Activity or inhibition	Plasmin	Streptokinase-plasmin	Streptokinase-plasminogen
Activator	0	1	∿3.5
Fibrinolytic	1	∿0.2 (at 25°C)	0
Caseinolytic	1	∿0.2 (at 25°C)	0
Tos-Arg-OMease	1	1	∿0.5
Ac-Lys-OMease	1	∿2.5	∿0.5
Gdn-Bz-ONpase	1 eq	1 eq	1 eq
Bovine pancreatic trypsin inhibitor			
Azocasein	Stoichiometric	Stoichiometric	No azocasein activity
Ac-Lys-OMe	Stoichiometric	Stoichiometric	Not stoichiometric
Soybean trypsin inhibitor			
Azocasein	Stoichiometric	Not stoichiometric	No azocasein activity
Ac-Lys-OMe	Stoichiometric	Very weak	None

[a] The property of plasmin, when present, was assigned the value of 1.

From Reddy, K. N. N. and Markus, G., *J. Biol. Chem.*, 249, 4851, 1974. American Society of Biological Chemists, Inc., Bethesda, Md., with permission.

VII. TRANSFORMATION OF STREPTOKINASE-PLASMINOGEN TO STREPTOKINASE-PLASMIN

A. Changes in Plasminogen

The SK-plasminogen complex exists transiently in a reaction mixture of SK and human plasminogen and is rapidly converted to the SK-plasmin complex, due to the proteolytic activity of the complex. Although the most significant change in the plasminogen molecule is the cleavage of an arginyl-valyl peptide bond, Taylor and Botts[57] have reported that a peptide of approximately 6000 daltons was also cleaved from the plasminogen molecule during activation. An analysis of the sequence of events that occurs during the transformation of SK-plasminogen to the SK-plasmin complex was carried out independently by McClintock et al.[58] and by Summaria et al.[59] The first bond to be cleaved in the plasminogen moiety of the SK-plasminogen complex was the arginyl-valyl peptide bond, giving rise to the two-chain structure of plasmin consisting of a heavy chain (56,000 daltons) and a light chain (20,000 daltons). Next, a peptide moiety of approximately 5000 daltons was cleaved from the NH_2-terminal part of the heavy chain of plasmin. Thus, the first step in the activation of human plasminogen by stoichiometric levels of SK involves the cleavage of an internal peptide bond catalyzed by the active site of the SK-plasminogen complex. McClintock et al. have also reported the interesting finding that when a catalytic amount of SK was used to activate human plasminogen, the plasminogen was found to be rapidly converted to an intermediate form of plasminogen of approximately 80,000 mol wt which was then transformed to plasmin. The loss of a peptide from the native plasminogen to give rise to the intermediate was ascribed to the activity of plasmin initially formed in the activation mixture. Later Bajaj and Castellino[60] arrived at the same conclusions regarding peptide bond cleavages in the plasminogen molecule upon activation by equimolar amounts of streptokinase.

It is of interest to note here that the ability of plasmin to split off the NH_2-terminal peptide of plasminogen can offer an explanation for the finding that some plasminogen preparations have lysine as their N-terminal amino acid residue instead of glutamic acid, as in native human plasminogen.[61] Chan and Mertz[62] had shown earlier that native plasminogen is altered during fractionation procedures. Therefore, if one wishes to obtain pure native human plasminogen, it is prudent to avoid contamination with plasmin during purification procedures, as well as during storage of the samples, since plasminogen is known to be spontaneously activated to plasmin slowly. However, since both Glu-plasminogen and Lys-plasminogen are activated by SK and even if one starts with Glu-plasminogen, the final activation product will be Lys-plasmin; the necessity for using Glu-plasminogen obviously depends upon the type and nature of investigations to be carried out.

B. Changes in Streptokinase

Earlier workers have recognized the fact that when SK is added to human plasminogen two reactions occur: (1) the activation of plasminogen to plasmin and (2) transformation of SK to a modified derivative, since it was found that while native SK was stable to acid treatment (pH 2.0), the SK after it had interacted with plasminogen was not. The modified SK showed a different electrophoretic mobility from that of native SK, indicating structural alterations in the molecule.[25,28] Thus, the SK moiety in the SK-plasminogen complex also undergoes proteolytic cleavages during the activation process.[50,58,59,63] The native molecule of SK of 47,000 daltons is very rapidly cleaved to a 43,000-dalton fragment which is then slowly converted to an SK derivative of 37,000 mol wt. Prolonged incubation leads to further fragmentation of SK to pieces of 10,000 daltons or less. The major fragment in complex with human plasmin which exhibits activator activity towards plasminogen from different species appears to be the 37,000 mol wt fragment. Recently, Chesterman et al.[64] found that considerable activator activity was present, even when the SK in the complex with human plasmin was degraded to peptides less than 10,000 mol wt.

The SK-plasminogen complex initially formed as a result of the interaction of SK with plasminogen is transformed to a relatively stable modified SK-plasmin complex as the final product. During this transformation, complexes of plasminogen and plasmin containing various forms of modified SK exist transiently in the activation mixture.

The activator activity of the various intermediates that form when the SK-plasminogen complex undergoes proteolytic cleavages was recently investigated by Markus et al.,[65] using bovine plasminogen as the substrate. Although these degradations of the protein molecules occur rapidly by a judicious use of inhibitors, various temperatures, and methods of analysis, they were able to study the activator activity of these intermediate complexes. The relative activator activities of the varius complexes are in Table 3. SKa, SKb, etc. denote progressively degraded forms of native SK. The relative activator activity was defined by these authors as the ratio of the activator activity of the complex to that of a fully developed SK-plasmin complex which contains the 37,000-dalton SK fragment. It can be seen that native SK when in complex with plasminogen or plasmin exhibits the highest activator activity. Fragmentation of only the SK moiety in the SK-plasminogen complex results in weak activator activity, for example with SKc and SKf fragments. However, it is interesting to note that this weak activity is enhanced more than two fold when the arginylvalyl peptide bond is cleaved in the plasminogen moiety of the same complex. Thus, fluctuations in activator activity

TABLE 3

Relative Activator Activities of Complexes of Plasminogen and Plasmin With Streptokinase at Progressive Stages of Fragmentation

Streptokinase	Plasminogen	Plasmin
SKa	"Native"[a] 1.3 (1.6)[b] "Modified":2.0 (2.6) 3.2*[d]	2.5(2.3)[c]
SKb	1.8 (1.8, 1.7, 1.6, 1.7, 2.1, 1.9)	n.d.[e]
SKc	0.3 (0.28, 0.36)	1.0 (0.8, 0.9, 1.0, 1.0)
SKd, SKe	n.d.	n.d.
SKf	0.4 (0.46)	(1.0)[f]

Note: Relative activator activity is defined as the ratio of the activator activity of the complex in question to that of a fully developed plasmin streptokinase complex (plasmin-SKf) of the same concentration.

[a] "Native" and "modified" refer to preparations with a predominantly glutamic acid NH_2-terminal end and to those with lysine or other NH_2-terminal ends.

[b] Numbers (outside parentheses) are felt to be the most reliable vluaes and are not necessarily the averages of all determined values for the species.

[c] Since the plasmin preparations used here were fully activated with urokinase, they must have been "modified", i.e., they must have lost the NH_2-terminal glutamic acid.

[d] This value for the activator activity of native SK-modified plasminogen complex has been reported recently.

[e] n.d., not determined.

[f] The value for this species is, by definition, 1.0.

From Markus, G., Evers, J. C., and Hobika, G. H., *J. Biol. Chem.*, 251, 6495, 1976. American Society of Biological Chemists, Inc., Bethesda, Md., with permission.

occur in the reaction mixture when the SK-plasminogen complex is transformed through transient intermediates to the relatively stable SK′-plasmin complex.

From the studies described above, it is clear that the interaction of SK with human plasminogen results in extensive changes in the polypeptide chains of both protein molecules. The molecule of SK loses peptides totalling at least 10,000 daltons from its polypeptide chain. (Henceforth, this modified form of SK will be represented as SK′). The single polypeptide chain of plasminogen is converted to the two-chain structure of plasmin (Lys-plasmin) accompanied by the loss of a peptide fragment from the NH_2-terminal portion of its polypeptide chain. The important point to be noted from the various studies on the transformation of the SK-plasminogen complex to the SK′-plasmin complex is that when SK is added to a solution of human plasminogen, the nature and properties of the transient products in the reaction mixture depends on various factors, such as the pH of the reaction mixture, the relative ratios of the reactants, the time of incubation, the temperature of the reaction, presence or absence of inhibitors, the type of inhibitors, and the presence of appropriate substrates during the activation process.

In the mechanism of activation of human plasminogen by SK described by Reddy and Markus, the catalytic step involves an intermolecular reaction, i.e., the SK-plasminogen activator cleaves the arginyl-valyl peptide bond present on another molecule of plasminogen. An alternate mechanism can also be considered in which the active site on the SK-plasminogen complex cleaves the arginyl-valyl bond within its own polyeptide chain. According to this mechanism, when catalytic amounts of SK are used to activate plasminogen, SK will combine with plasminogen and convert it to plasmin by intramolecular bond cleavage, dissociate from the newly formed plasmin, and repeat the process with other plasminogen molecules. Reddy and Markus ruled out this mechanism in view of the very well-known stability of the SK′-plasmin complex and the higher rate of activation obtainable with this complex than by using SK alone. However, Kosow[66] recenty proposed that the activation of plasminogen by SK proceeds by cleavage of the peptide bond within the complex itself, based on his measurement of the kinetics of plasminogen activation by SK, using the substrate *Nα*-CBZ-L-lysine- *p*-nitrophenyl ester. He claimed that in his assay system, only plasmin was being measured. However, Wohl et al.[54] showed that the SK-plasminogen complex also hydrolyzes the synthetic substrate with the same catalytic efficiency as that of plasmin itself. Markus et al.[65] recently pointed out that Kosow's inability to observe an initial burst of esterase activity in his studies can be explained by the simple fact that "a burst, i.e., a sudden release of product equivalent to the amount of enzyme present is observed only when one of the reaction products irreversibly blocks the active center, as in the case with NPGB".

VIII. SPECIES SPECIFICITY OF STREPTOKINASE

Wulf and Mertz studied the SK activation of plasminogens from several species using purified preparations, thus minimizing the possible contribution of factors other than SK and plasminogen to the activation process.[67] The purified preparations from all the species studied by them were found to contain two major activatable forms of plasminogen. They showed that the plasminogens from different species can be divided into three groups based on their response to SK:

1. Plasminogens that are activated by catalytic amounts of SK (human, cat, and monkey)
2. Plasminogens that require large amounts of SK for activation (dog and rabbit)
3. Plasminogens not at all activatable by SK (cow, sheep, pig, mouse, and rat)

All these plasminogen, however, were found to be activated by the SK′-plasmin complex and by urokinase. Thus, it appears that any structural differences between the plasminogens are reflected mainly in their ability to interact with SK. Since the activation of plasminogen by SK involves:

1. The formation of a complex between SK and plasminogen
2. The appearance of a functional catalytic site in the complex
3. The cleavage of a peptide bond in the plasminogen molecule. The inability of SK to activate some species of plasminogen may be due to a block in any of these steps.

For those species in which plasminogen is activatable by SK, the steps involving complex formation and active site generation were found to be involved in the activation as were shown in the case of cat, dog, and rabbit plasminogens.[51,59,68] In fact activation of rabbit plasminogen by SK was reported to be exclusively catalyzed by the SK-plasminogen complex, and rabbit plasmin was found to be unable to form a stable complex with SK.[51]

Studies were carried out in the author's laboratory to find an explanation as to why the quantitative activation of some plasminogen species require high concentrations of SK. Dog plasminogen was used as the model in these studies.[68] When the rate of activation of dog plasminogen by different concentrations of SK was measured, it was found that the concentration of SK affected the activation in two ways:

1. With low levels of SK, plasmin formation proceeded rapidly and reached a plateau with only a fraction of the plasminogen activated.
2. With concentrations of SK higher than equimolar with plasminogen, all of the plasminogen was activated following a significant lag period, during which no plasmin was formed.

The incomplete activation observed in the former case was found to be due to loss of activator activity in the reaction mixture. Polyacrylamide gel electrophoresis experiments showed that native SK, when added to dog plasminogen, was degraded rapidly to a fragment of approximately 25,700 mol wt. The loss in activator activity was found to occur when all of the added SK was converted to this modified SK in the reaction mixture. Thus, a major difference in the interaction of SK with human and dog plasminogen is that when human plasminogen is activated by catalytic amounts of SK, although the SK is cleaved rapidly to give the 37,000-dalton fragment the resulting SK′-plasmin complex itself carries on further activation of plasminogen. In contrast, in the dog plasminogen system, the modified SK-plasmin complex formed during the activation process is unable to activate the dog plasminogen. However, when the modified SK was dissociated from the SK dog plasmin complex and isolated free from dog plasmin, it exhibited significant activator activity towards human and dog plasminogens.[69]

Studies on the appearance of the active center in the SK-plasminogen complex revealed another significant difference between human and dog plasminogen.[68] When human plasminogen reacts with a stoichiometric amount of SK, 1.0 mol of active site is produced in 15 sec at room temperature, as seen by the NPGB "burst" assay. However, when 1.0 mol of dog plasminogen reacts with 1.0 mol of SK, only 0.13 mol of active sites are produced in 15 sec, and a much longer time (10 min) is required for the formation of 1.0 mol active center. The fraction of active centers formed in dog plasminogen in 15 sec was low at various ratios of SK and remained so even when a large excess of SK was used. This behavior of dog plasminogen is quite different from that of rabbit plasminogen, where the fraction of active centers rises as the SK concentration is increased.[51]

Although the rate of active site formation is low in dog plasminogen when high concentrations of SK are used, activation proceeds to completion following a lag period. Gel electrophoretic analysis showed that the activation of plasminogen was completed before all of the added SK was converted to the major degraded form. Moreover, the rate of this modification was found to be slow and proceeded through the formation of higher molecular weight fragments of SK. The activation of dog plasminogen by a high concentration of SK can be viewed as a race between the degradation of SK and the activation of plasminogen. When activation is carried out in the presence of excess SK, sufficient intact SK will be available to replace the loss in activator activity as a result of the fragmentation of SK. Moreover, due to the stepwise degradation of SK, the higher molecular weight fragments of SK formed in the reaction mixture may also contribute to and maintain activator activity.

Based on the information available so far from the studies on the interaction of SK

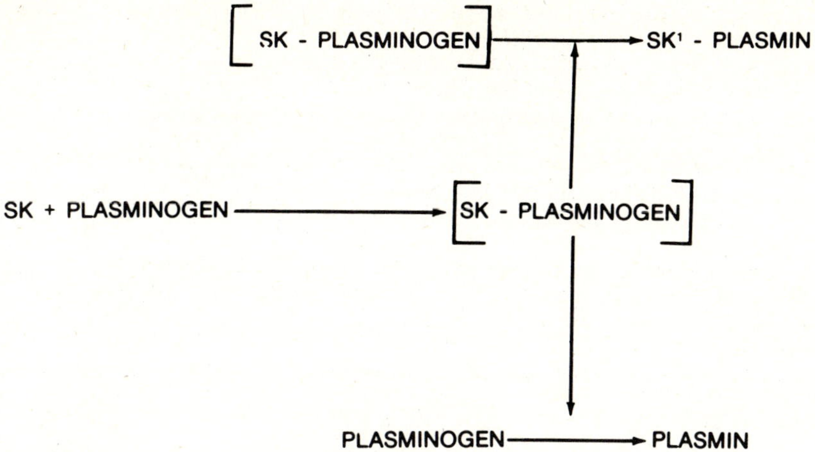

FIGURE 5. Activation of plasminogen. (From Reddy, K. N. N., and Markus, G., *J. Biol. Chem.*, 247, 1683, 1972. American Society of Biological Chemists, Inc., Bethesda, Md. With permission.)

with plasminogen, the important factors that govern the activation process can be identified as follows. The rate and extent of complex formation and active center development in the SK-plasminogen complex, the stability of the complex, and the rate at which the arginyl-valyl peptide bond is cleaved in the plasminogen moiety of the complex control the overall generation of plasmin. The rate of activation would also be dependent upon whether activation is being carried out solely by the SK-plasminogen complex, other intermediate molecular species, or by the modified SK-plasmin complexes. As soon as the active center appears in the SK-plasminogen complex, this center has the alternatives of attacking plasminogen or SK or both. The plasmin formed during the activation can exist as a complex with SK or dissociate from it or, being a protease, can degrade SK, plasmin, and plasminogen (See Figure 5). Since these reactions are dependent on time and the concentration of reactants as well as temperature, it is obvious that the moment SK is added to a solution of plasminogen, the amount and nature of the products formed depend on the parameters stated above, as well as on the species of plasminogen used.

REFERENCES

1. **Tillett, W. S. and Garner, R. L.,** The fibrinolytic activity of hemolytic streptococci, *J. Exp. Med.*, 58, 485, 1933.
2. **Tillett, W. S., Edwards, L. B., and Garner, R. L.,** Fibrinolytic activity of hemolytic streptococci. Development of resistance to fibrinolysis following acute hemolytic streptococcus infections, *J. Clin. Invest.*, 13, 47, 1934.
3. **Garner, R. L. and Tillett, W. S.,** Biochemical studies on the fibrinolytic activity of hemolytic streptococci. I. Isolation and characterization of fibrinolysin, *J. Exp. Med.*, 60, 239, 1934.
4. **Milstone, J. H.,** A factor in normal human blood which participates in streptococcal fibrinolysis, *J. Immunol.*, 42, 109, 1941.
5. **Denys, J. and de Marbaix, H.,** Les peptonisations provoquees par le chloroforme, *La Cellule*, 5, 197, 1889.
6. **Kaplan, M. H.,** Nature and role of lytic factor in hemolytic streptococcal fibrinolysis, *Proc. Soc. Exp. Biol. Med.*, 57, 40, 1944.

7. **Christensen, L. R.**, Streptococcal fibrinolysis: a proteolytic reaction due to a serum enzyme activated by streptococcal fibrinolysin, *J. Gen. Physiol.*, 28, 363, 1945.
8. **Christensen, L. R. and Macleod, C. M.**, A proteolytic enzyme of serum: characterization, activation, and reaction with inhibitors, *J. Gen. Physiol.*, 28, 559, 1945.
9. **Geiger, W. B.**, Involvement of a complement like factor in the activation of blood protease, *J. Immunol.*, 69, 597, 1952.
10. **Müllertz, S. and Lassen, M.**, An activator system in blood indispensible for formation of plasmin by streptokinase, *Proc. Soc. Exp. Biol. Med.*, 82, 264, 1953.
11. **Troll, W. and Sherry, S.**, The activation of human plasminogen by streptokinase, *J. Biol. Chem.*, 213, 881, 1955.
12. **Kline, D. L.**, The purification and crystallisation of plasminogen (profibrinolysin), *J. Biol. Chem.*, 204, 949, 1953.
13. **Sherry, S.**, The fibrinolytic activity of streptokinase activated human plasmin, *J. Clin. Invest.*, 33, 1054, 1954.
14. **Ablondi, F. B. and Hagan, J. J.**, Stability of the activator of bovine plasminogen, *Proc. Soc. Exp. Biol. Med.*, 93, 414, 1956.
15. **Ablondi, F. B. and Hagan, J. J.**, Comparison of certain properties of human plasminogen and "proactivator", *Proc. Soc. Exp. Biol. Med.*, 95, 195, 1957.
16. **Kline, D. L. and Fishman, J. B.**, Plasmin. The humoral protease, *Ann. N.Y. Acad. Sci.*, 68, 25, 1957.
17. **Hagan, J. J., Ablondi, F. B., and DeRenzo, E. C.**, Purification and biochemical properties of human plasminogen, *J. Biol. Chem.*, 235, 1005, 1960.
18. **Zylber, J., Blatt, W. F., and Jensen, H.**, Mechanism of bovine plasminogen activation by human plasmin and streptokinese, *Proc. Soc. Exp. Biol. Med.*, 102, 755, 1959.
19. **Kline, D. L. and Fishman, J. B.**, Proactivator function of human plasmin as shown by lysine esterase assay, *J. Biol. Chem.*, 236, 2807, 1961.
20. **Alkjaersig, N., Fletcher, A. P., and Sherry, S.**, The mechanism of clot dissolution by plasmin, *J. Clin. Invest.*, 38, 1086, 1959.
21. **Baumgarten, W.**, Interaction of plasminogen with SK, *Thromb. Diath. Haemorrh.*, 6 (Suppl. 1), 132, 1961.
22. **DeRenzo, E. C.**, Ultracentrifuge studies, *Thromb. Diath. Haemorrh.*, 6 (Suppl. 1), 134, 1961.
23. **Heimburger, N. and Schwick, G.**, Die fibrinagar-Elektrophorese. II. Mitteilung: untersuchungen zum wirkungsmechanismus der streptokinase, *Thromb. Diath. Haemorrh.*, 7, 444, 1962.
24. **Davies, M. E., Englert, M. E., and DeRenzo, E. C.**, Interaction of Streptokinase and plasminogen observed in the Ultracentrifuge under a variety of experimental conditions, *J. Biol. Chem.*, 239, 2651, 1966.
25. **Ling, C-M., Summaria, L., and Robbins, K. C.**, Isolation and characterization of bovine plasminogen activator from a human plasmingen-streptokinase mixture, *J. Biol. Chem.*, 242, 1419, 1967.
26. **Blatt, W. F., Segal, H., and Gray, J. L.**, Purification of streptokinase and human plasmin and their interaction, *Thromb. Diath. Haemorrh.*, 11, 393, 1964.
27. **Barg, W. F., Jr., Boggiano, E., and DeRenzo, E. C.**, Interaction of streptokinase and human plasmingen. II. Starch gel electrophoretic demonstration of a reaction product with activator activity, *J. Biol. Chem.*, 240, 2944, 1965.
28. **DeRenzo, E. C., Boggiano, E., Barg, W. F., Jr., and Buck, F. F.**, Interaction of streptokinase and human plasminogen. IV. Further gel electrophoretic studies on the combination of streptokinase with human plasminogen or human plasmin, *J. Biol. Chem.*, 242, 2428, 1967.
29. **Tomar, R. H. and Taylor, F. B., Jr.**, The streptokinase-human plasminogen activator complex. Composition and identity of a subcomponent with activator activity, *Biochem. J.*, 125, 793, 1971.
30. **Summaria, L., Ling, C-M., Groskopf, W. R., and Robbins, K. C.**, The active site of bovine plasmigen activator. Interaction of streptokinase with human plasminogen and plasmin, *J. Biol. Chem.*, 243, 144, 1968.
31. **Buck, F. F., Hummel, B. C. W., and DeRenzo, E. C.**, Interaction of streptokinase and human plasminogen. V. Studies on the nature and mechanism of formation of the enzymatic site of the activator complex, *J. Biol. Chem.*, 243, 3648, 1968.
32. **Groskopf, W. R., Hsieh, B., Summaria, L., and Robbins, K. C.**, Studies on the active center of human plasmin. The serine and histidine residues, *J. Biol. Chem.*, 244, 359, 1969.
33. **Markus, G. and Werkheiser, W. C.**, The interaction of streptokinase with plasminogen. I. Functional properties of the activated enzyme, *J. Biol. Chem.*, 239, 2637, 1964.
34. **Sherry, S., Alkjaersig, N., and Fletcher, A. P.**, Activity of plasmin and streptokinase-activator on substituted arginine and lysine esters, *Thromb. Diath. Haemorrh.*, 16, 18, 1966.
35. **Kline, D. L. and Ts'ao, C. H.**, Activation of human plasminogen by streptokinase in absence of plasmin-SK activator, *Am. J. Physiol.*, 220, 440, 1971.
36. **Summaria, C., Hsieh, B., Groskopf, W. R., and Robbins, K. C.**, Direct activation of human plasminogen by streptokinase, *Proc. Soc. Exp. Biol. Med.*, 130, 737, 1969.

37. **Werkheiser, W. C. and Markus, G.**, The interaction of streptokinase with plasminogen. II. The kinetics of activation, *J. Biol. Chem.*, 239, 2644, 1964.
38. **Ling, C-M., Summaria, L., and Robbins, K. C.**, Mechanism of formation of bovine plasminogen activator from human plasma, *J. Biol. Chem.*, 240, 4213, 1965.
39. **Gajewski, J. and Markus, G.**, Anion-specific effects on the streptokinase activation of human plasminogen, *J. Biol. Chem.*, 243, 6210, 1968.
40. **Gutman, M. and Rimon, A.**, Studies on the activation of plasminogen. II. On the nature of the proactivator, *Can. J. Biochem.*, 42, 1339, 1964.
41. **Rimon, S., Stupp, Y., and Rimon, A.**, Studies on the activation of plasminogen. III. Soluble derivatives of the proactivator and the activator, *Can. J. Biochem.*, 44, 415, 1966.
42. **Takada, A., Takada, Y., and Ambrus, J. C.**, Streptokinase-activatable proactivator of human and bovine plasminogen, *J. Biol. Chem.*, 245, 6389, 1970.
43. **Kline, D. L. and Bowlds, C. A.**, Possible isolation of an active derivative of streptokinase, *Fed. Proc. Fed. Am. Soc. Exp. Biol.*, 30, 984, 1971.
44. **Taylor, F. B., Jr. and Beisswenger, J. G.**, Identification of modified streptokinase as the activator of bovine and human plasminogen, *J. Biol. Chem.*, 248, 1127, 1973.
45. **Robbins, K. C., Summaria, L., Hsieh, B., and Shah, R. J.**, The peptide chains of human plasmin. Mechanism of activation of human plasminogen to plasmin, *J. Biol. Chem.*, 242, 2333, 1967.
46. **Chase, T., Jr., and Shaw, E.**, Comparison of the esterase activities of trypsin, plasmin, and thrombin on guanidinobenzoate esters. Titration of the enzymes, *Biochemistry*, 8, 2212, 1969.
47. **Reddy, K. N. N.**, Evidence for the presence of an active center in SK-plasminogen complex, *Fed. Proc. Fed. Am. Soc. Exp. Biol.*, 30, 982, 1971.
48. **McClintock, D. K. and Bell, P. H.**, Human plasminogen activator studies, *Fed. Proc. Fed. Am. Soc. Exp. Biol.*, 30, 981, 1971.
49. **Taylor, F. B., Jr. and Beisswenger, J.**, Localization of activator activity to the streptokinase portion of the streptokinase-plasminogen complex, *Fed. Proc. Fed. Am. Soc. Exp. Biol.*, 30, 983, 1971.
50. **Reddy, K. N. N. and Markus, G.**, Mechanism of activation of human plasminogen by streptokinase. Presence of active center in Streptokinase-plasminogen complex, *J. Biol. Chem.*, 247, 1683, 1972.
51. **Schick, L. A. and Castellino, F. J.**, Interaction of streptokinase and rabbit plasminogen, *Biochemistry*, 12, 4315, 1973.
52. **Reddy, K. N. N. and Markus, G.**, Further evidence for an active center in streptokinase-plasminogen complex; interaction with pancreatic trypsin inhibitor, *Biochem. Biophys. Res. Commun.*, 51, 672, 1973.
53. **Reddy, K. N. N. and Markus, G.**, Esterase activities in the zymogen moiety of the streptokinase-plasminogen complex, *J. Biol. Chem.*, 2119, 4851, 1974.
54. **Wohl, R. C., Arzadon, L., Summaria, L., and Robbins, K. C.**, Comparison of the esterase and human plasminogen activator activities of various activated forms of human plasminogen and their equimolar streptokinase complexes, *J. Biol. Chem.*, 252, 1141, 1977.
55. **Neurath, H.**, Limited proteolysis and zymogen activation, in *Proteases and Biological Control*, Vol. 2, Cold Spring Harbor Conferences on Cell Proliferation, Reich, E., Rifkin, D. B., and Shaw, E., Eds., Cold Spring Harbor Laboratory, Cold Spring Harbor, N.Y., 1975, 51.
56. **Buck, F. F. and Boggiano, E.**, Interaction of streptokinase and human plasminogen. VI. Function of the streptokinese moiety in the activator complex, *J. Biol. Chem.*, 246, 2091, 1971.
57. **Taylor, F. B., Jr. and Botts, J.**, Purification and characterization of streptokinase with studies of streptokinase activation of plasminogen, *Biochemistry*, 7, 232, 1968.
58. **McClintock, D. K., Englert, M. E., Dziobkowski, C., Snedeker, E. H., and Bell, P. H.**, Two distinct pathways of the streptokinase-mediated activation of highly purified human plasminogen, *Biochemistry*, 13, 5334, 1974.
59. **Summaria, L., Arzadon, L., Bernabe, P., and Robbins, K. C.**, The interaction of streptokinase with human, cat, dog and rabbit plasminogens. The fragmentation of streptokinase in the equimolar plasminogen-streptokinase complexes, *J. Biol. Chem.*, 249, 4760, 1974.
60. **Bajaj, S. P. and Castellino, F. J.**, Activation of human plasminogen by equimolar levels of streptokinase, *J. Biol. Chem.*, 52, 492, 1977.
61. **Rickli, E. E. and Cuendet, P. A.**, Isolation of plasmin-free human plasminogen with N-terminal glutamic acid, *Biochem. Biophys. Acta*, 250, 447, 1971.
62. **Chan, J. Y. S. and Mertz, E. T.**, Studies on plasminogen. IV. Alteration of bovine and human plasminogens during isolation, *Can. J. Biochem.*, 44, 469, 1966.
63. **Brockway, W. J. and Castellino, F. J.**, A Characterization of native streptokinase isolated from a human plasminogen activator complex, *Biochemistry*, 13, 2063, 1974.
64. **Chesterman, C. N., Cederholm-Williams, S. A., Allington, M. J., and Sharp, A. A.**, The degradation of streptokinase during the production of plasminogen activator, *Thromb. Res.*, 5, 413, 1974.
65. **Markus, G., Evers, J. L., and Hobika, G. H.**, Activator activities of the transient forms of the human plasminogen-streptokinase complex during its proteolytic conversion to the stable activator complex, *J. Biol. Chem.*, 251, 6495, 1976.

66. **Kosow, D. P.**, Kinetic mechanism of the activation of human plasminogen by streptokinase, *Biochemistry*, 14, 4459, 1975.
67. **Wulf, R. J. and Mertz, E. T.**, Studies on plasminogen. VIII. Species specificity of streptokinase, *Can. J. Biochem.*, 47, 927, 1969.
68. **Reddy, K. N. N.**, Kinetics of active center formation in dog plasminogen by streptokinase and activity of a modified streptokinase, *J. Biol. Chem.*, 251, 6624, 1976.
69. **Reddy, K. N. N. and Kline, D. L.**, Isolation of an active derivative produced from native streptokinase by dog plasmin, *Thromb. Res.*, 9, 407, 1976.

Chapter 5

SYNTHETIC FIBRINOLYTIC AGENTS

Kurt N. von Kaulla

TABLE OF CONTENTS

I. INTRODUCTION

A. Reasons for Searching for a Replacement for Urokinase by Synthetic Compounds

When in 1954 we obtained the first urokinase preparations from human urine,[1] the question arose as to how much of it would be needed for induction of a thrombolytic effect. In order to obtain this information, an in vitro thrombosis model was developed[2] which imitated a vessel completely occluded by a thrombus which exposed only one small side to the thrombolytic agent and which permitted reading on a scale the progress of the thrombolysis at any time, thus providing a time-related curve reflecting the intensity of thrombolysis. This gives much more precise information than can be obtained from one fibrinolytic value only. The tubes being utilized are shown in Figure 1. The progress of clot dissolution is read on the graduated hollow stem, where the clot is formed by recalcification of human citrated plasma (relation of plasma to citrate Na, 4:1 citrated plasma to $CaCl_2$ 0.5 *M*, 10:1). The plasma to be tested for "thrombolytic" activity is placed in the enlarged upper part of the tube on top of the plasma clot in its stem. The tubes are slowly rotated in an oblique position and incubated at 37°C.[2] Fibrinolytic dissolution of a clotted human plasma containing fibrinolytic material does not reflect the thrombolytic potential of such material. For instance, a plasma which after being clotted lysed after 204 min when placed as an unclotted specimen on top of the aforementioned preformed "thrombotic" clot, induced within 24 hr of incubation time a lysis of only 4 $\mu\ell$. In contrast, the unclotted specimen of an actively "fibrinolytic" plasma which after clotting dissolved within 60 min induced lysis of 44 $\mu\ell$ of the preformed clot, a marked fibrinolytic activity which clearly reflects a thrombolytic potential. Using human urokinase dissolved in human plasma, it was found that very large amounts of urokinase are required for inducing even very little dissolution of this preformed plasma clot. From this observation, it was concluded that urokinase would be a very expensive thrombolytic agent. At that time, it was not yet known that urokinase is not the plasminogen activator of the human blood and that, as was shown much later, the urine production for 1 year of one human being is required for an average thrombolytic treatment. Enhancement of urokinase-induced fibinolytic activity by synthetic compounds thus permitting reduction of the required amounts of urokinase was considered the next goal.

B. Discovery of Synthetic In Vitro Fibrinolysis-Inducing Compounds

There were no indications about the types of compounds to be used for exerting this enhancing effect. There was, however, a drug combination available in ampules called Cibalgin which had already been taken off the market at that time, but which, accord-

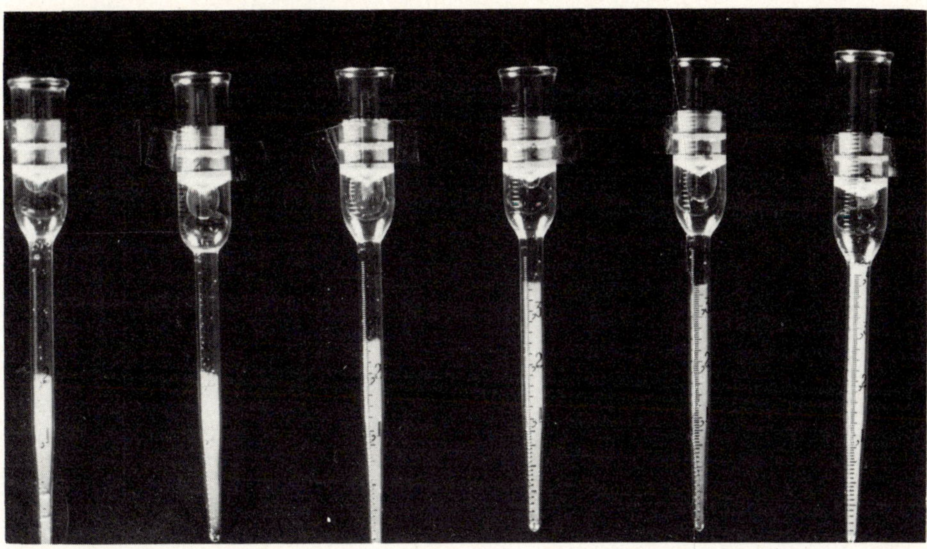

FIGURE 1. Tubes used for the rotating cylinder-shaped clots obtained from recalcified human plasma imitating an occluded vessel. The tubes show varied progress of "thrombolysis". Compound-less control tube on the right side.

ing to some physicians, would dissolve the thrombotic occlusions when injected into smaller thrombosed human superficial veins. It turned out that addition of Cibalgin to the plasma containing urokinase clearly enhanced the clot-dissolving potential of this plasma. However, controls using Cibalgin alone in the plasma without urokinase revealed that this plasma exerted a marked "thrombolytic" effect. It turned out that three of four compounds which were contained in the Cibalgin induced fibrinolytic activity in human plasma, as assessed with the hanging clot (this method will be described later). The required molarities expressed in millimols were as follows: monoethylurea, 1500, urethan, 700, and aminopyrine (pyramidon), 200. The hanging clot figures are given to permit a comparison with the fibrinolytic activity of the numerous other compounds tested with this method. The fourth compound, allobarbital, exerted no fibrinolysis-inducing activity. Figure 2 shows the kinetics of the fibrinolytic dissolution of the preformed "thrombotic" clot formed from recalcified human plasma by plasma containing Cibalgin, urethan, ethylurea, or urea at identical concentrations. It becomes evident that the lysis of the preformed clot induced by compounds dissolved in human plasma continues for days and that urethan at these concentrations is the most active compound. Several urethan and urea derivates were next tested by the simple plasma clot method, i.e., human citrated plasma containing a compound to be tested was clotted by calcium chloride and the clot dissolution time was recorded. The results are in Table 1. Ethylurethan proved to be the most active compound in this series. This compound then was used for further studies. When ethylurethan was dissolved in buffered saline and applied onto a "thrombotic" clot formed by thrombin not originating from human plasma but from bovine fibrinogen, no clot dissolution was observed. However, when increasing amounts of human plasma were added to buffered saline containing the ethylurethan, the resulting lysis intensity of the preformed clot of bovine fibrinogen increased with the increasing amounts of the plasma added (Figure 3). From this observation, it became quite evident that "something contained in human plasma" was required for lysis induction by the urea and urethan derivatives. With ethylurethan it was furthermore demonstrated that this fibrinolysis-

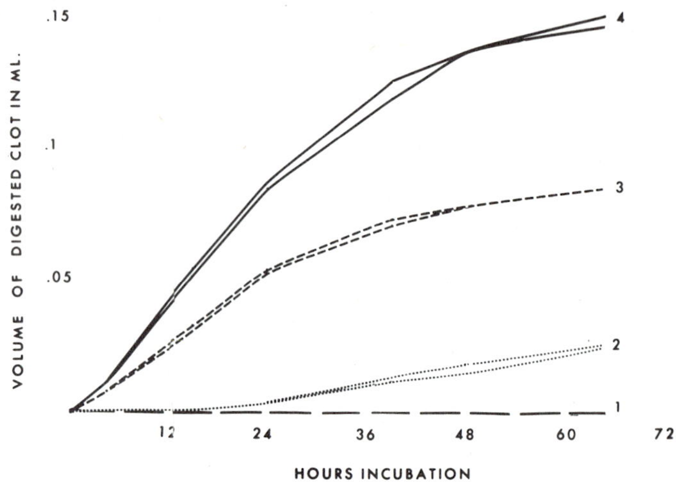

FIGURE 2. Progressive lysis induced on preformed cylinder-shaped "thrombotic" clots from human plasma by urethan, Cibalgin, and ethylurea dissolved at 8.1% in human plasma.

TABLE 1

Spontaneous Dissolution of Human Plasma Clots Formed in Presence of Various Urea Derivatives

Compound	Conc (%)	Amount (millimols)	Dissolution time (hr)
Urethan	4	449	40
Methylurethan	3	291	40
Ethylthiurea	3	288	16
Butylurea	3	258	16
Allylthiurea	3	258	21
Ethylurethan	2	171	24
None	—	—	>72

inducing compound very markedly enhanced the activity of urokinase. In fact, when concentration of urokinase and of ethylurethan were used which, when applied alone, induced no fibrinolytic activity at all, there was a very marked fibrinolytic activity induced in human plasma, as assessed with the preformed thrombotic clot when these two ineffective concentrations of urokinase and ethylurethan were combined (Figure 4).

C. Hydrotropism, an Indication for Evaluating Other Compounds

The next logical step was to search for more active compounds. A common property of the urea and urethan derivatives is hydrotropism. Hydrotropic substances are compounds whose aqueous solutions dissolve substances which are generally either insoluble or only slightly soluble in water of the same temperature as the compound solution.[3] Although hydrotropism later was shown not to be the only explanation for the

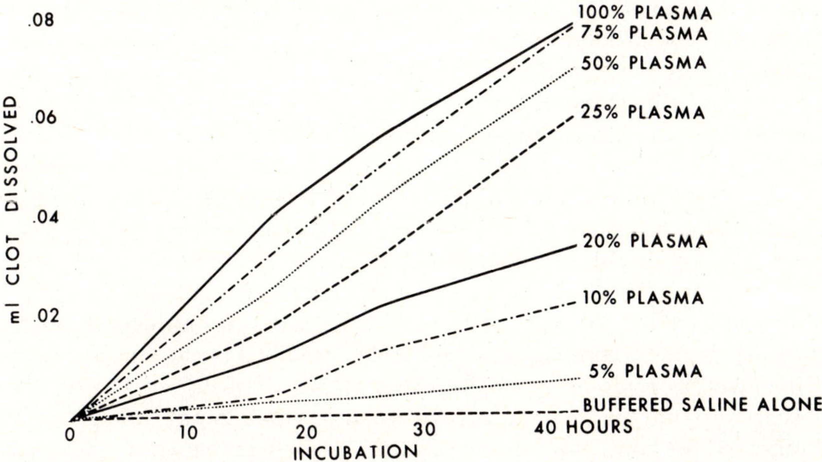

FIGURE 3. Progressive lysis of a preformed cylinder-shaped clot made from bovine fibrinogen by ethylurethan dissolved in buffered saline containing various amounts of human plasma. Increase of induced fibrinolytic activity with increasing amounts of human plasma present.

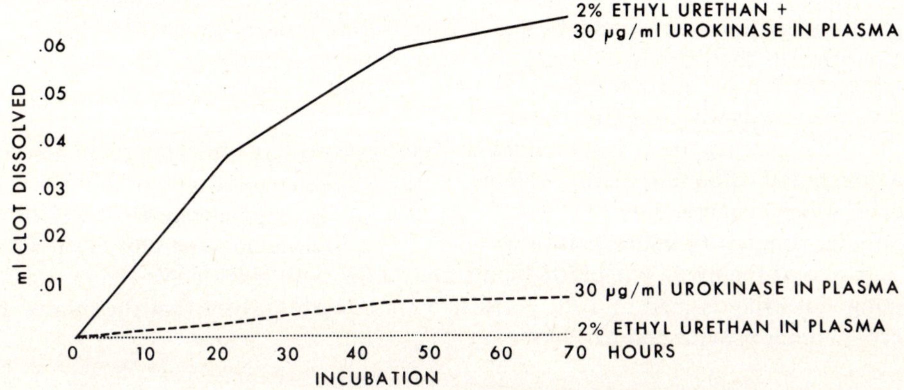

FIGURE 4. Synergistic lytic effect of the combination of individually ineffective concentrations of ethylurethan and urokinase. Preformed "thrombolytic" clot.

fibrinolysis-inducing capacity of synthetic compounds (we found large hydrotropic cations to be without any fibrinolysis-inducing effect), we checked other compounds with hydrotropic properties; 2,4-dimethylbenzene sulfonate[4] and 2-naphthalene sulfonate[5] were such compounds. Both were found to induce marked fibrinolytic activity in human plasma at lower concentrations than ethylurethan,[6] naphthalene sulfate being the most active compound. These observations opened the door for a further search for synthetic fibrinolysis-inducing organic compounds. In order to test large numbers of compounds, a simpler test had to be developed which would also permit studies at high concentrations. This and other tests are described in the next section.

II. METHODS FOR SERIAL TESTING OF POTENTIAL FIBRINOLYSIS-INDUCING SYNTHETIC COMPOUNDS

A. Hanging Clot

This method uses a preformed clot obtained from human plasma, thus permitting the testing of compounds at rather high concentrations.[7] A cylinder-shaped clot (0.5 mℓ) is formed from citrated human plasma (mostly obtained from outdated blood bank plasma) by its recalcification in a siliconized cylinder-shaped small glass tube with a flat bottom. Immediately after recalcification (0.05 mℓ $CaCl_2$, 0.5 *M*), a glass rod is inserted into the plasma to the bottom of the tube. In 30 min after the plasma has been clotted, the glass rod with the cylinder-shaped plasma clot attached is removed from the tube and suspended in 2.5 mℓ of a buffered saline solution pH 7.42 of the compound to be tested at 37°C. The solution is adjusted to pH 7.42 if necessary. The active molarity of the compound is determined by finding the lowest molarity which induces clot lysis within 24 hr of incubation. This method proved to be well adapted to serial testing. It is (and this is very essential) not influenced much by the binding of the synthetic compounds to albumin contained in the clot because the volume of the solution being tested is five times greater than that of the clot to be dissolved. Therefore, the binding of the compound to albumin has little effect upon the concentration of the compound in the solution into which the clot is submerged. The results with various types of synthetic asymmetric organic anions are given in the tables of the next section. Practically all compounds were active within a certain concentration range, inducing no fibrinolytic activity in a higher and a lower range. The range of activity was quite different. To give two examples: 5-benzylsalicylic acid was active from 10 to 4 m*M*: 5-(1,1,3,3-tetramethylbutyl) salicylic acid was active only at 3 m*M*. The compound diffuses into the preformed clot and is, as will be shown in the section on pathways of fibrinolysis induction, very firmly bound to fibrin where the induction of activation of the fibrinolytic system occurs. After several hours of incubation, the hanging clot can be transferred into a buffered saline solution containing no compound, where lysis will continue.

For testing plasma from small animals such as rats or when only very small amounts of a compound to be tested are available, a micro-hanging clot method has been developed which requires only 0.02 mℓ plasma for the hanging clot and 0.1 mℓ of the compound solution in which it is suspended.[8] The routine hanging clot is shown on the left side of Figure 5. The plasma clots are on the right side of this figure. For the hanging clot using human and rat plasma, it was clearly proven that the micro- and macro-methods provide comparable results (Table 2).

B. Plasma Clot

Citrated human plasma in which the compound to be tested was dissolved (pH adjusted to 7.42, if necessary) was clotted by recalcification. The calcium chloride added increased the volume of the plasma by only 10%. The lowest molarity which induced complete clot dissolution within 24 hr was determined. The plasma clot lysis procedure is being used when the compound-inducing fibrinolytic activity is present at rather low concentration and therefore does not interfere with the coagulation process. The differences between the required molarity as can be seen in Figure 5 with 5-cinnamyl salicylic acid for hanging clot and plasma clot are caused by the binding of the compounds to albumin which binding is quite different from compound to compound (see section on binding of compounds to albumin). For the plasma clot, animal plasma can

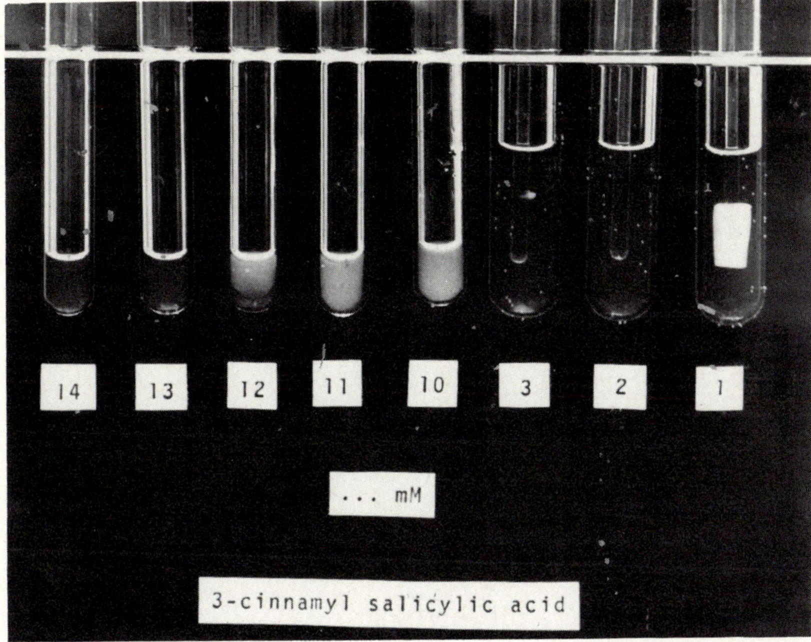

FIGURE 5. Clots made from human plasma for testing potentially synthetic fibrinolysis-inducing agents. Left side: plasma clots, complete lysis at 14 and 13 m*M*, partial lysis at 12 m*M*. Right side: hanging clots, complete lysis at 3 and 2 m*M*, no lysis at 1 m*M*.

also be used. The effects with animal plasma are somewhat different from human plasma as seen from Table 3 for flufenamic acid.

The preformed "thrombotic" rotating clot has already been described.

C. Serum-Free Clot

The serum-free human flat clot was designed to obtain some information on the fibrinolysis-inducing mechanism of the synthetic compounds. Clots obtained from recalcified human plasma were centrifuged at 35,000 g. By this centrifugation, they became very flat and all serum was expressed. Subsequently, these flat clots were washed three times with buffered saline. When exposed to solutions containing active compounds, they lysed after several hours at very low compound concentrations (Figure 6). The lysis mechanism will be described in the section on the pathway of fibrinolysis induction. Urokinase is completely ineffective with these serum-free clots. It is also less effective with the hanging clot than with the plasma clot in which the urokinase was added to the plasma before it was clotted. Urokinase penetrates very poorly into preformed clots, i.e., the hanging clots, in contrast to the synthetic fibrinolysis-inducing agents. These differences between the efficiency of urokinase and synthetic fibrinolytic agents are shown in Table 4.

III. OBSERVATIONS ON STRUCTURE-ACTIVITY RELATIONSHIP

Many organic anions of various structures induce fibrinolytic activity in human plasma and particularly in preformed human plasma clots into which they penetrate very easily. In the following, examples are given for such compounds. All of them have been tested with the hanging clot method. Figure 7 makes clear that the fibrinolysis-inducing capacity of salicylic acid is very markedly enhanced by various substitu-

TABLE 2

Fibrinolysis Induction In Vitro. Results with the Hanging Clot Method, Including a Micro-Method, Using Clots Made from Human and Rat Plasma

Plasma	Compound	HC[a] or MHC	BS[a] or Plasma	Millimoles[b]															
				16	15	14	13	12	11	10	9	8	7	6	5	4	3	2	1
Human	Flufenamic acid	HC	BS						−	−	−	(+)	(+)	(+)	+	+	+	(+)	−
Rat	Flufenamic acid	MHC	BS						−	−	−	−	−	(+)	+	+	(+)	−	−
Human	Flufenamic acid	HC	Plasma	−	(+)	(+)	(+)	+	+	+	(+)	−	−	−					
Rat	Flufenamic acid	MHC	Plasma	−	(+)	(+)	(+)	+	+	+	+	−	−	−					

Note: Clots were suspended in compound containing buffered saline or in compound containing plasma of the same species.

[a] HC = hanging clot (0.5 mℓ); MHC = micro hanging clot (0.02 mℓ); and BS = buffered saline.
[b] + Clot completely dissolved within 24 hr; (+), clot partially dissolved; −, clot not dissolved.

TABLE 3

Fibrinolysis Induced by Flufenamic Acid Na in Plasma of Animals and Man

Species	m*M*
Pig	6
Dog	6
Mouse (pooled)	6
Rat	8
Guinea pig	9
Man	12

Note: Lowest active concentration given in m*M*.

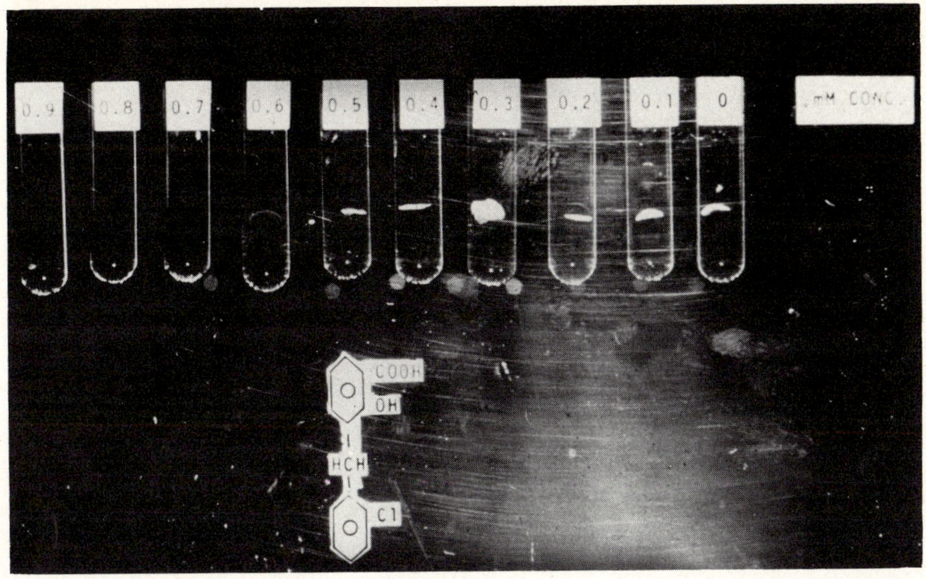

FIGURE 6. Fibrinolysis induced in serum-free human flat clots by (as one example of many) a synthetic fibrinolysis-inducing compound.

TABLE 4

Urokinase- vs. Compound-Induced Fibrinolysis of the Three Types of Clots Originating From Human Plasma used for Testing

	Urokinase (CTA units/mℓ)	*N*-(4-isopropylphenyl) anthranilic acid (m*M*)
Plasma clot	40	13
Hanging clot	90	8
Serum-free clot	up to 2000:0	0.9

Note: Lowest effective concentration given.

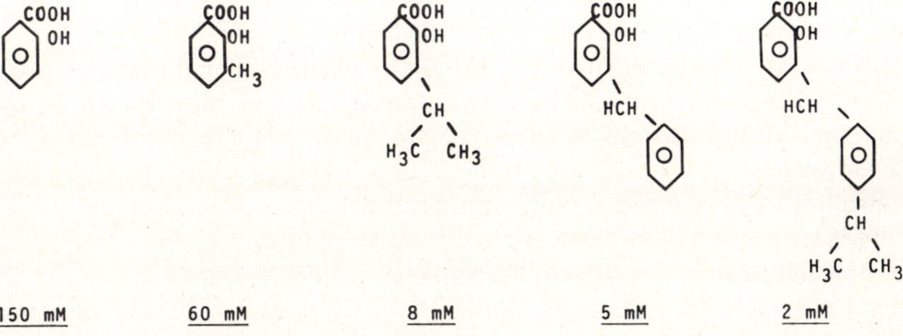

FIGURE 7. Increase of fibrinolysis-inducing capacity of salicylic acid derivatives with the increasing length of the substitutions.

tions. The activity increases with the increasing length of substitution. Figure 8 gives another example of the increasing fibrinolysis-inducing capacity of substitutions of

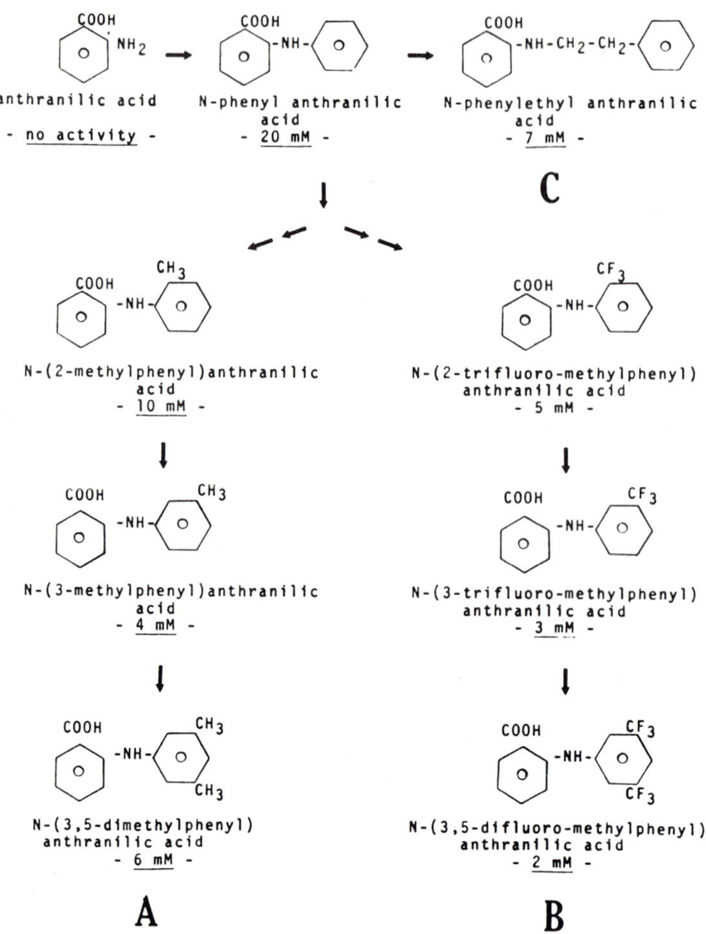

FIGURE 8. Induction of fibrinolysis-inducing capacity into the inactive molecule of anthranilic acid by various substitutions.

anthranilic acid. Anthranilic acid without substitutions does not exert any fibrinolysis-inducing activity. Of interest is the fact that trifluoro-substitutions enhance the fibrinolytic activity more than do methyl-substitutions in the same position. To give other examples: a number of derivatives of diaryl-carboxylic acid were found to induce marked fibrinolytic activity in vitro. For instance, simple diphenyl-carboxylic acid was inactive, but when the carboxyl group was attached to the ring through an alkyl or alkylene chain, but not through an alkoxy chain, there was a rather high fibrinolysis-inducing capacity.[9]

It has also been observed that a number of anti-inflammatory compounds (and many of their derivatives, including benzopyrazone, phenylbutazone, ketophenylbutazone, and indomethacin; for indomethacin derivatives, see Table 5) induce marked fibrinolytic activity in the test tube (hanging clot method),[10,11] and this effect is obtained with some pyrazolidine derivatives (Table 6). There exists some parallelism between their anti-inflammatory effectiveness and their fibrinolysis-inducing capacity.[10]

For studies of structure-activity relationship to cite just one example, alkylated 3-enol tautomers were used in order to hinder the keto-enol tautomerism. This hindrance did not cause loss of fibrinolytic activity, suggesting that the keto-enol tautomerism is not a major factor in rendering compounds fibrinolytically active. Furthermore, with

TABLE 5

Fibrinolytic Activity Induced by Indomethacin Derivatives

Indomethacin derivatives	Conc range of induced clot dissolution (m*M*)
1-(*p*-Chlorobenzoyl)-5-methoxy-2-methyl-3-indole acetic acid	5—7
1-(*p*-Chlorobenzoyl)-5-methoxy-2-methyl-3-indole-α-propionic acid	5—6
1-(*p*-Chlorobenzoyl)-5-methoxy-2-methyl-3-indole-β-propionic acid	7—8
1-(*p*-Chlorobenzoyl)-5-methoxy-2-methyl-3-indole-γ-butyric acid	8—10
1-(*p*-Chlorobenzoyl)-5-hydroxy-2-methyl-3-indole acetic acid	7—10
2-Methyl-5-methoxy-3-indole acetic acid	40—50 (partial)

Note: Activity range in m*M*; hanging clot.

TABLE 6

Fibrinolytic Activity Induced by Pyrazolidine-3,5-dione Derivatives

	(m*M*)
4-Butyl-1-phenyl-	80
4-(3′-Oxybutyl)-1,2-diphenyl-	40
1,2-Diphenyl-	30
4-Butyl-1-(*p*-hydroxyphenyl)-2-phenyl-	20
4-Phenylsulfonylethyl-1,2-diphenyl-	10
4-Butyl-1,2-diphenyl-	8
4-(2-Butene)-1,2-diphenyl-	6
4-Butyl-2-(*p*-hydroxyphenyl)-1-phenyl-	6
4-(4,4-Diphenyl-3-oxo-pentyl)-1,2-diphenyl-	3

Note: Lowest activity in m*M*, hanging clot.

substitution changes of the trimethazone related kebuzone (1,2-diphenyl-3,5-dioxo)-4-(3-oxobutyl)pyrazolidine, for instance, it could be shown that branching on the carbon atom next to the carboxyl group substantially enhanced the fibrinolytic activity of the compound. The fibrinolytic activity was further enhanced when the terminal methyl group was substituted by phenyl or furyl groups. Substitution of the terminal phenyl group by an alpha-substituted benzyl group resulted in an additional enhancement of fibrinolytic activity, although the activity was exerted within a rather narrow range.[12] To give an additional example of the relation of substitution to the increase of fibrinolysis-inducing capacity (Table 7), substitution of the benzene ring increases the fibrinolytic activity in the following order: 4 — F, 4 — CH_3, 4 — Cl, 2 — CH_3, 4 — Br, and 3 — Cl.[13] Another group of active compounds are derivatives of azopropazon (5-dimethylamino-9-methyl-2-propyl-1-H pyrazolo[1,2a][1,2,4]benzotriazone-1,3(2H·)-dione. The parent compound itself is inactive, but replacement of the methyl group on the benzene ring by trifluoromethyl induces a marked fibrinolytic activity which is further enhanced by additional substitutions.[14] Appropriate substitutions which result in an asymmetric molecule are very effective as indicated for anthranilic acid in Figure 8 (one example of many). Here, as can be seen from this figure, in

TABLE 7

Fibrinolytic Activity Induced by Derivatives of Phenylethynylene cyclopropane-1-carboxylic Acid

	24 hr	48 hr
4-Fluoro-	—	18
4-Methyl-	20	15
4-Chloro-	(20)[a]	12
2-Methyl-	(12)	9
4-Bromo-	(12)	6
3-Chloro-	12	6

Note: Lowest activity in m*M*, hanging clot.

[a] ( ) = Partial lysis.

X

TABLE 8

Fibrinolytic Activity Induced by 4-Aminothiophene-3-carboxylic Acid Derivatives

	(m*M*)
N-(2,3-xylyl)-	7
N-(2,4,6-trimethylphenyl)-	7
N-(2,3-dimethylphenyl)-	7
N-(3-trifluoromethylphenyl)-	6
N-(2,6-dimethylphenyl)-	5
N-(2,6-xylyl)-	5
N-(2-chloro-6-methylphenyl)-	4
N-(2-chloro-5-methylphenyl)-	4
N-(2-chloro-3-methylphenyl)-	3
N-(2,4,6-trichloro)phenyl-	2
N-(2,4,6-trichloro)-3-methylphenyl-	2

Note: Lowest active molarity in m*M*, hanging clot.

addition to the effect of asymmetry of the compounds, the position of a methyl group or of the more efficient tri-fluoro methyl group on the substituting benzyl ring plays a clear-cut role in the extent of the enhancement of fibrinolytic activity. The following tables with derivatives of 4-aminothiophene-3-carboxylic acid (Table 8), anthranilic acid (Table 9), benzoic acid (Table 10), indole carboxylic acid (Table 11), maleamic acid (Table 12), nicotinic acid (Table 13), resorcylic acid (Table 14), and salicylic acid (Table 15) indicate the marked effect of various types of substitution on the fibrinolysis-inducing capacity of the various compounds. In Figure 9, other examples of various quite different structures are shown which induce fibrinolytic activity in human plasma as assessed with the hanging clot method.

IV. REMARKS ON COMMON PROPERTIES OF THE SYNTHETIC FIBRINOLYTIC COMPOUNDS

Looking for some sort of common denominator, it appears as if the anionic acid, in particular the lipophilic character of the compounds, has a clear-cut relation to their fibrinolytic activity as shown by mathematical analysis.[15] Cepelak et al.[16] came to a similar conclusion. They stated that fibrinolytic activity significantly increases with

TABLE 9

Fibrinolytic Activity Induced by Anthranilic Acid Derivatives

Anthranilic acid, tested up to 300 m*M*	0
5-Iodo-	40
N-(4-*tert*-butylphenyl)-	40
N-(3,4-xylyl)-	30
N-phenyl-	20
N-(2,6-xylyl)-	20
N-(2,4-xylyl)-	20
N-(2-tolyl)-	10
4-Chloro-*N*-(2,5-xylyl)-	8
4-*tert*-Butyl-*N*-(3-trifluoromethylphenyl)-	8
N-(3,5-xylyl)-	7
N-(2-trifluoromethylphenyl)-	6
3,5-Diiodo-	6
N-(2,5-xylyl)-	5
N-(2,3-xylyl)-	5
N-hexanoyl-3,5-diiodo-	5
4-Chloro-*N*-(3-chlorophenyl)-	5
N-(3-tolyl)-	4
N-(3,5-di-(trifluoromethylphenyl)-	4
N-(3-trifluoromethylphenyl)-	3
N-(3-trifluoromethyl-4-chlorophenyl)-	3
N-(3-trifluoromethyl-6-chlorophenyl)-	3

Note: Lowest active molarity in m*M*, hanging clot.

TABLE 10

Fibrinolytic Activity Induced by Benzoic Acid Derivatives

	(m*M*)
3,5-Di-iodo-hydroxy-	0
2,4-Di-chloro-	150
4-Ethyl-	100
Pentafluoro-	100
4-Chloro-	90
2-Iso-propyl-4-propoxy-6-methyl-	70
4-Iso-propyl-	60
4-Iodo-	50
4-Allyloxy-3,5-di-idopropyl-	50
4-Propyl-	40
2-(4-Ethyl-formanilino)-	40
4-Dimethylamino-3,5-di-nitro-	30
2-(3-Trifluoromethylformanilino)-	30
4-*tert*-Butyl-	30
4-*tert*-Butyl-2-bromo-	30
4-Allyloxy-3-propyl-	30
4-Allyloxy-3,5-dichloro-	30
4-Allyloxy-3,5-diethyl-	30
3,5-Di-bromo-	8
4-(α,α-Diethylethyl)-	6
3,5-Di-iodo-	2

Note: Lowest active molarity in m*M*, hanging clot.

TABLE 11

Fibrinolytic Activity Induced by Indole Carboxylic Acid Derivatives

1-(*p*-Chlorobenzyl)-2-methyl-5-methoxy-3-indole-γ-butyric acid	8
1-(*p*-Chlorobenzoyl)-2-methyl-5-hydroxy-3-indole acetic acid	7
1-(*p*-Chlorobenzyl)-2-methyl-5-methoxy-3-indole-β-propionic acid	4
1-(*p*-Chlorobenzoyl)-2-methyl-5-methoxy-3-indole acetic acid	4
1-(*p*-Methylmercaptobenzyl)-2-methyl-5-methoxy-3-indole-α-propionic acid	4

Note: Lowest molarity in m*M*, hanging clot.

TABLE 12

Fibrinolytic Activity Induced by Maleamic Acid Derivatives

N-(2,4-xylyl)-	100
N-(4-nitrophenyl)-	80
N,N-diphenyl-	60
N-(2,4-dichlorophenyl)-	60
N-(2-bromo-4-methylphenyl)-	60
N-(2-chlorophenylethyl)-	60
N-(4-chlorophenyl)-	60
N-(3-trifluoromethylphenyl)-	50
N-[β-(-*p*-chlorophenyl)-α,α-dimethylphenylethyl]-	40
N-(4-iodophenyl)-	30
N-(4-phenoxyphenyl)-	8

Note: Lowest active molarity in m*M*, hanging clot.

TABLE 13

Fibrinolytic Activity Induced by Nicotinic Acid Derivatives

Nicotinic acid (up to 80)	0
2-Anilino-	(30)
2-(2-Methyl-3-chloro-anilino)- (clonoxin)	9
2-(3-Trifluoro-methylanilino)- (niflumic acid)	8

Note: Lowest active molarity in m*M*, hanging clot.

TABLE 14

Fibrinolytic Activity Induced by Resorcylic Acid Derivatives

Resorcylic acid	50
4-Methyl-γ-	40
3-Benzyl-γ-	3
5-Cyclohexyl-γ-	3
3-(β-Phenethyl)-γ-	3
3,5-Dibenzyl-γ-	(2)
3,5-Di-tert-butyl-γ-	(0.9)

Note: Lowest active molarity in m*M*, hanging clot.

TABLE 15

Fibrinolytic Activity Induced by Salicylic Acid Derivatives

Salicylic acid	(150)
4-Hydroxy-	140
5-Methyl-	70
3-Methyl-	60
5-Hydroxy-	50
5-Ethyl-	50
3-Hydroxy-	30
3-Methyl-6-isopropyl-	20
3-Isopropyl-methyl- (thymotic acid)	20
4-Trifluoromethyl-	20
5-Iodo-	20
5-*tert*-Butyl-	10
3,4-Dichloro-	9
3-Isopropyl	8
3-*sec*-Butyl-	8
3-Phenyl-	8
5-(2-Cyclopentenyl)-	8
5-Benzyloxy-	8
5-*sec*-Butyl	7
3-*n*-Butyl	7
3-*tert*-Butyl-5-methyl-	7
3-Isopropyl-5-allyl-6-methyl-	6
3-*tert*-Butyl-	6
3-*tert*-Butyl-6-methyl-	6
4-Phenyl-	6
5-Phenyl-	6
5-(1,1 Dimethyl-p-hydroxybenzyl)-	5
3-Cyclohexyl-	5
3-Benzyl-	5
3,5-Diisopropyl-	5
5-(2-Chlorobenzyloxy)-	5
5-Benzyl-	4
3,5-Dibromo-	4
3-(1,1-Dimethylpropyl)-	4
5-Cyclohexyl	3
5-(3-Chlorobenzyloxy)-	3
3-(3′-Chlorobenzyl)-	3
3-Cinnamyl-	3
3,5-Diiodo-	2

TABLE 15 (continued)

Fibrinolytic Activity Induced by Salicylic Acid Derivatives

3-(4-Chlorobenzyl)-	2
3-(2′-Chlorobenzyl)-	2
3-(4′-Isopropylbenzyl)-	2
5-(1,1,3,3-Tetra-methylbutyl)-	2
3-(1,1,3,3-Tetra-methylbutyl)-	0.9

Note: Lowest active molarity in m*M*, hanging clot.

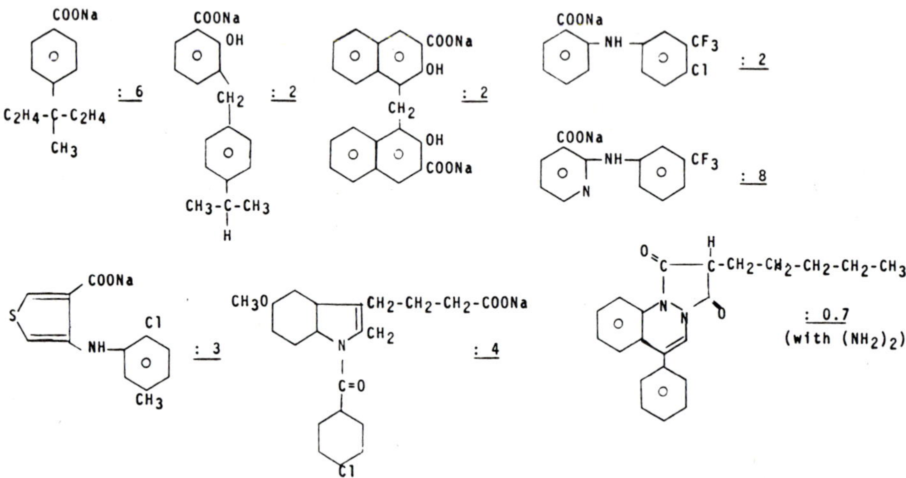

FIGURE 9. Various organic anionic structures which induce fibrinolytic activity.

increasing lipophilia of either aromatic or beta-alkyl substituents and that the steric effect of beta-alkyls merely plays an accessory role. However, it was also proposed that the steric effect might be of importance for designing more active compounds. To study this, it was proposed to lengthen all three chains of Deriphat 160 C to see if one could maximize a steric difference.[17] The electronic effect of aromatic substituents does not influence the fibrinolytic activity. These findings will assist in the search for more active compounds.

The fibrinolysis-inducing synthetic compounds are ineffective at higher concentrations than the ones at which fibrinolysis is induced in human and animal plasma. This is shown in Table 5. Some of them, when the concentration is further increased, even inhibit the fibrinolytic activity.

V. DIFFERENCE OF UROKINASE AND COMPOUND-INDUCED FIBRINOLYTIC ACTIVITY

Urokinase is not the plasminogen activator occurring in circulating blood. This was biochemically proven by Aoki and von Kaulla,[18] who developed a method of extracting from human cadavers sufficient human vascular activator for its characterization.[19] The properties are in Table 16. The synthetic fibrinolytic compounds, by a mechanism described in the following section, "permit" the vascular activator to induce fibrino-

TABLE 16

Parameters Which Differentiate Urokinase from Vascular Activator

There is a difference in molecular weights.
Antisera against urokinase do not react with vascular activator.
Acetylglycyllysine methylester is hydrolyzed at different kinetics.
L-valyl-glycyl-L-arginine-β-naphthylamide is only a substrate for urokinase, but not for vascular activator.
Stability in salt solution is different.
Vascular activator induces clot lysis at less CTA units than urokinase does.
Vascular activator-induced fibrinolytic activity does not result in destruction of clottable proteins in human plasma, whereas urokinase-induced one does.
Vascular activator is very much stronger bound to fibrin than urokinase is.

lysis. One of the clinically most important differences between the vascular activator and urokinase is the adsorption of the vascular activator onto the fibrin strands. Urokinase is much less adsorbed to the fibrin strands.[20,21] This results clinically in a high percentage of complications, primarily in bleeding tendency, which, for instance, has been found to reach 45% in urokinase-treated patients,[22] the main reason being the induction of fibrinolytic activity in circulating blood and not primarily on the fibrin strands in contrast to the fibrinolysis induced by the vascular activator.

VI. PATHWAYS OF FIBRINOLYSIS INDUCTION BY SYNTHETIC FIBRINOLYTIC COMPOUNDS

A. The Fibrinolytic Compounds Diffuse into the Preformed Clot

This diffusion can be demonstrated by various approaches. For instance, a hanging clot is incubated for 3 hr in 5 m*M* (2,2-dimethylpropyl)salicylic acid Na and subsequently transferred into a buffered saline solution pH 7.4 at 37°C. The transferred hanging clot will dissolve. Also, if a synthetic fibrinolytic compound inducing UV fluorescence is dissolved in human plasma and this plasma is placed in a narrow tube upon a clot made from the same plasma which completely fills the lower part of the tube, it diffuses into this clot with concentration-dependent intensity and induces at the higher concentrations its lysis, starting from the top. This is shown in Figure 10. Niflumic acid is the compound used for this figure, its concentration in the plasma placed on the preformed clot increases from the left to the right: 0, 2, 4, 6, 8, 10 m*M*. The extent of diffusion into the clot is indicated by the progression of the fluorescence into the preformed clot. There is a fibrinolytic effect at 8 and 10 m*M*. At 10 m*M* there is also an inhibition of fibrinolysis on top of the preformed clot. This is due to the high concentration of the diffused compound at this point.[23]

B. Strong Adsorption onto Fibrin

The compounds are very strongly adsorbed onto fibrin which also adsorbs vascular activator, plasminogen, antiactivator, and antiplasmin. The compounds inactivate the adsorbed inhibitors, thus permitting the activators to activate plasminogen which subsequently results in fibrinolysis. This pathway is clearly proven by the previously mentioned fact that the synthetic fibrinolysis-inducing compounds induce lysis of serum-free highly centrifuged flat human clots. Further evidence for the adsorption of the compounds onto fibrin is in Table 17. To understand Point 4 in this table, the following details are essential. Human citrated plasma was clotted on a slide. After complete clotting, a solution of 3 m*M* pamoic acid in buffered saline (B.S.) was added. After 15 min, the clot was intensely rinsed three times with compound-free B.S. and then incubated at 37°C. Several hours later, the fibrin network was photographed in the

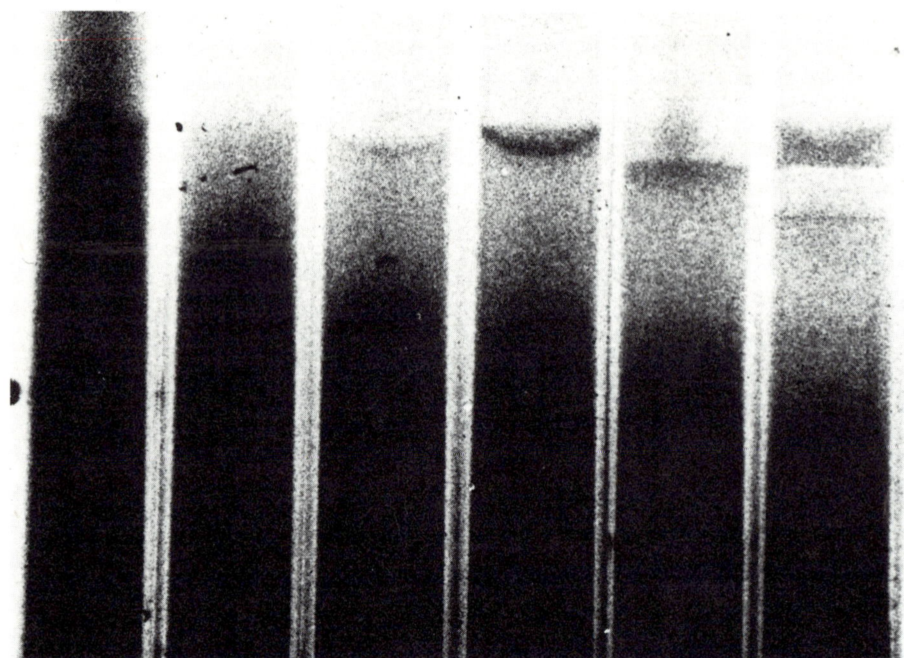

FIGURE 10. Diffusion of fibrinolysis-inducing niflumic acid, dissolved in human plasma, into preformed clots made from the same plasma. Niflumic acid concentrations from the left to the right are 0, 2, 4, 6, 8, and 10 m*M*. Incubation time 18 hr.

TABLE 17

Evidence for Adsorption of the Synthetic Fibrinolytic Compounds onto Fibrin Strands

1. Hanging clot incubated in BS[a] containing synthetic fibrinolytic compounds, transferred into compound-free BS, incubated — clot dissolves
2. Compound dissolved in human plasma, plasma clotted, centrifuged at 36,000 g, clot washed three times, incubated in BS — clot dissolves
3. As in Number 2 above, amount of compound adsorbed on serum-free clot, 3-(1,1-dimethyl-propyl)salicylic acid as example — 14.9 μg/mg
4. Fluorescent compound added to plasma clotted on a slide, clot washed three times with BS — fluorescent fibrin strands

[a] BS, buffered saline.

dark using UV light. The adsorption of the fluorescent pamoic acid onto the fibrin strands is obvious and makes the fibrin strands distinctly visible. This is in Figure 11. It is obvious from this figure that a partial lysis of this fibrin network had already taken place.

C. Suppression of Antiplasmin Activity

The synthetic fibrinolysis-inducing compounds suppress the antiplasmin activity of human plasma, serum, and in particular, of the antiplasmin adsorbed onto the fibrin strands. This effect develops within 1 hr on incubation and reaches its maximum after several hours. The antiplasmin effect can be assessed, for instance, by using bovine fibrinogen clots which were exposed to human plasmin together with human serum

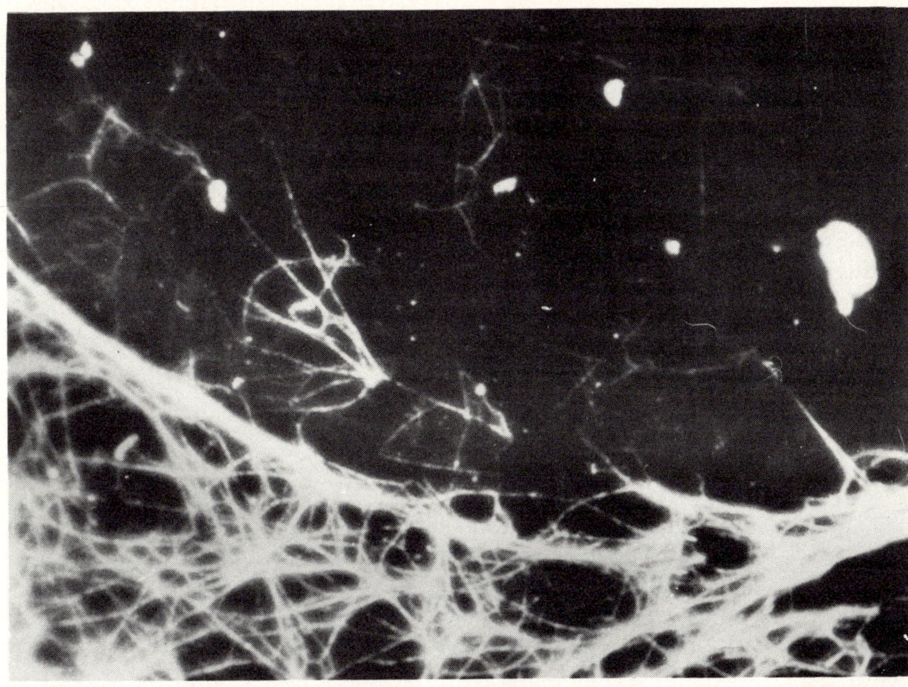

FIGURE 11. Adsorption of the fluorescent fibrinolysis-inducing pamoic acid on the fibrin strands of a human clot. Partial lysis has already occurred. For technical details see text.

which had been preincubated with the compounds except for the control. The compounds reduce or eliminate antiplasmin activity of the serum with a concentration-dependent time reaction. Minor structural changes which abolish fibrinolysis-inducing capacity of the compounds also eliminate their ability to reduce antiplasmin activity.[24,25] α-2-Macroglobulin also inhibits fibrinolytic activity; thus immunologically pure preparations inhibit the dissolution of bovine fibrin clots by plasmin. With pilot studies, it has been found that this inhibition was completely abolished by preincubation of the α-2-macroglobulins with various synthetic fibrinolysis-inducing compounds.[25]

D. Suppression of Antiactivator Activity

Aoki and von Kaulla[26] showed that the antiactivators in the blood are quite dissimilar from antiplasmin. They inhibit urokinase and, in particular, vascular activator. The antiurokinase activity is suppressed by the synthetic fibrinolysis-inducing compounds. This has been demonstrated for all compounds tested.[25] It has further been shown that the amount of urokinase required to dissolve human plasma clots within 15 min is reduced from 200 CTA (Committee on Thrombolytic Agents) units to 20 CTA units in the presence of 5 m*M* of the fibrinolysis-inducing 3,5-diiodo salicylic acid by blocking the binding of urokinase to the inhibitor.[27] It was also shown that substituted benzoates block the inhibition of urokinase by plasma antiactivators.[28] These and other findings point to probably the most important effect of the synthetic fibrinolytic compounds: suppression of antiactivator activity in human plasma or serum. This suppression was also proven by various compounds, including flufenamic acid for the antiactivator which inhibits the vascular activator, the body's own plasminogen activator. The inhibition of antiactivator by the compounds is irreversible. Minor structural changes which abolish the fibrinolysis-inducing capacity of the compound also abolish their effect on the human serum or plasma antiactivator activity.[29] A suppression of antiactivator in regard to vascular activator could also be demonstrated for dog plasma using *o*-thymotic acid. With this plasma, it was furthermore observed that compounds which in high concentrations do not induce fibrinolysis (an effect observed with all compounds tested) do not reduce, but instead potentiate the activity of antiactivator.[30] This effect may explain the inhibitory effect of compounds in high concentrations.

It has also been claimed that the fibrinolysis-inducing flufenamic acid liberates a plasminogen activator from a latent activator. This latent activator is distributed among euglobulin precipitate and euglobulin supernatant of serum in a relation 3:7. This effect of the compound is supposed to be different from its suppression of antiactivator and antiplasmin activity.[31]

VII. IN VIVO AND IN VITRO INDUCTION OF FIBRINOLYTIC ACTIVITY BY THE SAME SYNTHETIC COMPOUNDS

Various vasoactive drugs induce in human beings and in animals in vivo after i.v. injection a rather short-lasting, but marked fibrinolytic activity. These drugs are not active in vitro. Nicotinic acid is one example of this type of compound. However, a derivative of nicotinic acid, 3-fluoromethyl-3-phenylamino-2-nicotinic acid, niflumic acid, is active both in vitro (hanging clot at 8 m*M*, and plasma clot at 12 m*M*, both types of clots made from human plasma) and in vivo after i.v. injection in rats. Thus, this compound is able to induce fibrinolytic activity by two different pathways: the inactivation of antiactivator and of antiplasmin (in vitro) and by inducing release of vascular activator into the circulation. Niflumic acid therefore represents a prototype of an optimal synthetic fibrinolytic agent. The in vivo fibrinolysis-inducing capacity is demonstrated with rats using a micro-euglobulin lysis technique, permitting a number of blood specimens to be obtained from a tail vein of the same rat, thus enabling one to follow the trend of fibrinolytic activity in an individual animal without reducing its circulating blood volume very markedly.[32] After i.v. injection of 10 mg/kg niflumic acid, the euglobulin lysis time in the rat is considerably but transitorily shortened.[33] This is in Figure 12. The in vitro enhancement of niflumic acid induced fibrinolytic activity by plasma from rats injected with niflumic acid is demonstrated with the use of the micro-hanging clot method.[23] Here, plasma clots (from 0.2 mℓ blood) obtained from rats 5 min after i.v. injection of niflumic acid suspended in rat plasma containing niflumic acid dissolve at a lower molarity than do plasma clots obtained from untreated rats.[34] Bencyclane, *N*-[3-(1-benzyl-cycloheptyl-oxy)-propyl]-*N,N*-dimethyl-hydrogenfumarate, induces a marked but brief increase of fibrinolytic activity in the rat (see Figure 13). It also induces fibrinolytic activity in vitro at 7 m*M* (hanging clot method), but usually only in the presence of hydrazine. For the enhancing effect of hydrazine on compound-induced fibrinolytic activity, see the next section. It has also been claimed that some other compounds, active in vitro, induce in vivo fibrinolytic activity of short duration in the rat after oral administration (100 mg/kg) or after i.v. injection (1/10 of LD_{50}; approximately 10 mg/kg). The most active compound in this regard was 2-hydroxy-5-(2′-methyl-4-thiazolyl) benzoic acid.[35] It was also observed that regional infusion of trimethazone, 4-(4,4-dimethyl-3-oxopentyl)1,2-diphenyl-pyrazolidin-3,5-dion (in vitro activity at 3 m*M*) into rabbits with artificial thrombi reduced the size of the thrombi by more than 50%, as compared with clots in animals receiving saline only. Systemic infusion had no effect.[36] In earlier studies, we found that after 10 hr of oral treatment with 2 g of *p*-aminobenzoic acid (2 g every 2 hr), a dissolution of a diluted plasma clot (1:20) occurred within 24 hr in 40% of the patients; in 64% of the patients such a dissolution resulted after 48 hr of incubation.[37]

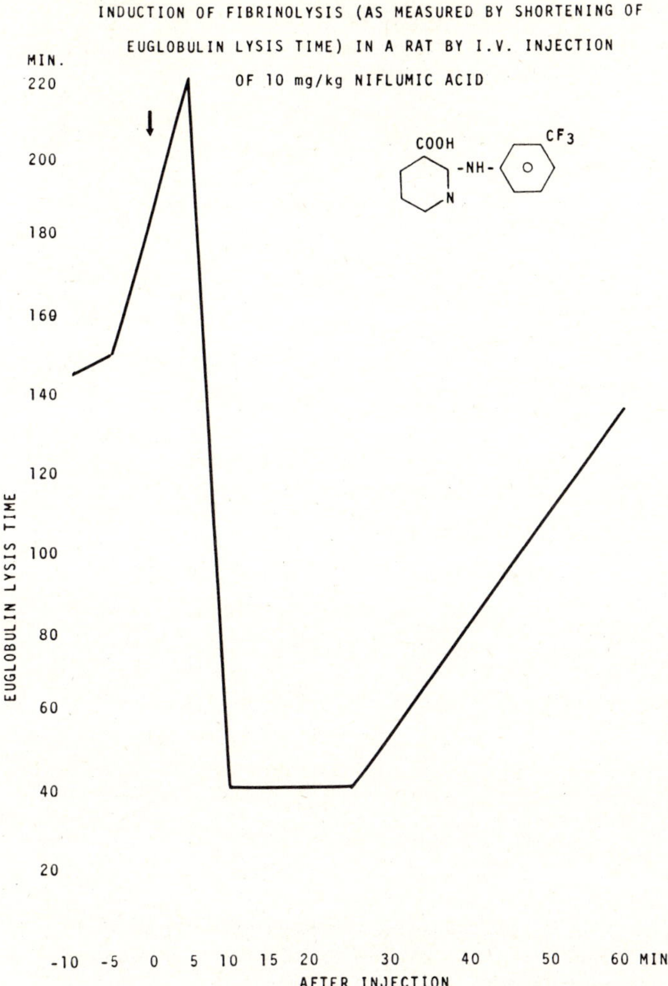

FIGURE 12. Induction of transitorily increased fibrinolytic activity in a rat after i.v. injection of 10 mg/kg niflumic acid, Microeuglobulin lysis time.

azolidin-3,5-dion (in vitro activity at 3 m*M*) into rabbits with artificial thrombi reduced the size of the thrombi by more than 50%, as compared with clots in animals receiving saline only. Systemic infusion had no effect.[36] In earlier studies, we found that after 10 hr of oral treatment with 2 g of *p*-aminobenzoic acid (2 g every 2 hr), a dissolution of a diluted plasma clot (1:20) occurred within 24 hr in 40% of the patients; in 64% of the patients such a dissolution resulted after 48 hr of incubation.[37]

VIII. GENERAL ASPECTS

A. Inhibition of Compound-Induced Fibrinolytic Activity by ε-Aminocaproic Acid and Its Marked Enchancement by Hydrazine

ε-Aminocaproic acid inhibits the fibrinolytic activity induced by the compounds in human plasma to varying degrees. This inhibition and the differences are in Table 18. The ε-aminocaproic acid concentration required to inhibit the 3-*o*-chlorobenzyl salicylic acid-induced fibrinolysis is, for instance, more than ten times higher than that required to block indomethacin-induced fibrinolysis. The reasons for these differences have not been investigated.

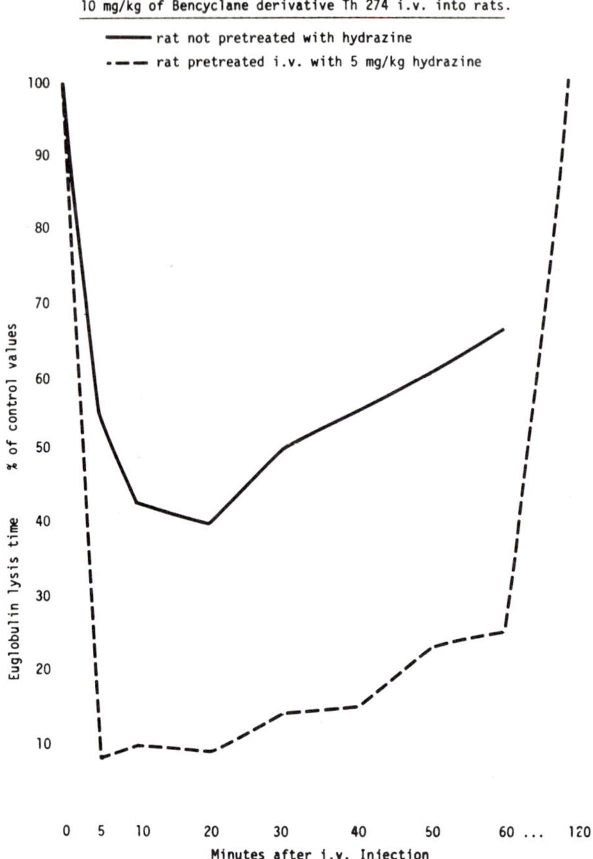

FIGURE 13. Marked enhancement by hydrazine (dotted lines) of the fibrinolytic activity induced in a rat by a bencyclane derivative.

TABLE 18

Inhibition of Compound-Induced Fibrinolysis (Plasma Clot) by ε-Aminocaproic Acid

	mM ε-Aminocaproic acid[a]				
Compound and concentration	0	1	5	10	50
3-(α,α-Dimethylpropyl)salicylic acid 6 mM	+	(+)	(+)	−	−
3-p-Isopropylbenzylsalicylic acid 2 mM	+	+	+	(+)	−
3-o-Chlorobenzylsalicylic acid 2 mM	+	+	+	+	−
Flufenamic acid 3 mM	+	+	(+)	−	−
Indomethacin 7 mM	+	−	−	−	−

[a] Lysis in 24 hr: +, complete; (+), partial; −, none.

Hydrazine enhances compound-induced fibrinolysis in vitro and in vivo as assessed with both the plasma clot and the hanging clot methods.[38] Hydrazine does not exhibit

TABLE 19

Enhancement by Preincubation (60 min) of Plasma with 2.5 m*M* Hydrazine of Fibrinolytic Activity Induced by Synthetic Organic Compounds

Compound	Without N_2H_4 (m*M*)	With N_2H_4 (m*M*)	Activity increase (%)
Niflumic acid	12	8	66
3-(3,5-Ditrifluoro-methyl-anilino)-4-thiophene COOH	8	5	75
3-(4-Isopropylbenzyl)salicylic acid	12	7	83
n-(3,5-Dimethylphenyl)anthranilic acid	11	6	91
4-(*n*-Decyl)benzene sulfonic acid	Not active	11	—
5-*n*-Nonyl salicylic acid	Not active	7	—
Lauryl sulfate	Not active	7	—

Note: Lowest molarity inducing complete clot lysis within 24 hr is given, plasma clot method (human).

any fibrinolysis-inducing capacity of its own. Preincubation with hydrazine of the hanging clot or of the plasma to be clotted considerably reduced the compound concentration required to lyse the clots. This is in Table 19 with the plasma clot method. As shown with the last three compounds in this table, hydrazine also unmasks the potential for fibrinolysis induction of apparently inactive compounds which theoretically — based on their structure — should be quite potent fibrinolysis inducers. Hydrazine diffuses into preformed clots. Hanging clots preincubated for 4 hr with hydrazine, subsequently removed from the hydrazine solution and then transferred into the solutions of the synthetic fibrinolytic agents, still show the enhancing effect of hydrazine. The optimal concentration was found to be 2.5 m*M* hydrazine; increase of the hydrazine concentration does not further enhance the effect, and lowering of the concentration reduces its lysis-enhancing activity. The enhancing effect of hydrazine is not yet clearly understood, but it was shown that preincubation of plasma with 2.5 m*M* hydrazine reduces its antiplasmin activity. Hydrazine has also been reported to reduce the α-2-macroglobulin content of human plasma.[39] Hydrazine does not enhance the fibrinolytic activity of streptokinase or urokinase.[23] It is of great interest that hydrazine enhances the fibrinolysis-inducing effect of synthetic compounds in vivo. This has been shown, for instance, for niflumic acid. Pretreatment of rats with i.v. injection of 5 mg/kg hydrazine intensifies and prolongs the fibrinolytic activity induced by niflumic acid and reduces the rebound effect which may occur. The enhancing effect of hydrazine both in vivo and in vitro was also shown for bencyclane derivatives[8] which also exerted fibrinolytic activity both in vitro at 7 m*M* and in vivo. The in vitro effect, however, was only observed when hydrazine was present. The marked enhancing effect of hydrazine on the fibrinolytic activity induced in vivo by this compound is in Figure 13. Here, pretreatment of the rat with hydrazine increased and prolonged very considerably the compound-induced fibrinolytic activity. The enhancing effect of hydrazine and its clinical potential are of importance, but require further investigation.

B. Enhancement of Endogenously Increased Fibrinolytic Activity in the Test Tube by Synthetic Fibrinolytic Agents

The best procedure to increase the endogenous fibrinolytic activity of the circulating blood is to exclude the liver from the circulation. Within a few minutes, its exclusion leads to a very pronounced increase of fibrinolytic activity. This increase was observed during the first liver transplants in human beings[40] and after exclusion of the liver from

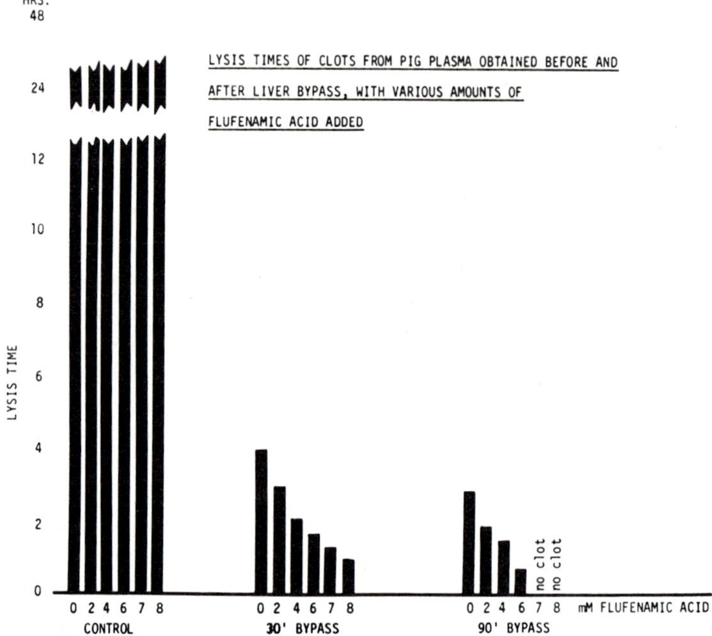

FIGURE 14. Enhancement of liver bypass-induced fibrinolytic activity in pig plasma by flufenamic acid at concentrations which do not induce fibrinolysis. Control values before bypass on the left side. Lysis times of plasma clots obtained after 30 min bypass are shown in the center and those obtained after 90 min are on the right side. Note the marked enhancing enhancing effect of flufenamic acid.

the circulation by various methods in animals,[41] as measured by a modification of the micro-euglobulin lysis time.[8] This phenomenon has not been investigated to any great extent. It has been claimed that the liver removes vascular activator from the circulation.[42] Thus, liver bypass would prevent the removal of the activator from the circulation. Using plasma from pigs with liver bypass, the synergistic effect of the synthetic compounds with endogenous activator on fibrinolytic activity was clearly demonstrated. Figure 14 indicates that clots made from pig plasma do not dissolve within 24 hr, and no lysis occurs even when these clots contain flufenamic acid (tested up to 8 m*M*) (columns on the left). After liver bypass of 30-min duration, the compound-free clotted plasma lyses in approximately 4 hr. This lysis time is progressively shortened with increasing concentrations of flufenamic acid (columns in the center). After 90-min bypass, the fibrinolytic activity is further increased in the control sample and is markedly enhanced by the flufenamic acid to a point that with the two highest concentrations (7 and 8 m*M*), no clot can be obtained because it dissolves as fast as it is being formed.[34]

A marked synergistic effect is also obtained when the preformed rotating clot is used as substrate. Example: pig plasma obtained before bypass containing 9 m*M* flufenamic acid did not induce any lysis of the rotating standard clot (which imitates a vessel completely occluded by a thrombus) after 24 and 48 hr of incubation time. The fibrinolytic plasma (without compound) obtained after 30 min of bypass also has no effect on this type of performed clot. However, addition of 9 m*M* flufenamic acid to this bypass plasma very markedly enhances its fibrinolytic activity to a point that it dissolves the preformed clot: 40 $\mu\ell$ are lysed within 24 hr, and 60 $\mu\ell$ are lysed within 48 hr, which actually results from a shortening of 4 and 6 mm, respectively, of this cylinder-shaped preformed clot which can be fibrinolytically attacked from one small side only. In this connection, it should be stated that compounds tested for a thrombolytic (in contrast to a fibrinolytic) potential should always be tested with preformed clots obtained from human plasma, such as the ones described herein, the rotating standard clot (see Figure 1). Lysis time only can give very misleading results in regard to the thrombolytic effect. Liver bypass plasma with a lysis time between 2 and 3 hr does not "shorten" the preformed "thrombotic" clot, but when by addition of a synthetic fibrinolytic compound the lysis time is reduced to 1 hr or less, it does. From these observations, one can conclude that for clinical use, an intermediate step for the development of synthetic fibrinolytic compounds may well be their enhancement of the fibrinolytic activity induced by enzymatic plasminogen activators. This potential is of practical interest because in the foregoing section, it has been demonstrated that synergism can be obtained with activator and compound concentrations, either of which alone is too low for fibrinolytic activity induction.

C. Binding of Synthetic Fibrinolysis-Inducing Compounds to Albumin — Suggestion for Reduction of This Effect

The differences of the required molarity of a given compound to induce fibrinolytic dissolution of hanging clot and of plasma clot indicate that a portion of the compounds is adsorbed onto proteins unrelated to fibrinolysis induction. The difference is primarily due to the fact that with the hanging clot, the compound is present in excess and its adsorption to the proteins does not reduce its concentration to a great extent. This is not the case with the plasma clot; here, the compounds are dissolved in the plasma before clot formation, and their adsorption to inert proteins markedly reduces the amount available for fibrinolysis induction after clotting. Albumin is the primary inert compound-binding protein. Thus, using ^{125}I-labeled 3,5-diiodo salicylic acid, it was found that about 85% of this compound was bound to albumin.[25] The concentration of flufenamic acid required for lysis induction of a clot made from human plasma containing 4.1 g albumin per 100 mℓ plasma is 10 m*M*. In the same plasma with an albumin content reduced to 0.4 mg/100 mℓ, only 3 m*M* is required. Blocking of the binding sites of albumin with oxacillin has a similar effect: the flufenamic acid concentration required to lyse hanging human plasma clots is 4 m*M*; flufenamic acid required to lyse hanging clots made from plasma containing 20 mg/mℓ oxacillin which binds more firmly to albumin than the flufenamic acid is 0.9 m*M*. For the fibrinolysis-inducing flufenamic acid, it has been reported that the aromatic portion of the compound is inserted into a hydrophobic crevice of the albumin, while the carboxylate group of the compound interacts with the cationic site of the protein surface.[43] The binding of the compounds to albumin represents an undesirable property of these agents because the amount bound is "lost" for fibrinolysis induction. The greater the difference between the molarity required to induce fibrinolysis of the hanging clot and of the plasma clot, the more intensive is the binding of the compound to albumin. However, these differences vary greatly from compound to compound. The smaller the difference the less the binding of the compound to albumin, and this suggests a possibility to overcome the albumin binding of the compounds.

Table 20 indicates the very marked differences of albumin binding between various compounds, as indicated by the relation of the molarity required for lysis of hanging clot (H.C.) and plasma clot (P.C.). For the first compound it is 1:13, indicating a very pronounced binding to albumin, whereas the compounds at the bottom of the list by a ratio close to one indicate a very reduced binding of the compounds onto albumin. Here is an indication that fibrinolysis-inducing compounds with very reduced binding to albumin can be developed. In fact, the last compound in this table, Deriphat 160 C (*N*-lauryl-*β*-dipropionic acid Na), although not the most active one, shows a relation

TABLE 20

Ratio of the Molarity (m*M*) of the Synthetic Fibrinolysis-Inducing Compounds Required to Induce Within 24 hr Lysis of Hanging Clots (HC) and of Plasma Clots (PC), Both Made From the Same Human Plasma

Compound	HC	PC	Ratio HC to PC
3,5-Di-*tert*-butyl-γ-resorcylic acid	0.9	12	1: 13
3-*tert*-Octyl salicylic acid	1	11	1: 11
3-(4′-Isopropylbenzyl)salicylic acid	2	12	1: 6
3-(2,4,6-Trimethylanilino)4-thiophene COOH	3	15	1: 5
5-(Cyclohexyl)salicylic acid	3	13	1: 4.3
Methylene-di-β-hydroxynaphthoic acid	2	7	1: 3.5
3,5-Diiodo anthranilic acid	6	16	1: 2.7
Niflumic acid	8	12	1: 1.5
3-(2,3-Xylyl-anilino)-4-thiophene COOH	7	10	1: 1.4
3-Isopropyl-6-methylsalicylic acid	20	25	1: 1.25
N-Lauryl-β-dipropionic acid Na (Deriphat 160 C)	14	14	1: 1

of 1:1, reflecting no difference between protein binding in hanging clots and plasma clots. This shows that there is a clear-cut possibility of developing more active compounds with little binding to albumin.

D. Inhibition of Aggregation of Human Thrombocytes, an Additional Potentially Antithrombotic Effect of Synthetic Fibrinolysis-Inducing Compounds

Collagen-induced aggregation of human platelets in their own plasma was inhibited at various concentrations by most of the synthetic fibrinolytic compounds tested for this particular effect. These observations reveal the possibilities of designing drugs with a dual antithrombotic action: prevention of thrombus formation and induction of thrombolysis. There is some correlation between the structural features which enhance the fibrinolysis-inducing activity of the compounds and those which enhance their ability to prevent thrombocyte aggregation. The prevention of collagen-induced platelet aggregation was observed, for instance, with fibrinolytic derivatives of anthranilic acid, salicylic acid, and of thiophenecarboxylic acid,[44] with fibrinolytic pyrazolidine derivatives,[45] as well as many other compounds. The parent compounds have little or no activity, either for the prevention of platelet aggregation or for fibrinolysis induction. Table 21 lists examples of fibrinolysis-inducing derivatives of phenyl-4-aminothiophene-3-carboxylic acid which at various concentrations inhibits collagen-induced thrombocyte aggregation. Furthermore, a particular structural change can enhance the inhibitory effect on platelet aggregation, but also abolish the fibrinolytic effect. For instance, *N*-(2,3-dimethylphenyl)-4-aminothiophene carboxylic acid induced fibrinolysis at 7 m*M* (hanging clot) and inhibited collagen-induced platelet aggregation at 0.2 m*M*. Combination of the carboxylic group of this compound with an aliphatic chain completely abolishes the fibrinolysis-inducing capacity yet enhances the aggregation inhibition by a factor of ten to 0.02 m*M*. However, substitution of the benzyl ring of the compound with free carboxylic group with Cl in Position 2 together with a methyl group in Position 4 endows it with both fibrinolysis-inducing (at 3 m*M*) and platelet aggregation-preventing (at 0.05 m*M*) capacity.[23] With salicylic acid derivatives it has been found, to give other examples of the effects of structure modifications, that substitution in the 3 or 5 position with cyclohexyl enhances fibrinolytic activity, but not platelet aggregation inhibition, whereas substitution in Position 3 with 2-chlorobenzyl

TABLE 21

Fibrinolysis Induction (Hanging Clot) and Inhibition of Collagen-Induced Aggregation of Human Thrombocytes Left in Their Plasma by Derivatives of Phenyl-4-aminothiophene-3-carboxylic Acid

Derivatives of phenyl-4-aminothiophene-3 COOH	Lower limit of Fibrinolytic (Molarity)	Lower limit of Aggregation inhibiting (50%) (Molarity)
Thiophene-3-carbonic acid	5×10^{-2}	4×10^{-3}
N-2,6-dimethyl-	5×10^{-3}	1×10^{-3}
N-2-chloro-5-methyl-	3×10^{-3}	1×10^{-3}
N-2-chloro-6-methyl-	4×10^{-3}	5×10^{-4}
N-2,3-dimethyl-	7×10^{-3}	5×10^{-4}
N-2,4,6-trichloro-	2×10^{-3}[a]	5×10^{-4}
N-2,4,6-trichloro-3-methyl	5×10^{-3}[a]	5×10^{-4}
N-2,4,6-tri-methyl-	3×10^{-3}	4×10^{-4}
N-3-tri-fluoromethyl-	6×10^{-3}	4×10^{-4}
N-2-chloro-3-methyl-	3×10^{-3}	5×10^{-5}

[a] Partial lysis.

increases the fibrinolysis-inducing activity and reduces by a factor of ten the molarity required for aggregation inhibition.[44]

Figure 15 gives some examples for the effect of structural changes of salicylic acid derivatives on the concentrations required for induction of fibrinolysis of hanging clots and for the inhibition of collagen-induced platelet aggregation. For pyrazolidine it was observed that an α-substitution in the side chain of 1,2-diphenyl-3,5-dioxopyrazolidine always enhanced the activity of the parent compound both for fibrinolysis induction and for thrombocyte aggregation inhibition.[45] It has also been claimed that the lipophilic effect with the fibrinolytic β-substituted phenylaliphatic acid, as another example, is as important for the platelet aggregation inhibition as it is for the fibrinolytic activity, whereas the steric effect plays a less important role.[12]

Niflumic acid, the fibrinolytic compound which induces fibrinolytic activity both in vitro and in vivo, is in addition effective in reducing collagen-induced platelet aggregation. Actual measurements of this effect with niflumic acid are shown with four different molarities in Figure 16, using the dual-sample aggregometer.[46] Although with this compound a higher concentration is required for inhibition of platelet aggregation as compared to some of the other compounds, this additional activity of niflumic acid indicates that it might well be possible to develop multiaction antithrombotic drugs, inducing fibrinolytic activity by two different pathways and also preventing platelet aggregation. At present, the mechanism involved in the inhibition of collagen-induced platelet aggregation by synthetic fibrinolytic compounds has not been established.

Two compounds were tested and found to inhibit an entirely different type of thrombocyte aggregation, the aggregation of pig platelets suspended in saline or in pig plasma by dog serum. Dog serum contains a powerful preformed humoral antibody against porcine tissue. It is assumed that the antigens on the surface of pig platelets are the same as those in other porcine cells. The dog serum was incubated for 30 min with 12 mM flufenamic acid or with 7 mM pamoic acid and subsequently dialyzed for 15 hr in the cold for removal of the unbound compounds in order to avoid reduction

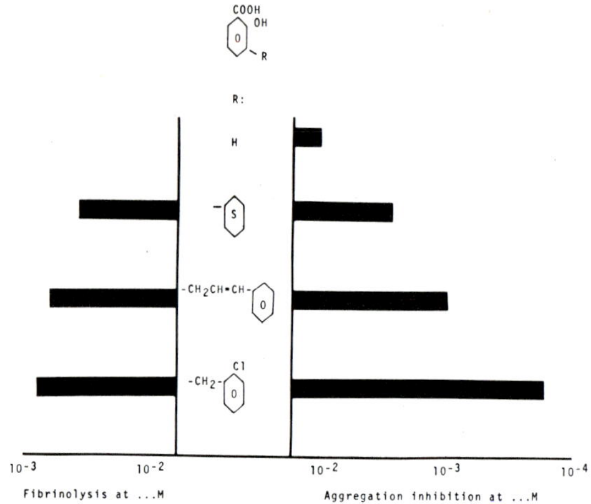

FIGURE 15. Effect of structural changes of salicylic acid derivatives on their molarity required to induce dissolution of hanging clots and for inhibition of collagen-induced aggregation of thrombocytes left in their citrated human plasma.

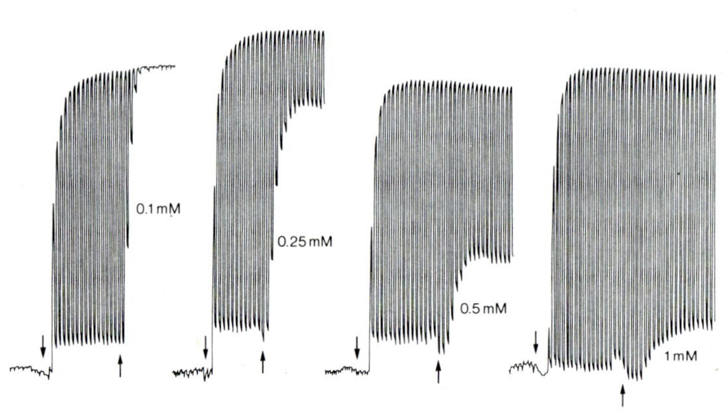

FIGURE 16. Effect of four concentrations of the fibrinolysis-inducing niflumic acid on collagen-induced human platelets left in their citrated plasma. Dual-sample aggregometer running a compound-free control simultaneously.

of the complement activity of the pig plasma (for effect of synthetic fibrinolytic compounds on complement see following section). After this treatment, the dog plasma had lost most of its ability to aggregate pig platelets. Within 5 min, both compounds also reduced the complement activity of the dog serum of <5 CH_{50}. Whether or not the elimination of complement activity is the mechanism by which the two synthetic fibrinolysis-inducing compounds abolish the ability of the dog serum to aggregate pig platelets is not quite clear because pamoic acid exhibited the same abolishing effect on complement activity as flufenamic acid, but did not inhibit the dog serum-induced pig platelet aggregation[47] as much as was found with flufenamic acid.

E. Reduction of C′-Complement Activity by Synthetic Fibrinolysis-Inducing Compounds

Fibrinolysis-inducing synthetic compounds also reduce on incubation the C′-complement activity of human plasma at concentrations which are practically identical to those that induce fibrinolytic activity in the plasma.[24] Minor modification of the molecule, such as shifting of the substituent from the *p* to *o* position or introduction of a second carboxylic group into the molecule that would abolish the fibrinolytic activity of a given compound, also abolishes its ability to inactivate complement C′ and to suppress antiplasmin activity. Further studies revealed that the compounds actually inactivate β_1C-globulin in the serum without interaction with other components of the complement system. Whether or not this inactivation has a relation to fibrinolysis induction is an open question. Blocking of the fibrinolytic activity induced by the compounds with ε-aminocaproic acid does not inhibit their effect on β_1C-globulin.[48]

F. Inhibition of Increased Sedimentation Rate and Experimentally Induced Aggregation Tendency of Human Erythrocytes by Synthetic Fibrinolytic Compounds

The inhibition of increased sedimentation tendency of erythrocytes may reflect a potential secondary antithrombotic function. Based on clinical observations and on experimental evidence, many investigators suggest a role of erythrocytes in thromboembolism. For description of the role of erythrocytes in enhancing a thrombosis tendency, both terms have been used, increased aggregability and increased sedimentation rate. The inhibitory function of the compounds on the increased sedimentation role of erythrocytes has been shown in two ways: inhibition of increased sedimentation of erythrocytes left in their plasma obtained from citrated blood and inhibition (measured as sedimentation rate) of aggregation of erythrocytes suspended in buffered saline induced by fibrinogen and also by dextran and gelatine. As typical examples, Figure 17 shows the difference in the inhibiting effect of four fibrinolytic compounds at 0.5 m*M* concentration on the very markedly enhanced erythrocyte sedimentation rate of a patient with an acute myocardial infarction. Experimentally, it was shown to what extent the following compounds at 0.1 m*M* inhibit the bovine fibrinogen-induced (final concentration 0.77%) sedimentation of human erythrocytes. The inhibition is expressed in percent: niflumic acid, 98%; 3-(2-chlorobenzyl)salicylic acid, 83%; flufenamic acid, 62% and 3-(2-methyl-3-chloro-3-methyl)-anilino-4-thiophene COOH, 0%. A correlation of this inhibiting activity of the compounds with the extent of their ability to prevent collagen-induced platelet aggregation could not be demonstrated.[49] The mechanism of the compound-induced inhibition of the sedimentation or aggregation of human erythrocytes is unknown, although it might have something to do with interaction of the compounds with the erythrocyte membrane. For flufenamic acid, for instance, it has been shown that this compound is adsorbed on the erythrocyte membrane.[50] It was further shown that membrane stabilization by synthetic fibrinolytic agents (β-aryl aliphatic acid, for instance) prevents the osmotic hemolysis of the erythrocytes.[16] The membrane-stabilizing effect of the compounds was claimed to be correlated primarily with the lipophilic and, in contrast to the fibrinolysis-inducing capacity, with an electronic effect and, to a lesser degree, with a steric effect.[12] It should be added that of all 13 compounds tested, niflumic acid which induces fibrinolytic activity by two pathways, exerted the most marked inhibition of fibrinogen-, dextran-, and gelatine-induced sedimentation of human erythrocytes. At 0.05 m*M*, only niflumic acid was effective with gelatine. Here again, niflumic acid appears to be one of the most interesting types of synthetic fibrinolytic agents.

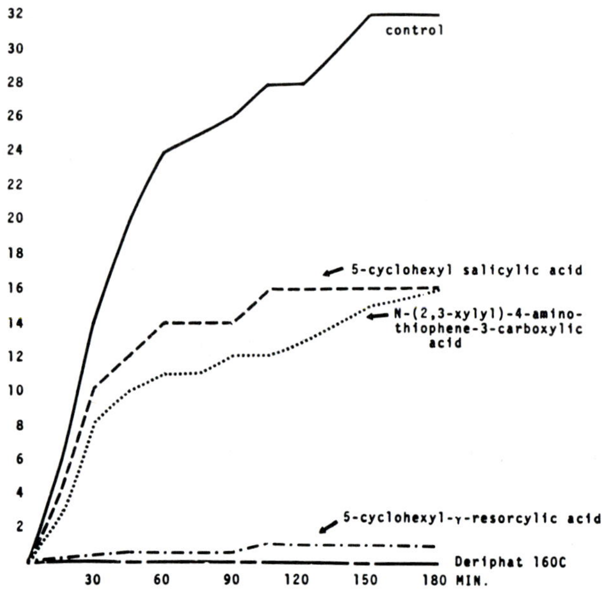

FIGURE 17. Inhibition of the sedimentation of erythrocytes left in the citrated plasma of a patient with acute myocardial infarction by synthetic fibrinolytic compound at a concentration of 0.5 m*M*. Note the complete inhibition by Deriphat 160 C, the compound with the lowest binding to albumin.

G. Antihemophilic Globulin (Factor VIII) Activity of Certain Synthetic Fibrinolysis-Inducing Compounds

In hemophilic plasma, Factor VIII activity is considerably enhanced when the plate-free plasma is exposed at 4°C to certain synthetic fibrinolytic agents (others are without effect). The Factor VIII activity increase by synthetic compounds is a time reaction with a maximum effect developing mostly after 1 to 2 hr. Thus, to give a few examples: with 90 min of exposure time, flufenamic acid increased Factor VIII activity in the plasma of hemophiliacs from 1 to 33%; 3-cinnamyl salicylic acid, from 1 to 35%; and *N*-(2-chloro-6-methylphenyl)-4-aminothiophene-3 carboxylic acid, from 2.5 to 48%.[51,52] The 4-aminothiophene derivative was one of the most active compounds, whereas closely related derivatives, such as *N*-(4-chloro-6-methylphenyl)-COOH and *N*-(2-chloro-4-methylphenyl)-4-aminothiophene-3 COOH, induced no activity. Once the Factor VIII activity in the plasma has been generated by active compounds, it is relatively stable when the compound-plasma mixture at its peak activity is stored in the frozen state. It was also observed that hydrazine added to the same hemophilic plasma enhanced the Factor VIII-increasing effect of the active fibrinolytic compounds. The active compounds were also able — and this is very important — to increase the in vitro Factor VIII activity in the plasma of some patients with a Factor VIII inhibitor of high titer which made blood transfusions useless. For example: Factor VIII activity in a plasma of a patient with a Factor VIII inhibitor was ±1%. After 5 min of incubation with *N*-(2-chloro-6-6-methylphenyl)-4-aminothiophene-3 carboxylic acid, the activity rose to 16% (and with the same compound plus hydrazine, to 30%).

After 90 min of incubation at 4°C, the activity rose to 51% (and with hydrazine added, over 100%). After 90 min of incubation of the same plasma with addition of 3-cinnamyl salicylic acid, Factor VIII activity rose to 40% (and with hydrazine to 100%). Interestingly enough, an increase of Factor VIII activity was obtained with the same compounds in several cases of von Willebrand disease.[54] The mechanism by which some of the synthetic compounds improve Factor VIII activity in hemophilic plasma is not yet known, but removal of an inhibitor might be the pathway.

IX. CONCLUSION

It should be pointed out that synthetic organic anions inducing fibrinolytic activity in vitro represent an important potential for the development of multiaction antithrombotic drugs, a potential which deserves further intensive investigation. It might be added that some foods, like cayenne pepper and certain onions (active compound cyclo-alliin), after ingestion induce in human beings a marked shortening of the euglobulin lysis time (see von Kaulla).[53] Isolation and structural analysis of the active compounds might offer an additional possibility for the development of synthetic fibrinolytic agents.

X. ACKNOWLEDGMENT

The very helpful assistance of Mrs. E. von Kaulla in preparing this manuscript is gratefully acknowledged.

REFERENCES

1. **von Kaulla, K. N.,** Urine adsorbate with fibrinolytic and thromboplastic properties, *J. Lab. Clin. Med.,* 44, 944, 1954.
2. **von Kaulla, K. N.,** The standard clot, *Thromb. Diath. Haemorrh.,* 5, 489, 1961.
3. **McBain, M. E. L. and Hutchinson, E.,** *Solubilization and Related Phenomena,* Academic Press, New York, 1955.
4. **Booth, H. S. and Everson, H. E.,** Hydrotropic solubilities, *Ind. Eng. Chem.,* 41, 2627, 1949.
5. **Osol, A. and Kilpatrick, K. M.,** The "salting out" and "salting in" of weak acid, *J. Am. Chem. Soc.,* 55, 4430, 1933.
6. **von Kaulla, K. N.,** Fibrinolysis induction in vitro by aromatic derivatives, *Arch. Biochem. Biophys.,* 96, 4, 1962.
7. **von Kaulla, K. N.,** A simple test tube arrangement for screening fibrinolytic activity of synthetic organic compounds, *J. Med. Chem.,* 8, 164, 1965.
8. **von Kaulla, K. N. and von Kaulla, E.,** Remarks on the euglobulin lysis time in *Progress in Chemical Fibrinolysis and Thrombolysis,* Vol. 1, Davidson, J. F., Samama, M. M., and Desnoyers, P. C., Eds., Raven Press, New York, 1975, 131.
9. **Gryglewski, R. J. and Eckstein, M.,** Fibrinolytic activity of some biaryl-carboxylic acids, *Nature (London),* 214, 626, 1967.
10. **Roubal, Z. and Nemecek, O.,** Antiinflammatory compounds exhibiting fibrinolytic activity, *Med. Chem. N.Y.,* 9, 840, 1966.
11. **von Kaulla, K. N.,** Structure-dependent fibrinolytic (clot-dissolving) activity of antiinflammatory drugs and related compounds, *Arzneim.-Forsch.,* 18, 407, 1968.
12. **Roubal, Z., Gromova, J., Kuchar, M., Nemecek, O., and Cepelak, V.,** An investigation into the interrelationship between structure and fibrinolysis activating capacity of some non-steroidal anti-inflammatory drugs in vitro, in *Synthetic Thrombolytic Agents: Chemical, Biochemical, Pharmacological and Clinical Aspects,* von Kaulla, K. N. and Davidson, J. F., Eds., Charles C Thomas, Springfield, Ill., 1975, 133.
13. **Yoshimoto, M., von Kaulla, K. N., and Hansch, C.,** Structure-activity relationship in synthetic fibrinolytic 2-phenethynyl-cyclopropan-carboxylates, *J. Med. Chem.,* 18, 950, 1975.

14. **Wagner-Jauregg, Th., Jahn, U., and Bürlimann, W.,** Fibrinolytische Antirheumatika. Vergleich von Substanzen der Flufenamsaurereihe mit Trifluormethyl-Analogen des Azopropazons, *Arzneim.-Forsch.*, 23, 911, 1973.
15. **Hansch, C. and von Kaulla, K. N.,** A structure-activity model for certain synthetic fibrinolytics, in *Synthetic Fibrinolytic Thrombolytic Agents: Chemical, Biochemical, Pharmacological and Clinical Aspects,* von Kaulla, K. N. and Davidson, J. F., Eds., Charles C Thomas, Springfield, Ill., 1975, 227.
16. **Cepelak, V., Roubal, Z., and Kuchar, M.,** Fibrinolysis induction by synthetic organic acid. Chemical structure and biological activity relationship, *Folia Haematol. (Leipzig),* 103, 343, 1976.
17. **Hansch, C.,** personal communication.
18. **Aoki, N. and von Kaulla, K. N.,** Dissimilarity of human vascular plasminogen activator ahd human urokinase, *J. Lab. Ciin. Med.*, 78, 354, 1974.
19. **Aoki, N.,** Preparation of plasminogen from vascular trees of human cadavers. Its comparison with urokinase, *J. Biochem. (Tokyo),* 75, 731, 1974.
20. **Gurewich, V., Hyde, E., and Lipinski, B.,** The resistance of fibrinogen and soluble fibrin monomers in blood to degeneration by a potent plasminogen activator derived from cadaver limbs, *Blood,* 46, 555, 1975.
21. **Thorsen, S., Glas-Greenwalt, P., and Astrup, T.,** Differences in the binding to fibrin of urokinase and tissue plasminogen activator, *Thromb. Diath. Haemorrh.*, 28, 65, 1972.
22. **Six, P., Marbet, G. A., Walter, M., Nyman, A., Duckert, F., Madar, G., da Silva, A., Widmer, L. K., and Ritz, R.,** Nebenwirkung bei verschiedenen Thrombolysemethoden, in *Blutgerinnung und Antikoagulantien. Aktuelle Probleme fur Klinik und Praxis,* Neuhaus, K. and Duckert, F., Eds., Schattauer-Verlag, Stuttgart, 1976, 164.
23. **von Kaulla, K. N.,** Synthetische Fibrinolytika. Eigene Erfahrungen und Vorschlage, *Folia Haematol. (Leipzig),* 103, 313, 1976.
24. **von Kaulla, K. N.,** Inactivation of antiplasmin and complement C′ in human plasma rendered fibrinolytic by synthetic organic compounds, *Thromb. Diath. Haemorrh.*, 10, 151, 1963.
25. **von Kaulla, K. N.,** On the in vitro mechanism of synthetic fibrinolytic agents, in *Chemical Control of Fibrinolysis-Thrombolysis. Theory and Clinical Applications,* Schor, J. M., Ed., Wiley-Interscience, New York, 1970, 1.
26. **Aoki, N. and von Kaulla, K. N.,** Human serum plasminogen antiactivator, its distinction from antiplasmin, *Am. J. Physiol.*, 220, 1137, 1971.
27. **Nanninga, L. B.,** Blocking of urokinase binding to plasma inhibitor by diiodosalicylate, *Fed. Proc. Fed. Am. Soc. Exp. Biol.*, 34 (Abstr.), 290, 1975.
28. **Nanninga, L. B. and Guest, M.,** Blocking of fibrinolytic antiactivator by substituted benzoates, *Life Sci.*, 14, 2507, 1974.
29. **Aoki, N. and von Kaulla, K. N.,** Inactivation of human serum plasminogen antiactivator by synthetic fibrinolysis inducers, *Thromb. Diath. Haemorrh.*, 22, 251, 1969a.
30. **Daver, J. and Desnoyers, P.,** Nouvelle hypothese concernant le mecanisme de la fibrinolyse et de la coagulation, *Anesth. Anal. Reanim.*, 31, 539, 1974.
31. **Tomikawa, M. and Abiko, Y.,** The plasminogen-plasmin system. VIII. On the mechanism of chemical induction of fibrinolysis. Isolation of a latent plasminogen activator from human plasma, *Thromb. Diath. Haemorrh.*, 29, 50, 1973.
32. **Wasantapruek, S. and von Kaulla, K. N.,** A serial micro-fibrinolysis test and its use in rats with liver-bypass, *Thromb. Diath. Haemorrh.*, 15, 284, 1966.
33. **von Kaulla, K. N.,** The synthetic approach to fibrinolysis/thrombolysis, in *Synthetic Fibrinolytic Thrombolytic Agents: Chemical, Biochemical, Pharmacological and Clinical Aspects,* von Kaulla, K. N. and Davidson, J. F., Eds., Charles C Thomas, Springfield, Ill., 1975, 53.
34. **von Kaulla, K. N., Ostendorf, P., and Leppke, L.,** In vitro synergism of endogenously increased fibrinolysis with compound-induced fibrinolysis, in *Progress in Chemical Fibrinolysis and Thrombolysis,* Vol. 1, Davidson, J. F., Samama, M. M., and Desnoyers, P. C., Eds., Raven Press, New York, 1975, 385.
35. **Desnoyers, P. C.,** Experimental study of synthetic chemical agents with fibrinolytic activity, in *Chemical Control of Fibrinolysis-Thrombolysis. Theory and Clinical Applications,* Schor, J. M., Ed., Wiley-Interscience, New York, 1970, 73.
36. **Cepelak, V., Chudacek, Y., Muratova, J., Roubal, Z., and Nemecek, O.,** Effect of some non-steroidal antiinflammatory drugs on fibrinolysis activation in vitro and thrombosis in vivo, in *Synthetic Fibrinolytic Thrombolytic Agents: Chemical, Biochemical, Pharmacological and Clinical Aspects,* von Kaulla, K. N. and Davidson, J. F., Eds., Charles C Thomas, Springfield, Ill., 1975, 148.
37. **von Kaulla, K. N.,** Gibt es Wege zur therapeutischen Verwertung der Fibrinolyse?, *Wien. Z. Inn. Med. Ihre Grenzgeb.*, 8, 329, 1952.

38. **von Kaulla, K. N.,** In vitro enhancement by hydrazine and Cobra venom factor of fibrinolytic activity induced by synthetic organic anions, in *Synthetic Fibrinolytic Thrombolytic Agents: Chemical, Biochemical, Pharmacological and Clinical Aspects,* von Kaulla, K. N. and Davidson, J. F., Eds., Charles C Thomas, Springfield, Ill., 1975, 166.
39. **Desnoyers, P. C. and Samama, M. M.,** Synthetische Verbindungen mit fibrinolytischer und thrombolytischer Aktivitat. 2.Teil. Untersuchungen zum Wirkungsmechanismus, *Folia Haematol. (Leipzig),* 103, 357, 1976.
40. **Starzl, T. E., Marchioro, T. L., von Kaulla, K. N., Herman, G., Brittain, S., and Waddell, W.,** Homotransplantation of liver in humans, *Surg. Gynecol. Obstet.,* 117, 657, 1963.
41. **von Kaulla, K. N., von Kaulla, E., and Wasantapruek, S.,** Rapid increase of fibrinolytic activity in pig and rat after exclusion of the liver from the circulation and its control by various organs, *Acta Hepato-Gastroentol.,* 26, 4, 1979.
42. **Tytgat, G., Collen, C., de Vreker, R., and Verstraete, M.,** Investigations on the fibrinolytic system in liver cirrhosis, *Acta Haematol.,* 40, 265, 1968.
43. **Chignell, C. F.,** Optical studies of drug-protein complexes. III. Interaction of flufenamic and other *N*-arylanthranilates with serum albumin, *Mol. Pharmacol.,* 5, 955, 1969.
44. **Thilo, D. and von Kaulla, K. N.,** Structure-dependent inhibition by synthetic fibrinolytic anions of collagen-induced aggregation of human platelets, *J. Med. Chem.,* 13, 503, 1970.
45. **Roubal, Z., Cepelak, V., and Nemecek, O.,** Newly synthesized pyrazolidine derivatives as potential activators of fibrinolysis and antiaggregating agents, *Acta Univ. Carol. Med. Monogr.,* 52, 49, 1972.
46. **Gerloff, J. and von Kaulla, K. N.,** The dual-sample aggregometer. A new instrument adapted for serial testing of antiaggregating agents, *Thromb. Diath. Haemorrh.,* 27, 246, 1972a.
47. **Gerloff, J. and von Kaulla, K. N.,** Prevention of dog serum-induced aggregation of pig platelets, *Proc. Soc. Exp. Biol. Med.,* 141, 298, 1972b.
48. **Aoki, N. and von Kaulla, K. N.,** β_1C-globulin and synthetic fibrinolytic agents, *Proc. Soc. Exp. Biol. Med.,* 130, 101, 1969b.
49. **von Kaulla, K. N.,** In vitro inhibition of aggregation of human erythrocytes by synthetic fibrinolytic compounds, *Arzneim.-Forsch.,* 25, 152, 1975.
50. **Tanaka, K., Kobayashi, K., and Kazui, S.,** Temperature dependent reaction of flufenamic acid with rat erythrocyte membrane, *Biochem. Pharmacol.,* 22, 879, 1973.
51. **von Kaulla, E. and von Kaulla, K. N.,** Factor VIII activity in hemophilic plasma unmasked by synthetic organic anions, *Nature (London) New Biol.,* 240, 144, 1972.
52. **von Kaulla, E. and von Kaulla, K. N.,** Is inhibitor removal the mechanism for unmasking factor VIII activity in hemophilic plasma by certain synthetic fibrinolytic agents?, in *Synthetic Fibrinolytic Thrombolytic Agents: Chemical, Biochemical, Pharmacological and Clinical Aspects,* von Kaulla, K. N. and Davidson, J. F., Eds., Charles C Thomas, Springfield, Ill., 1975, 176.
53. **von Kaulla, K. N.,** Anticoagulants, antithrombotics and haemostatics, in *Burger's Medicinal Chemistry,* 4th ed., John Wiley & Sons, New York, 1979, 1081.
54. **von Kaulla, E. and von Kaulla, K. N.,** unpublished.

Chapter 6

INHIBITORS OF FIBRINOLYSIS

D. Collen

TABLE OF CONTENTS

I. INTRODUCTION

Substances inhibiting fibrinolysis have been recognized at least since the beginning of this century. There are two main types of inhibitors: those which inhibit plasmin (plasmin inhibitors or antiplasmins) and those which inhibit the activation of plasminogen (antiactivators). Many substances derived from biological fluids, tissues, plants, or microorganisms inhibit fibrinolysis. Some active-site titrants of serine proteases are potent inhibitors of fibrinolytic enzymes and certain amino acids, such as lysine, 6-aminohexanoic acid, or tranexamic acid, inhibit the digestion of fibrin. Reviews on the inhibitors of fibrinolysis have been published in a number of recent monographs.[1-5] The main new development in the field of fibrinolytic inhibitors during the last few years has been the characterization of a new and physiologically most important inhibitor of plasmin in human blood, which has been called antiplasmin,[6,7] α_2-plasmin inhibitor,[8] or primary plasmin inhibitor.[9] The present presentation also gives a detailed account of our present knowledge of the biochemistry and physiological role of this inhibitor.

II. INHIBITORS OF PLASMIN

A. Plasmin Inhibitors Occurring in Human Blood

Human plasma exerts a very important inhibitory action on plasmin. There are at least five well-defined plasma proteins which inhibit plasmin in a purified system, namely α_2-macroglobulin, α_1-antitrypsin, inter-α-trypsin inhibitor, antithrombin III — heparin complex, and C1-esterase inhibitor, but the role of these inhibitors in the inactivation of plasmin, formed in its natural environment, plasma, has been poorly understood. For a long time, it was accepted that there were essentially two functionally important plasmin inhibitors in plasma, an immediately reacting one and a slow-reacting one,[10] identical with α_2-macroglobulin and α_1-antitrypsin, respectively.[11,12]

Recently, however, a new plasmin inhibitor occurring in human plasma has been described[6-9] which we have called antiplasmin. Upon activation of plasminogen in plasma, the formed plasmin is first preferentially bound to antiplasmin; only upon complete activation of plasminogen, resulting in saturation of the antiplasmin, is the excess plasmin neutralized by α_2-macroglobulin. In the presence of normal concentrations of these two inhibitors, the other plasma protease inhibitors do not play a role in the inactivation of plasmin.[7,9,13]

1. Antiplasmin, the Fast-Acting Plasmin Inhibitor in Human Plasma

a. Identification

Müllertz[13,14] studied the activation products of human plasminogen in postmortem and urokinase-activated human plasma and found a compound which reacted with antiplasminogen antisera, but not with antisera against the known protease inhibitors. One of the explanations which he suggested was that this compound might represent plasmin in complex with a strong (unknown) inhibitor. Müllertz and Clemmensen[9] later purified this compound and provided unequivocal evidence for the existence of a plasmin inhibitor in plasma, different from the known protease inhibitors, which they called the primary plasmin inhibitor.

Aoki and von Kaulla[15] identified a fibrinolytic inhibitor in human serum which they thought acted mainly at the level of plasminogen activation. Later work by Moroi and Aoki[8] indicated, however, that this inhibitor acts primarily at the level of formed plasmin, and they therefore called it α_2-plasmin inhibitor.

In the course of our studies on the turnover of labeled plasminogen during fibrinolytic therapy, we observed the in vivo formation of radioactive complexes which were initially assumed to represent plasmin-α_2-macroglobulin and plasmin-α_1-antitrypsin complexes.[16] Further work, however, indicated that the presumed plasmin-α_1-antitrypsin complex did not react with antisera against this inhibitor. By isolating this complex and raising antibodies against its inhibitor part, we obtained the first positive evidence for the existence of a fast-acting plasmin inhibitor in human plasma which we called antiplasmin.[6]

With the use of antisera, it was shown that the primary plasmin inhibitor, α_2-plasmin inhibitor, and antiplasmin are identical.[9,17] The Task Force on Inhibitors of the International Society on Thrombosis and Hemostasis has suggested calling this inhibitor α_2-antiplasmin (meeting at the 6th Congress, Philadelphia, Pa., 1977).

In several recent reviews, it is assumed that the inhibitors described by Aoki and von Kaulla[15] and by Hedner[18] are identical because both were initially thought to act at the level of plasminogen activation. It has, however, clearly been shown that these two substances are different.[19]

Gallimore[20] partially purified a fibrinolytic inhibitor from human serum which he called inter-α-antiplasmin. Recent data[17] suggest that this preparation may be a mixture of antiplasmin and the inhibitor of plasminogen activation described by Hedner.

b. Purification

Up to now, four methods have been described for the purification of antiplasmin from plasma.

Moroi and Aoki[8] used a combination of ammonium sulfate precipitation, DEAE-Sephadex chromatography, affinity chromatography on plasminogen-Sepharose, and chromatography on hydroxylapatite and purified the inhibitor to homogeneity. Wiman and Collen[21] developed a modified purification method consisting of chromatography on insolubilized plasminogen, followed by chromatography on DEAE-Sephadex® and concanavalin-A-Sepharose which resulted in a higher yield and a more stable inhibitor preparation. Müllertz and Clemmensen[9] partially purified the inhibitor by ammonium sulfate precipitation, DEAE-Sephadex chromatography, chromatography on insolubilized concanavalin A, gel filtration, and again DEAE-Sephadex chromatography. Collen et al.[22] isolated the inhibitor (mostly in an inactive form, however) by immunoabsorption chromatography and gel filtration.

c. Quantitative Determination

Antiplasmin can be accurately determined in plasma, either with enzymatic assays based on the very fast inhibition of plasmin or with immunochemical assays using specific antisera. In the enzymatic assays, residual plasmin can be measured with natural or with synthetic substrates.[23-25] The normal level of the inhibitor in plasma is around 70 mg/ℓ plasma or 1 μmol/ℓ.[8,9,21]

d. Physicochemical Properties

Antiplasmin is a single-chain polypeptide with a molecular weight of 65,000 to 70,000 estimated by SDS-gel electrophoresis and ultracentrifugation.[8,21] On electrophoresis it migrates as an α_2-globulin. The amino acid composition reported by Moroi and Aoki[8] and that reported by Wiman and Collen[21] correspond well for most amino acids, and the estimated carbohydrate content of the molecule was 11.7 and 13.7%, respectively. The inhibitor is immunochemically different from α_1-antitrypsin, α_2-macroglobulin, C1-esterase inhibitor, antithrombin III, α_1-antichymotrypsin and inter-α-trypsin inhibitor,[8,21] and from the inhibitor of plasminogen activation described by Hedner.[19,21] The inhibitor is stable in solution at pHs above 6.3, but is rapidly inactivated at pHs below 6.0.[21]

e. Interaction with Enzymes

In purified systems[8,21] and in plasma,[7,13] antiplasmin forms a 1:1 stoichiometric complex with plasmin which is devoid of protease or esterase activity and which cannot be dissociated with denaturing agents, such as urea, guanidinium hydrochloride, or dodecylsulfate. Dodecylsulfate polyacrylamide gel patterns indicate that complex formation occurs by strong interaction between the light-(B) chain of plasmin and the inhibitor. A polypeptide with a molecular weight of 11,000 to 14,000 may be released during formation of the complex.[7-9] This has led to the assumption that inhibition occurs by hydrolysis of a specific peptide bond in the inhibitor followed by esterification between the newly formed COOH-terminal residue of the inhibitor and the active-site serine residue of plasmin. Recently, however, it has been shown that the release of this polypeptide is not an essential step in complex formation, but the result of hydrolysis of the inhibitor by free plasmin.[21] It is possible that antiplasmin reacts with plasmin through formation of an ester bond between the carbonyl group of a specific (basic) residue of the inhibitor and the hydroxyl group of the active center serine of plasmin. Moroi and Aoki[26] indeed observed several bands on dodecylsulfate polyacrylamide gel electrophoresis of plasmin-antiplasmin complex following treatment with hydrazine. One of these bands had a molecular weight of 25,000, comparable with the light-(B) chain of plasmin, but no further positive identification of this fragment was made. Antiplasmin has also been shown to react rapidly with trypsin and chymotrypsin and slowly with urokinase, kallikrein, Factor X_a, and thrombin in purified systems.[8,27] Antiplasmin plays a role in the binding of plasmin and, to a lesser extent, trypsin, but not thrombin or chymotrypsin when these enzymes are added to normal plasma.[28] Neither does antiplasmin play a role in the inhibition of purified granulocyte collagenase, elastase, or chymotrypsin-like enzyme.[29]

f. Kinetics of the Reaction Between Plasmin and Antiplasmin

The reaction between plasmin and antiplasmin proceeds in at least two steps: a very fast reversible second-order reaction, followed by a slower irreversible first order reaction,[30,31] and may be represented by:

$$P + A \underset{}{\overset{k_1}{\rightleftarrows}} PA \xrightarrow{k_2} PA'$$

The rate constant k_1 at pH 7.5 is 3.8×10^7 $M^{-1}s^{-1}$ and 1.8×10^7 M^{-1} s^{-1} for the two plasmin forms with different affinities for lysine-Sepharose.[31] This reaction rate is the fastest so far described for protein-protein interactions and is one order of magnitude higher than the reaction rate of trypsin with its inhibitors. The dissociation constant of the reversible step is approximately 2×10^{-10} *M*, and the rate constant of the second step is 4×10^{-3} s^{-1}.[31] Plasmin which as 6-aminohexanoic acid[31] or lysine[30] bound to its lysine binding sites or substrate bound to its active site reacts only very slowly with antiplasmin.

The reaction between antiplasmin and a low molecular weight form of plasmin (LMW-plasmin) was also found to follow the same type of kinetics.[32] The LMW-plasmin, obtained by limited elastase digestion,[33] was composed of an intact B-chain and a small A-chain lacking the lysine binding sites. The k_1 was found to be 30 to 60 times smaller than for normal plasmin and antiplasmin, and the dissociation constant was found to be 10 times higher. LMW-plasmin with substrate bound to its active site reacted only very slowly with antiplasmin. The reaction rate in the first step was only slightly influenced by 6-aminohexanoic acid.

These findings indicate that free lysine binding sites and a free active site in the plasmin molecule are of great importance for the rate of its reaction with antiplasmin. As discussed further, these interactions are most probably of great importance for the regulation of fibrinolysis in vivo.

g. Variation in Health and Disease

The normal plasma level of antiplasmin determined either enzymatically or immunologically is between 80 and 120% (mean ± 2 SD), 100% being the value obtained for a pool of normal plasma.[24,25] The concentration may be below 30% in severe cases of liver disease or intravascular coagulation,[24,25] but is normal in patients with cardiovascular, renal, or malignant disease. The inhibitor is temporarily exhausted during thrombolytic therapy with streptokinase[25,34] when measured with the enzymatic assay. With the immunologic method, residual antigen may be found representing complexed and/or degraded inhibitor.[34] Antiplasmin is a weak acute phase reactant.[25] It is possible that some of the antiplasmin in plasma is inactive.[9]

h. Role of Antiplasmin in the Regulation of In Vivo Fibrinolysis[35]

Human plasminogen and plasmin contain at least two structures known as lysine binding sites which are responsible for their interaction not only with amino acids, such as lysine or 6-aminohexanoic acid,[36-38] but also with fibrin[39] and with antiplasmin.[8,21] In purified systems, native plasminogen (with NH_2-terminal glutamic acid) has a weak affinity for fibrin, whereas the partially degraded form of plasminogen (with NH_2-terminal lysine) has a much stronger affinity.[40] When whole plasma is clotted, approximately 4% of the plasminogen is specifically bound to fibrin through its lysine binding sites.[41]

Antiplasmin interferes with the binding of plasminogen to fibrin, since it also has an affinity for the lysine binding sites.[42] In plasma, however, this interference seems to be very small.[41] Furthermore, it appears that antiplasmin cannot efficiently displace fibrin-bound plasminogen.[41]

These findings, taken in conjunction with the kinetics of the plasmin-antiplasmin reaction, suggest that antiplasmin acts as a very rapid and irreversible inhibitor of plasmin formed in the circulation. Plasmin formed on the fibrin surface, which is bound through its lysine binding site and with its active site involved in fibrin digestion, reacts very slowly with antiplasmin. The specific interactions between plasmin(ogen), fibrin, and antiplasmin thus provide a molecular basis for the classical hypothesis of in vivo thrombolysis which claims that plasminogen binds to fibrin and, following activation within the thrombus, exerts its action in a relatively inhibitor-free environment.[43]

This regulatory role of antiplasmin in in vivo fibrinolysis was confirmed in patients during thrombolytic therapy.[44] Depletion of antiplasmin, either by infusion of high doses of streptokinase (600,000 units over 30 min) or of human plasmin (8000 CTA units over 30 min), is accompanied by systemic fibrinogen breakdown, as evidenced by a fast drop of plasma fibrinogen and the generation of high amounts of fibrinogen degradation products in serum. Infusion of either urokinase or smaller amounts of plasmin which only resulted in decrease of antiplasmin to about 50% of the preinfusion value was not accompanied by systemic fibrinogen breakdown. Thus, the occurrence of systemic fibrinogenolysis depends on depletion of the circulating antiplasmin pool.

i. Turnover of Antiplasmin

The turnover of purified biologically intact iodine-labeled antiplasmin was studied in control subjects and in patients during thrombolytic therapy.[44] The main turnover parameters in the controls were: plasma radioactivity half-life, 2.64 ± 0.32 days; fractional catabolic rate, 0.53 ± 0.09 of the plasma pool per day; synthetic (catabolic) rate, 1.4 ± 0.3 mg/kg/day; and intravascular fraction, 0.51 ± 0.05. The half-life of the plasmin-antiplasmin complex, measured from the disappearance rate of labeled antiplasmin, plasmin, or plasmin-antiplasmin complex during thrombolytic therapy, was approximately 0.5 days. The disappearance rate of the complex was independent of its concentration in plasma.

j. Inhibition by Antiplasmin of the Fibrinolysis Associated with Oncogenic Transformation and Neoplasia

We have studied the role of antiplasmin in the inhibition of fibrinolysis associated with malignant cells.[45] When mixed cultures of mouse fibroblasts and mouse fibroblasts transformed with Kirsten murine sarcoma virus were grown in petri dishes and overlayed with casein, the appearance of focal lysis zones due to a plasminogen activator released by the malignant cells was inhibited by the addition of human plasma. Likewise, lysis of a fibrin clot by the culture fluid from a human melanoma cell line was inhibited by the addition of human plasma. Specific removal of antiplasmin from plasma by immunoabsorption completely abolished its inhibitory activity, both in the caseinolytic and fibrinolytic assays. Thus, antiplasmin is the only protein in human plasma capable of inhibiting the fibrinolytic activity associated with oncogenic transformation or neoplasia. Whether this effect is exclusively due to inhibition of formed plasmin or whether it is also due to interference with plasminogen activation remains unclear. Investigation of the influence of antiplasmin on the molecular events occurring during plasminogen activation by proteases from malignant tissues in purified systems may clarify this problem.

k. Plasmin-Antiplasmin Complex: Its Determination and Value as an Indicator of In Vivo Activation of the Fibrinolytic System

Activation of the fibrinolytic system results in the formation of plasmin which has a short lifespan in the blood, as it is very rapidly bound to and neutralized by antiplasmin. The plasmin-antiplasmin complex, however, contains new antigenic structures which render it immunochemically distinct from the precursor molecules.[46,47]

For the study of the occurrence in vivo and clinical relevance of this complex, we have developed a simple latex agglutination test for its rapid quantitation in plasma.[48] The purified complex was found to cause a distinct agglutination of the particles at a concentration of 0.1 to 0.2 mg/ℓ. Purified plasminogen and antiplasmin were over 100 times less reactive. Activation of fresh human plasma with urokinase caused progressive generation of agglutinating activity up to a plasma dilution of 1/480. I.v. injection of streptokinase into patients resulted in an increase of the plasmin-antiplasmin titer to at least 1/240. The titer remained high during the first 3 hr after injection and was still raised after 24 hr, indicating that the half-life of this complex in plasma is several hours.

Out of 101 male and 23 female control subjects, only three of the men had a plasmin-antiplasmin titer above 1/16. Plasmin-antiplasmin titers of 1/40 or more were detected in 25 of 230 hospitalized patients. Seven out of eight patients with diffuse intravascular coagulation of various origins had plasmin-antiplasmin titers of 1/80 or 1/160.

From these findings, it was concluded that primary activation of the fibrinolytic system in vivo or activation secondary to in vivo coagulation is associated with the appearance of circulating plasmin-antiplasmin complex which can be directly assayed in plasma on the basis of its neoantigenic expression.

2. α_2-Macroglobulin

a. Identification of α_2-Macroglobulin as an Inhibitor of Plasmin

Norman and Hill[10] detected a fast-acting plasmin inhibitor in the α_2-region on electrophoresis of human plasma, and Schwick et al.[11] later showed that the high molecular weight α_2-globulin which inhibited plasmin was identical with α_2-macroglobulin. It has long been accepted and is still claimed in most of the recent reviews that α_2-macroglobulin is the fast-acting and most important inhibitor of plasmin present in human plasma. However, it is now firmly established that α_2-macroglobulin represents the slower reacting plasmin inhibitor of plasma, and its role seems to be to inactivate any plasmin formed in excess of the inhibitory capacity of antiplasmin.[7,13] Indeed, when the plasma plasminogen (concentration approximately 1.5 μmol/ℓ) is activated, the formed plasmin is initially primarily bound to antiplasmin (concentration approximately 1 μmol/ℓ) until after its saturation, when the excess plasmin is neutralized by α_2-macroglobulin.[7,13]

A number of reviews on the physiology and biochemistry of α_2-macroglobulin have recently appeared.[49-52] α_2-Macroglobulin forms complexes not only with serine proteases, such as trypsin, plasmin, and thrombin, but also with thiol proteases, such as papain, ficin, and bromelain, carboxyl proteases, such as cathepsin D, and metal proteases, such as thermolysin and collagenase.[52]

b. Purification

Several methods have been described for the purification of α_2-macroglobulin. Harpel[53] isolated α_2-macroglobulin from human plasma by polyethylene glycol precipitation, ultracentrifugation in KBr, DEAE-cellulose chromatography, agarose (Biogel A5m) gel filtration, and pevicon block electrophoresis. His final material was homogeneous on cellulose acetate electrophoresis and on polyacrylamide gel electrophoresis.

TABLE 1

Physicochemical Properties of the Main Inhibitors of Fibrinolysis in Human Plasma[a]

Parameter	Antiplasmin	α_2-Macroglobulin	Inhibitor of plasminogen activation
Molecular weight	63,000—70,000	725,000	75,000
$s^{o}_{20,w}$	3.4—3.45	18.1—19.6	—
Electrophoretic mobility	α_2	α_2	α_2
Concentration in plasma (g/l)	0.07	2 (in adults)	—
pI	—	5.0—5.5	—
$A^{1\%}_{280nm}$	6.7—7.0	8.1	—
Number of polypeptide chains	1	4	—
Carbohydrate content (%)	11.7—13.7	8—11	—
Enzyme molecules bound (mol/mol)	1	1 or 2?	—
NH_2-terminal amino acid	Asn	—	—

[a] For references see text.

Roberts[54] delipoproteinized fresh serum with dextran sulfate and $MnCl_2$ and precipitated IgM by dialysis against 0.01 *M* sodium acetate buffer pH 5.2. α_2-Macroglobulin was isolated from the supernatant by gel filtration on two agarose (Biogel A5m) columns followed by gel filtration on Sephadex G-200. The resulting preparation had no detectable impurities by analytical centrifugation or polyacrylamide gel electrophoresis.

c. Quantitative Determination

α_2-Macroglobulin can be accurately quantitated by electroimmunoassay or radial immunodiffusion using commercially available antisera.[55] Alternatively, α_2-macroglobulin can be estimated from the esterase activity of its complex with trypsin.[56] This esterase activity is measured with synthetic substrates, following addition of trypsin in excess of the α_2-macroglobulin and neutralization of the remaining free trypsin by soybean trypsin inhibitor.

d. Physicochemical Properties

α_2-Macroglobulin is a glycoprotein with a molecular weight of 725,000 and containing 8% carbohydrate. It is composed of two half-molecules held together by noncovalent bonds. Each half-molecule is composed of two chains with a molecular weight of approximately 185,000 held together by disulfide bonds. Incubation of α_2-macroglobulin with trypsin-like enzymes results in the generation of fragments with a molecular weight of 85,000, apparently by hydrolytic cleavage somewhere in the middle of the polypeptide chains.[53] The amino acid composition of α_2-macroglobulin is well known,[57,58] but the results of NH_2-terminal and COOH-terminal amino acid determinations are not consistent, probably due to the sensitivity of the molecule to proteolytic degradation.

More detail on the physicochemical properties of α_2-macroglobulin can be found elsewhere[49,50] and in Table 1.

e. Interaction with Enzymes

α_2-Macroglobulin reacts with endopeptidases of several classes, including serine proteases, thiol proteases, metal proteases, and carboxyl proteases.[49-52] The active site of the enzymes is necessary for binding, but proteolysis is not completely inhibited by the linkage. The α_2-macroglobulin bound enzymes have a low or negligible residual proteolytic activity on large natural substrates, but a high to normal hydrolytic activity on small synthetic substrates. Pancreatic trypsin inhibitor (Trasylol®) and soybean trypsin inhibitor quickly neutralize free plasmin, but not the esterolytic activity of the α_2-macroglobulin-plasmin complex.

Barret and Starkey[51,52] have proposed the following working hypothesis for the molecular mechanism of the interaction between α_2-macroglobulin and enzymes. Binding is initiated by a proteolytic attack on the α_2-macroglobulin molecule, and this results in a conformational change such that the enzyme molecule is irreversibly trapped within the α_2- macroglobulin molecule. The inhibition of enzymic activity results from the steric hindrance of the access of substrates to the enzyme in its enclosed environment.

At present it is not clear whether α_2-macroglobulin binds one or two molecules of enzyme. Human α_2-macroglobulin has been claimed to bind 2-mol equivalents of trypsin and of plasmin, but equimolar binding ratios have also been reported.[49-52]

f. Variation and Biological Function

The concentration of α_2-macroglobulin in plasma is age dependent; it reaches a maximum of about 4.5 g/ℓ at 1 to 3 years of age and declines slowly to the adult level of about 2 g/ℓ at 25 years.[59] It is 10 to 20% higher in women than in men. Congenital deficiencies have not been reported, and increased values are found in nephrosis and liver cirrhosis.[60] Decreased levels have also been found during streptokinase therapy.[61,62] The restoration of a normal α_2-macroglobulin level following thrombolytic therapy requires several days.

It has been suggested that α_2-macroglobulin plays a key role in the inhibition and very fast elimination of endopeptidases released in the blood and that it therefore protects against autodigestion.[63] Depletion of α_2-macroglobulin by infusion of trypsin in dogs leads to irreversible shock. In addition it has been suggested that trypsin is transfered from α_1-antitrypsin to α_2-macroglobulin and then cleared with a half-life of 8 min.

Plasmin generated in man during thrombolytic therapy preferentially binds to antiplasmin, and this complex disappears with a half-life of approximately 0.5 days.[44,64] The bond in this complex is very strong, and it is therefore unlikely that it is dissociable by α_2-macroglobulin. The plasmin-α_2-macroglobulin complex generated in vivo has a half-life of several hours, as judged from the disappearance rate of plasma radioactivity during thrombolytic therapy with streptokinase.[64] In our view, α_2-macroglobulin acts as a second-line inhibitor of plasmin formed in excess of the neutralizing capacity of antiplasmin.

3. Other Plasma Protease Inhibitors

There are at least three plasma protease inhibitors in addition to antiplasmin and α_2-macroglobulin which inhibit plasmin in purified systems. These are α_1-antitrypsin, antithrombin III, and $C\bar{1}$-inactivator.[65] Inter-α-trypsin inhibitor is a polyvalent inhibitor and probably also reacts to some extent with plasmin.[65] In the presence of normal concentrations of antiplasmin and α_2-macroglobulin, however, none of these inhibitors play a role in the neutralization of plasmin formed in the blood.[7,13]

Purified antithrombin III is a progressive, time-dependent inhibitor of purified plasmin. Heparin accelerates the rate of this reaction 50- to 100-fold.[66] On the basis of these findings, it has been suggested that antithrombin-heparin complex may be a major inhibitor of in vivo fibrinolysis. The role of antithrombin III-heparin complex as an inhibitor of plasmin formed in plasma has been reevaluated in vitro and in vivo.[67,68]

It was found that in the absence of heparin and following complete activation of the plasma plasminogen, about 1% of the formed plasmin binds to antithrombin III. In the presence of therapeutic concentrations of heparin (1 to 2 IU per milliliter of plasma), this value increased to 2 to 5%, both in vitro and in vivo. These data suggest that the antithrombin III-heparin complex plays a very limited role in the inactivation of plasmin.

4. Plasmin Inhibitors from Platelets

Johnson and Schneider[69] reported on an antiplasmin activity of bovine platelets which accounted for a major part of the antiplasmin of bovine blood. In human blood, however, the platelets contributed only 1 to 3% of the antiplasmin activity.[70,71] The platelet contribution to the total antiplasmin activity of whole human blood is therefore probably small.

Antiplasmin materials in platelets have, however, been characterized to some extent. McDonagh et al.[72] found two antiplasmin activities, one of which was platelet Factor XIII and the other one was eluted earlier on Sephadex G-200. Ganguly et al.[73,74] described low molecular weight antiplasmins which were dialysable in extracts of human platelets. All these plasmin inhibitors are at present poorly characterized.

B. Inhibitors of Plasmin in Tissues and Secretions

Proteinase inhibitors in tissues (lung, spleen, liver, parotid gland, and pancreas) and body fluids (exudates, urine, seminal fluid, and amniotic fluid) have been described by many authors. Mostly these inhibitors are poorly characterized antiproteases of unknown physiological function. References to papers dealing with these substances can be found elsewhere.[1,75,76] Two of these inhibitors (aprotinin and the urinary trypsin inhibitor) have been studied in more detail and will be reviewed here.

1. Aprotinin

a. Identification

This inhibitor has also been called Kunitz inhibitor, bovine pancreatic trypsin inhibitor, basic pancreatic trypsin inhibitor, pulmin, bovine trypsin-kallikrein inhibitor, kallikrein inactivator of bovine parotid gland, and polyvalent inhibitor from bovine organs. It was first described in the bovine parotid gland by Kraut et al.[77] and isolated from bovine pancreas by Kunitz and Northrop.[78] This protein is now commercially available in a highly purified form, e.g., as Trasylol® (Bayer, Leverkusen, Federal Republic of Germany), Iniprol® (Choay, Paris, France), or Basic Pancreatic Trypsin Inhibitor (Worthington, Freehold, N.J.).

b. Purification

Following the earlier extraction and precipitation methods, the inhibitor has been purified to homogeneity by classic chromatography methods[79,80] and by chromatography on insolubilized trypsin.[81]

c. Quantitative Determination

The inhibitor may be assayed following incubation with trypsin followed by measurement of the remaining trypsin.[81]

The inhibitor may also be determined following incubation with kallikrein (from pi pancreas) by measuring the hydrolysis rate of *N*-α-benzoyl-L-arginin-ethyleste (BAEE).[82] One kallikrein inhibitor unit is defined as the amount of inhibitor whic under standard conditions (15 min incubation at 37°C and pH 8) neutralizes 50% c two kallikrein units of the enzyme, one kallikrein unit being the amount of enzyn which hydrolyzes 1 μmol of the substrate per minute.

d. Physicochemical Properties

The inhibitor is very stable towards heating, pH changes, and enzymatic degradation. Its molecular weight is 6512, and its isoelectric point is 10.5.

The sequence of the 58 amino acids has been determined by several groups of workers.[83-85]

e. Interaction with Enzymes

The inhibitor neutralizes serine proteases, such as trypsin, plasmin, kallikrein, and chymotrypsin by forming a 1:1 stoichiometric complex.

The mechanism of inhibition of trypsin by the pancreatic trypsin inhibitor has been elucidated.[86,87] The carbonyl group of the lysine-15 residue of the inhibitor forms a covalent bond with the active site seryl residue of the enzyme. This is, however, not associated with peptide bond cleavage in the inhibitor, since the carbonyl carbon acquires a tetrahedral intermediate configuration between that of the Michaelis complex and that of the acyl-enzyme. The combination of aprotinin with plasmin probably follows the same mechanism, but is characterized by different dissociation constants (6×10^{-14} *M* for trypsin and 2.3×10^{-10} *M* for plasmin). The complex of aprotinin with plasmin is dissociated below pH 3.0 and above pH 9.0.

f. Clinical Use of Aprotinin

Aprotinin has been used in the treatment of patients with diffuse intravascular coagulation (abruptio placentae, amniotic fluid embolism, septic abortion, and Gram-negative sepsis), postsurgical bleeding, acute pancreatitis, shock lung, myocardial infarction, etc. This work has recently been reviewed.[88] It was concluded that no definite evidence exists to date to prove that aprotinin can, by inhibiting plasmin, decrease blood loss. Since results from acceptable trials are not yet available, no definite guidelines can be given at present for the use of this drug in the management of excessive blood loss. Clinical benefit has been shown in acute pancreatitis[89] and in shock lung.[90]

2. Urinary Trypsin Inhibitor

Urine, and especially pregnancy urine, contains an inhibitor also known as mingin which has a potent trypsin inhibitory activity, but only a weak effect on plasmin.[91,92] This inhibitor is acid stable and is probably identical with the urinary trypsin inhibitors which are antigenically related to inter-α-trypsin inhibitor.[93] Nasal and bronchial mucus also contain inhibitors which are antigenically related to inter-α-trypsin inhibitor.[94]

Hochstrasser et al. have isolated two acid-stable inhibitors of mol wt 14,000 and 20,000 from bronchial mucus and two inhibitors of mol wt 22,000 and 44,000 from human urine and human plasma which all showed immunological cross-reaction with inter-α-trypsin inhibitor[94] and which all inhibited trypsin, chymotrypsin, and plasmin. The inhibitors isolated from mucus are, in addition, strong inhibitors of leucocyte proteases. The mucus inhibitors are structurally different from the plasma and urinary inhibitors.[94] The origin and the physiological role of these inhibitors are unknown.

C. Plasmin Inhibitors from Microorganisms, Plants, and Lower Animals

Protease inhibitors are widely distributed in bacteria, plants, and lower animals. Detailed information on these inhibitors can be found in recent books.[75,95,96] Some of these inhibitors are strong inhibitors of plasmin, and those which have been used in the field of fibrinolysis will be reviewed here.

1. Microbial Inhibitors

Several kinds of low molecular weight enzyme inhibitors are found in microbial culture filtrates.[96] Leupeptins are propionyl or acetyl-L-leucyl-L-leucyl-L-argininal or their analogues in which each leucine is replaced by L-isoleucine or L-valine. These substances have been found in several strains of streptomyces, and they inhibit trypsin, plasmin, papain, cathepsin B, kallikrein, and boar acrosin.

The purification and properties of leupeptins have been described. They inhibit the hydrolysis of TAME (*N-p*-toluene sulfonyl-L-arginine methyl ester) and BAEE (*N*-benzoyl-L-arginine methyl ester) by trypsin in a competitive fashion and that of BAPA (*N*-benzoyl-L-arginine-*p*-nitroanilide) in a noncompetitive way. Leupeptins inhibit chemically induced malignant transformation in vitro and in vivo.[97]

Antipain, (1-carboxy-2-phenylethyl)-carbamoyl-L-arginyl-L-valyl-argininal produced by actinomycetes inhibits papain, trypsin, thrombokinase, cathepsin A, cathepsin B, plasmin, acrosin, and kallikrein. Further information on these microbial inhibitors can be obtained from recent reviews.[75,95]

2. Plant Inhibitors

Several kinds of protease inhibitors with different specificities towards various proteolytic enzymes occur in plants. The molecular weights of these inhibitors vary between 3,000 and 25,000. Many of them have been purified and extensively characterized, both with respect to their physicochemical properties and mechanism of action. Detailed recent information on these inhibitors can be obtained elsewhere.[75,95] One of these inhibitors, soybean trypsin inhibitor, which has been extensively characterized[98] and used in fibrinolysis research, is briefly discussed here.

Soybean trypsin inhibitor has been purified by water extraction and DEAE cellulose chromatography. It is commercially available from a.o. Novo Industri A/S, Copenhagen, Denmark; Nutritional Biochemical Corporation, Cleveland, Ohio; Sigma Chemical Corporation, St. Louis, Mo., and Worthington Biochemical Corporation, Freehold, N.J. Its molecular weight is 22,000. It inhibits trypsin, chymotrypsin, and some kallikreins. Its inhibitory activity against plasmin has been established by several authors. The complete sequence of the 181 amino acids of the inhibitor has been determined.

The reaction of trypsin with soybean trypsin inhibitor comprises at least two steps, a reversible second order complex formation followed by an irreversible first order transition.

The reactive site of the inhibitor is localized around Arg-63 and Ile-64.[99] The inhibitor reacts with trypsin by formation of a covalent bond between the carbonyl carbon of Arg-63 and the oxygen of the side chain of the active site serine of the enzyme.[100]

3. Plasmin Inhibitors from Lower Animals

Protease inhibitors are also widely distributed in lower animals, such as snails, cuttlefish, mussels, leeches, sea anemones, and in snake venoms.[75,95] Some of these inhibitors, such as the bdellins from leeches, the inhibitor in the venoms of Russel viper and Cape cobra, and the inhibitors from sea anemones are potent plasmin inhibitors, but their use in the field of fibrinolysis is still very restricted. More information on these inhibitors is available in recent reviews.[75,95]

D. Active-Site Directed Synthetic Inhibitors of Plasmin

Trypsin-like serine proteases (including plasmin) are inhibited by substances which form covalent bonds with amino acids of the active center. Two types of active-site directed inhibitors have been designed, namely diisopropyl phosphorofluoridate[101] and esters of *p*-guanidinobenzoate[102] which react with the active center serine and chloromethylketones[103] which react with the active center histidine.

Both diisopropylphosphorofluoridate (DFP) and L-1-chloro-3-tosyl-amido-7-amino-2-heptanone (TLCK) are slow irreversible inhibitors of plasmin which have been used for localizing the active center serine and histidine in the light-(B) chain of plasmin.[104] *p*-Nitrophenyl-*p*′-guanidinobenzoate is a rapid acting, slowly reversible inhibitor of plasmin which has been used for titration of the active site serine.[102]

III. INHIBITORS OF PLASMINOGEN ACTIVATION

A. Physiological Inhibitors of Plasminogen Activation in Human Blood

The existence in blood of physiological inhibitors to the activation of plasminogen has been much disputed. The demonstration of activation inhibitors in plasma is indeed hampered by two obstacles. First, it is very difficult to measure antiactivator activity in the presence of antiplasmins. Antiactivator activity may, however, be demonstrated in the following ways: complex formation between activator and inhibitors, inhibition of activator-catalyzed hydrolysis of low molecular weight substrates, and inhibition of cleavage of the internal peptide bond in plasminogen.[5] Second, the various protease inhibitors in plasma may each have some affinity for plasminogen activators and in concert confer some inhibitory activity to the plasma, without actually being specific inhibitors. Despite these difficulties, it seems, however, that plasma contains components which act or may act as inhibitors of plasminogen activation. The physiological role of most of these inhibitors is, however, unknown.

1. Streptokinase Antibodies

Human plasma contains antibodies directed against streptokinase, the bacterial protein used for activation of the fibrinolytic system in vivo. These antibodies most probably result from previous infections with β-hemolytic streptococci and are responsible for the requirement of high doses of streptokinase to activate the fibrinolytic system and for allergic side reactions.

The amount of streptokinase antibodies varies over a wide range among individuals. Bachmann[105] reported antistreptokinase titers varying from 2 to 402 units per milliliter in 120 individuals. Verstraete et al.[106] found that 352,000 units of streptokinase were required to neutralize the circulating antibodies in 95% of a healthy population.

Since streptokinase reacts quickly with antibodies and is thereby rendered biochemically inert, sufficient streptokinase must be infused to neutralize the antibodies before fibrinolytic activation is obtained.[107] A few days after streptokinase injection, the antistreptokinase titer rises rapidly to 50 to 100 times the preinfusion value and remains high for 4 to 6 months, during which time renewed treatment is impracticable. Administration of corticosteroids commonly is used as adjuvant to streptokinase to prevent allergic side reactions.

2. The Inhibitor of Plasminogen Activation in Human Plasma Described by Hedner

Hedner[18] has identified an α_2-globulin with an estimated molecular weight of 75,000 in human plasma which inhibits plasminogen activation. The author has recently reviewed the available information on this inhibitor.[108] Immunochemical evidence indicates that it is different from antiplasmin.[19]

The inhibitor was partially purified by DEAE-Sephadex chromatography, Sephadex G-200 gel filtration, and preparative agarose electrophoresis of serum previously depleted of haptoglobin by chromatography on insolubilized hemoglobin.[18] This material which was devoid of other plasma protease inhibitors as judged by immunochemical analysis, inhibits the activation of plasminogen both by urokinase and streptokinase, but its activity is very labile. Increased levels have been found in patients with malignant diseases or uremia and in some patients with recurrent idiopathic deep vein thrombosis.[108] The inhibitor does not seem to form a stable complex with purified urokinase or plasmin,[109] but it seems to neutralize the amidolytic activity of urokinase.[110] These findings suggest that the inhibitor might react reversibly with the active site region of urokinase. Although there seems to be some correlation between increased levels of this inhibitor and recurrent deep vein thrombosis, the physiological role and reaction mechanism of this inhibitor remain unknown.

3. C$\bar{1}$-esterase Inhibitor

Activation of Factor XII (Hageman factor) in human blood results in enhanced fibrinolytic activity. Activated Hageman factor may directly convert plasminogen to plasmin or in the presence of a cofactor activate a plasminogen proactivator present in plasma. The plasminogen proactivator may be identical with prekallikrein. This pathway of fibrinolytic activation is discussed in more detail by Kaplan in another chapter of this book (see Chapter 3). The physiological importance of this intrinsic pathway of fibrinolysis is at present unclear.

Human serum contains C$\bar{1}$-esterase inhibitor, an α_2-globulin with a molecular weight of 104,000, occurring at a concentration of 18 ± 5 mg/100 mℓ which inhibits C1s, plasma kallikrein, plasmin, Factor XII_a, and Factor XI_a.[111]

Insofar as C$\bar{1}$-esterase inhibitor is the main inactivator of Hageman factor and kallikrein in human plasma, one might expect it to play a role as an inhibitor of plasminogen activation through the intrinsic pathway.

4. Other Plasma Protease Inhibitors

Several plasma protease inhibitors exert an effect on the activation of plasminogen when measured under certain conditions. Thus, α_1-antitrypsin has been found to slowly inactivate urokinase, but not porcine tissue activator or streptokinase-activator in human plasma.[112] It has also been shown that α_2-macroglobulin acts as a competitive inhibitor of urokinase[113] and enhances the antifibrinolytic effect of tranexamic acid.[114]

Antiplasmin has been shown to inhibit urokinase very slowly, but irreversibly.[8] In addition antiplasmin might have an inhibitory effect on fibrinolysis by decreasing the extent of binding of plasminogen to fibrin.[42] In plasma, however, this phenomenon seems to be of minor importance.[41]

Helle[115] and Bennet[116] have described a labile urokinase inhibitory activity which develops in plasma upon clotting. This inhibitory activity is more effective against porcine tissue activator than against urokinase.[117]

5. Clearance of Plasminogen Activator from the Circulation

The disappearance of plasminogen activator activity from human plasma is faster in vivo than in vitro.

Plasminogen activator released in the plasma by nicotinic acid injection in normal subjects has a half-life in vivo of 13 ± 5 min,[118,119] but in vitro of 78 ± 9 min.[118] In cirrhotic patients, the in vivo half-life is significantly longer,[118,119] but the in vitro half-life is similar to that of the normals. These findings suggest firstly that the liver is an important organ in the clearance of plasminogen activator and secondly that human plasma progressively inhibits the plasminogen activator. Likewise the disappearance rate of urokinase is faster in vivo (half-life of 9 to 16 min) than in vitro (half-life of 27 to 61 min).[120]

These data indicate that a significant amount of plasminogen activator in the circulation is removed by clearance through the liver and not by enzymatic inhibition in the blood.

6. *Inhibitors of Plasminogen Activation from Platelets*

Platelets contain inhibitors which have been claimed to primarily inhibit fibrinolysis induced by activators.[121-124] Washed platelets, at a concentration which does not inhibit plasmin, are capable of inhibiting plasminogen activators.[122] Murray et al.[123] partially purified an inhibitor of urokinase and tissue activator from human platelets with an estimated molecular weight of 45,000. Moore et al.[124] isolated a fraction possessing antiurokinase activity, but no antiplasmin activity, in addition to a fraction containing antiplasmin activity.

The physiological significance of these inhibitors is uncertain; they may have a role in the protection of thrombi from premature lysis.

B. Inhibitors of Plasminogen Activation in Tissues

Inhibitors of fibrinolysis have been found in many tissues, but due to methodological difficulties in distinguishing between antiplasmins and antiactivators, the site of action of these inhibitors is not always firmly established.

The bovine pancreatic trypsin inhibitor (aprotinin) was found to act as a competitive inhibitor of plasminogen activation by streptokinase and urokinase.[125]

Inhibitors of urokinase have been found in culture supernatants of human lung, kidney, heart, bladder, and skin muscle.[126] Two inhibitors of urokinase (and plasmin?) activity have been identified in human placenta extracts and partially characterized.[127,128] One of these inhibitors was found to also inactivate vascular plasminogen activator and tissue plasminogen activator.[129]

C. Active Site-Directed Synthetic Inhibitors of Plasminogen Activators

All plasminogen activators described so far are serine proteases and are to a variable extent sensitive to substances which react irreversibly or very slowly with the active-site serine (diisopropylphosphorofluoridate, DFP, and *p*-nitrophenyl-*p*′-guanidinobenzoate, NPGB) or histidine (peptide chloroketones) residues. Urokinase is inhibited by DFP[130] and derivatives of lysine chloroketone.[131] Pig heart activator is inhibited by DFP, but apparently not by tosyl-lysine-chloromethyl ketone (TLCK).[132] The plasminogen-streptokinase complex is inhibited by NPGB.[133]

IV. SYNTHETIC INHIBITORS OF FIBRINOLYSIS USED FOR CLINICAL APPLICATION

Certain amino acids, such as 6-aminohexanoic acid (ε-aminocaproic acid, EACA), *trans*-4-aminomethylcyclohexane-1-carboxylic acid (AMCHA, tranexamic acid), and *p*-aminomethylbenzoic acid (PAMBA) inhibit fibrinolysis, both in vitro and in vivo.[134] The relation between the structure of these substances and their antifibrinolytic effect has been studied in detail.[134] Their clinical usefulness has recently been reviewed.[135] In purified systems, however, these agents greatly accelerate the activation of native plasminogen.[136,137] This paradox has recently been elucidated.[138,139]

Native plasminogen (with NH_2-terminal glutamic acid) is slowly activated by urokinase, whereas partially degraded plasminogen (with NH_2-terminal lysine, valine, or methionine) is rapidly activated.[136,137] In the presence of EACA, however, the activation rate of native plasminogen is greatly increased and approaches that of the partially degraded plasminogen. This acceleration has been ascribed to conformational changes in the plasminogen molecule induced by the presence of EACA or removal of the NH_2-terminal part of the molecule. The conformational change is probably a result of the dissociation between a site in the NH_2-terminal part (Residues 45 to 51) and a structure in the plasminogen molecule which binds the antifibrinolytic amino acids ("lysine binding site").[140,141] The plasminogen molecule contains at least two such lysine binding sites.[33,38]

The antifibrinolytic effect of EACA and analogues appears to result from its interference with the binding of plasmin(ogen) to fibrin.[39-41] When whole plasma is clotted, approximately 4% of the plasminogen is specifically bound to fibrin through its lysine binding sites, and this interaction is abolished by EACA.[41] The specific affinity between plasminogen and fibrin seems to play an important role in the activation of plasminogen with tissue activator which is also specifically adsorbed to fibrin.[138,142] Indeed, fibrin markedly potentiates the activation of plasminogen, but this stimulating effect is completely lost in the presence of EACA.[138,139] EACA and its more active analogue tranexamic acid have been successfully used to reduce blood loss in essential menorrhagia, prostatectomy, and dental extraction in hemophiliacs.

V. PHYSIOPATHOLOGICAL CONDITIONS ASSOCIATED WITH INHIBITION OF FIBRINOLYSIS*

A number of physiopathological changes in the blood are associated with a delayed lysis of euglobulin clots or dilute blood clots. These include pregnancy, hyperlipidemia, smoking, wine and beer drinking, and possibly atherosclerosis. The molecular mechanism of inhibition of fibrinolysis by these factors is in most instances unknown. A detailed review of these phenomena is given by Dr. I. M. Nilsson in this book (Chapter 8).

* The author wishes that a note be added that this manuscript was completed in December 1977.

REFERENCES

1. **Konttinen, Y. P.,** *Fibrinolysis,* Oy Star AB, Tampere, Finland, 1968, chap. 5.
2. **McNicol, G. P. and Douglas, A. S.,** The fibrinolytic enzyme system, in *Human Blood Coagulation, Haemostasis and Thrombosis,* Biggs, R., Ed., Blackwell Scientific, Oxford, 1976, chap. 14.
3. **Davidson, J. F.,** Recent advances in fibrinolysis, in *Recent Advances in Blood Coagulation,* Vol. 2, Poller, L., Ed., Churchill Livingstone, Edinburgh, 1977, chap. 4.
4. **Ogston, D. and Bennett, B.,** Biochemistry of naturally occurring inhibitors of the fibrinolytic enzyme system, in *Haemostasis,* Ogston, D. and Bennett, B., Eds., John Wiley & Sons, London, 1977, chap. 12.
5. **Müllertz, S.,** Natural inhibitors of fibrinolysis, in *Progress in Chemical Fibrinolysis and Thrombolysis,* Vol. 3, Davidson, J. F., Rowan, R. M., Samama, M. M., and Desnoyers, P. C., Eds., Raven Press, New York, 1978, 213.
6. **Collen, D., De Cock, F., and Verstraete, M.,** Immunochemical distinction between antiplasmin and α_1-antitrypsin, *Thromb. Res.,* 7, 245, 1975.
7. **Collen, D.,** Identification and some properties of a new fast-reacting plasmin inhibitor from human plasma, *Eur. J. Biochem.,* 69, 209, 1976.
8. **Moroi, M. and Aoki, N.,** Isolation and characterization of alpha α_2-plasmin inhibitor in human plasma. A novel proteinase inhibitor which inhibits activator-induced clot lysis, *J. Biol. Chem.,* 251, 5956, 1976.
9. **Müllertz, S. and Clemmensen, I.,** The primary inhibitor of plasmin in human plasma, *Biochem. J.,* 159, 545, 1976.
10. **Norman, P. S. and Hill, B. M.,** Studies on the plasmin system. III. Physical properties of the two plasmin inhibitors in plasma, *J. Exp. Med.,* 108, 639, 1958.
11. **Schwick, H. G., Heimburger, N., and Haupt, H.,** Antiproteasen des Human-serums, *Z. Inn. Med.,* 21, 1, 1966.
12. **Rimon, A., Shamash, Y., and Shapiro, B.,** The plasmin inhibitor of human plasma. IV. Its action on plasmin, trypsin, chymotrypsin and thrombin, *J. Biol. Chem.,* 241, 5102, 1966.

13. **Müllertz, S.,** Different molecular forms of plasminogen and plasmin produced by urokinase in human plasma and their relation to protease inhibitors and lysis of fibrinogen and fibrin, *Biochem. J.*, 143, 273, 1974.
14. **Müllertz, S.,** Molecular forms of plasmin and protease inhibitors in human fibrinolytic post-mortem plasma, *Scand. J. Clin. Lab. Invest.*, 30, 369, 1972.
15. **Aoki, N. and von Kaulla, K. N.,** Human serum plasminogen antiactivator: its distinction from antiplasmin, *Am. J. Physiol.*, 220, 1137, 1971.
16. **Collen, D. and Vermylen, J.,** Metabolism of iodine-labeled plasminogen during streptokinase and reptilase therapy in man, *Thromb. Res.*, 2, 239, 1973.
17. **Gallimore, M. J. and Hedner, U.,** Further evidence for the presence of two plasma inhibitors of fibrinolysis distinct from α_2-macroglobulin, *Thromb. Res.*, 11, 267, 1977.
18. **Hedner, U.,** Studies on an inhibitor of plasminogen activation in human serum, *Thromb. Diath. Haemorrh.*, 30, 414, 1973.
19. **Hedner, U. and Collen, D.,** Immunochemical distinction between the inhibitors of plasminogen activation and antiplasmin in human plasma, *Thromb. Res.*, 8, 875, 1976.
20. **Gallimore, M. J.,** Serum inhibitors of fibrinolysis, *Br. J. Haematol.*, 31, 217, 1975.
21. **Wiman, B. and Collen, D.,** Purification and characterization of human antiplasmin, the fast-acting plasmin inhibitor in plasma, *Eur. J. Biochem.*, 78, 19, 1977.
22. **Collen, D., Nauwelaers, F., and Wiman, B.,** Isolation and partial characterization of antiplasmin, the fast-reacting plasmin inhibitor of human plasma, in *Progress in Chemical Fibrinolysis and Thrombolysis,* Vol. 3, Davidson, J. F., Rowan, R. M., Samama, M. M., and Desnoyers, P. C., Eds., Raven Press, New York 1978, 243.
23. **Edy, J., De Cock, F., and Collen, D.,** Inhibition of plasmin by normal and antiplasmin depleted human plasma, *Thromb. Res.*, 8, 513, 1976.
24. **Edy, J., Collen, D., and Verstraete, M.,** Quantitation of the plasma protease inhibitor antiplasmin with the chromogenic substrate S-2251, in *Progress in Chemical Fibrinolysis and Thrombolysis,* Vol. 3, Davidson, J. F., Rowan, R. M., Samama, M. M., and Desnoyers, P. C., Eds., Raven Press, New York, 1978, 315.
25. **Teger-Nilsson, A. C., Friberger, P., and Gyzander, E.,** Determination of a new rapid plasmin inhibitor in human blood by means of a plasmin specific tripeptide substrate, *Scand. J. Clin. Lab. Invest.*, 37, 403, 1977.
26. **Moroi, M. and Aoki, N.,** On the interaction of α_2-plasmin inhibitor and proteases. Evidence for the formation of a covalent crosslinkage and noncovalent weak bondings between the inhibitor and proteases, *Biochim. Biophys. Acta,* 482, 412, 1977.
27. **Moroi, M. and Aoki, N.,** Inhibition of proteases in coagulation kinin-forming and complement systems by α_2-plasmin inhibitor, *J. Biochem. (Tokyo),* 82, 969, 1977.
28. **Edy, J. and Collen, D.,** The interaction in human plasma of antiplasmin, the fast-reacting plasmin inhibitor, with plasmin, thrombin, trypsin and chymotrypsin, *Biochim. Biophys. Acta,* 484, 423, 1977.
29. **Ohlsson, K. and Collen, D.,** Comparison of the reaction of neutral granulocyte proteases with the major plasma protease inhibitors and with antiplasmin, *Scand J. Clin. Lab. Invest.*, 37, 345, 1977.
30. **Christensen, U. and Clemmensen, I.,** Kinetic properties of the primary inhibitor of plasmin from human plasma, *Biochem. J.*, 163, 389, 1977.
31. **Wiman, B. and Collen, D.,** On the kinetics of the reaction between human antiplasmin and plasmin, *Eur. J. Biochem.*, 84, 573, 1978.
32. **Wiman, B., Boman, L., and Collen, D.,** On the kinetics of the reaction between human antiplasmin and a low molecular weight form of plasmin, *Eur. J. Biochem.*, 87, 143, 1978.
33. **Sottrup-Jensen, L., Claeys, H., Zajdel, M., Petersen, T. E., and Magnusson, S.,** The primary structure of human plasminogen: isolation of two lysine-binding fragments and one "mini"-plasminogen (M.w. 38,000) by elastase-catalyzed-specific limited proteolysis, in *Progress in Chemical Fibrinolysis and Thrombolysis,* Vol. 3, Davidson, J. F., Rowan, R. M., Samama, M. M., and Desnoyers, P. C., Eds., Raven Press, New York, 1978, 191.
34. **Verstraete, M., Vermylen, J., and Schetz, J.,** Intermittent administration of streptokinase, *Thromb. Haemost.*, 39, 61, 1978.
35. **Wiman, B. and Collen, D.,** Molecular mechanism of physiological fibrinolysis, *Nature (London),* 272, 549, 1978.
36. **Alkjaersig, N.,** The purification and properties of human plasminogen, *Biochem. J.*, 93, 171, 1964.
37. **Abiko, Y., Iwamoto, M., and Tomikawa, M.,** Plasminogen-plasmin system. V. A stoichiometric equilibrium complex of plasminogen and a synthetic inhibitor, *Biochim. Biophys. Acta,* 185, 424, 1969.
38. **Iwamoto, M.,** Plasminogen-plasmin system. IX. Specific binding of tranexamic acid to plasmin, *Thromb. Diath. Haemorrh.*, 33, 573, 1975.

39. **Wiman, B. and Wallén, P.**, The specific interaction between plasminogen and fibrin. A physiological role of the lysine binding site in plasminogen, *Thromb. Res.*, 10, 213, 1977.
40. **Thorsen, S.**, Differences in the binding to fibrin of native plasminogen and plasminogen modified by proteolytic degradation. Influence of omega-amino-carboxylic acids, *Biochim. Biophys. Acta*, 393, 55, 1975.
41. **Rakoczi, I., Wiman, B., and Collen, D.**, On the biological significance of the specific interaction between fibrin, plasminogen and antiplasmin, *Biochim. Biophys. Acta*, 540, 295, 1978.
42. **Moroi, M. and Aoki, N.**, Inhibition of plasminogen binding to fibrin by α_2-plasmin inhibitor, *Thromb. Res.*, 10, 851, 1977.
43. **Alkjaersig, N., Fletcher, A. P., and Sherry, S.**, The mechanism of clot dissolution by plasmin, *J. Clin. Invest.*, 38, 1086, 1959.
44. **Collen, D. and Wiman, B.**, Turnover of antiplasmin, the fast-acting plasmin inhibitor of plasma, *Blood*, 53, 313, 1979.
45. **Collen, D., Billiau, A., Edy, J., and De Somer, P.**, Identification of the human plasma protein which inhibits fibrinolysis associated with malignant cells, *Biochim. Biophys. Acta*, 499, 194, 1977.
46. **Collen, D. and De Cock, F.**, Emergence in plasma during activation of the coagulation or fibrinolytic system of neoantigens associated with the complexes of thrombin or plasmin with their inhibitors, *Thrombos. Res.*, 5, 777, 1974.
47. **Collen, D. and De Cock, F.**, A tanned red cell hemagglutination inhibition immunoassay (TRCHII) for the quantitative estimation of thrombin-antithrombin III and plasmin-α_1-antiplasmin complexes in human plasma, *Thrombos. Res.*, 7, 235, 1975.
48. **Collen, D., De Cock, F., Cambiaso, L., and Masson, P.**, A latex agglutination test for rapid quantitative estimation of the plasmin-antiplasmin complex in human plasma, *Eur. J. Clin. Invest.*, 7, 21, 1977.
49. **Harpel, P. C.**, Human α_2-macroglobulin, in *Methods in Enzymology*, Vol. 45, Lorand, L., Ed., Academic Press, New York, 1976, chap. 52.
50. **Laurell, C.-B. and Jeppsson, J. O.**, Protease inhibitors in plasma, in *The Plasma Proteins*, Vol. 1, 2nd ed., Putnam, F. W., Ed., Academic Press, New York, 1975, chap. 5.
51. **Barret, A. J., Starkey, P. M., and Munn, E. A.**, The unique nature of the interaction of α_2-macroglobulin with proteinases, in *Proteinase Inhibitors*, Fritz, H., Tschesche, H., Greene, L. J., and Truscheit, E., Eds., Springer-Verlag, Berlin, 1974.
52. **Barret, A. J. and Starkey, P. M.**, The interaction of alpha 2-macroglobulin with proteinases. Characteristics and specificity of the reaction, and a hypothesis concerning its molecular mechanism, *Biochem. J.*, 133, 709, 1973.
53. **Harpel, P. C.**, Studies on human plasma alpha 2-macroglobulin-enzyme interactions. Evidence for proteolytic modification of the subunit chain structure, *J. Exp. Med.*, 138, 508, 1973.
54. **Roberts, R. C., Riesen, W. A., and Hall, P. K.**, Studies on the quaternary structure of human serum α_2-macroglobulin, in *Proteinase Inhibitors*, Fritz, H., Tschesche, H., Greene, L. J., and Truscheit, F., Eds., Springer-Verlag, Berlin, 1974, 63.
55. **Scolari, L., Picard, J. J., and Heremans, J. F.**, Quantitative determination of human alpha 2-macroglobulin by means of immunoelectrophoresis in antibody-containing gel, *Clin. Chim. Acta*, 19, 25, 1968.
56. **Ganrot, P. O.**, Determination of alpha-2-macroglobulin as trypsin-protein esterase, *Clin. Chim. Acta*, 14, 493, 1966.
57. **Heimburger, N., Heide, K., Haupt, H., and Schultze, H. E.**, Bausteinanalysen von Humanserumproteinen, *Clin. Chim. Acta*, 10, 293, 1964.
58. **Hamberg, U., Stelwagen, P., and Ervast, H. S.**, Human alpha-2-macroglobulin, characterization and trypsin binding. Purification methods, trypsin and plasmin complex formation, *Eur. J. Biochem.*, 40, 439, 1973.
59. **Ganrot, P. O. and Scherstén, B.**, Serum alpha-2-macroglobulin concentration and its variation with age and sex, *Clin. Chim. Acta*, 15, 113, 1967.
60. **Laurell, C.-B.**, A screening test of α_1-antitrypsin deficiency, *Scand. J. Clin. Lab. Invest.*, 29, 247, 1972.
61. **Niléhn, J. E. and Ganrot, P. O.**, Plasmin, plasmin inhibitors and degradation products of fibrinogen in human serum during and after intravenous infusion of streptokinase, *Scand. J. Clin. Lab. Invest.*, 20, 113, 1967.
62. **Arnesen, H. and Fagerhol, M. K.**, α_2-Macroglobulin, α_1-antitrypsin, and antithrombin III in plasma and serum during fibrinolytic therapy with urokinase, *Scand. J. Clin. Lab. Invest.*, 29, 259, 1972.
63. **Ohlsson, K.**, Interaction between endogenous proteases and plasma protease inhibitors in vitro and in vivo, in *Proteinase Inhibitors*, Fritz, H., Tschesche, H., Greene, L. J., and Truscheit, F., Eds., Springer-Verlag, Berlin, 1974, 96.

64. **Collen, D. and Vermylen, J.**, Metabolism of iodine-labeled plasminogen during streptokinase and reptilase therapy in man, *Thromb. Res.*, 2, 239, 1973.
65. **Steinbuch, M.**, Les antiproteases du plasma, *Rev. Fr. Transfus.*, 14, 61, 1971.
66. **Highsmith, R. F. and Rosenberg, R. D.**, The inhibition of human plasmin by human antithrombin-heparin cofactor, *J. Biol. Chem.*, 249, 4335, 1974.
67. **Semeraro, N., Colucci, M., Telesforo, P., and Collen, D.**, The inhibition of plasmin by antithrombin-heparin complex. I. In human plasma in vitro, *Br. J. Haematol.*, 39, 91, 1978.
68. **Collen, D., Semeraro, N., Telesforo, P., and Verstraete, M.**, The inhibition of plasmin by antithrombin III-heparin complex. II. During thrombolytic therapy in man, *Br. J. Haematol.*, 39, 101, 1978.
69. **Johnson, S. A. and Schneider, C. L.**, Existence of antifibrinolysin activity in platelets, *Science*, 117, 229, 1953.
70. **Den Ottolander, G. J., Leijnse, B., and Cremer-Elfrink, H. M.**, Plasmatic and platelet anti-plasmins and anti-activators, *Thromb. Diath. Haemorrh.*, 18, 404, 1967.
71. **Ekert, H., Friedlander, I., and Hardisty, R. M.**, The role of platelets in fibrinolysis. Studies on the plasminogen activator and anti-plasmin activity of platelets, *Br. J. Haematol.*, 18, 575, 1970.
72. **McDonagh, J., Kiesselbach, T. H., and Wagner, R. H.**, Factor 13 and antiplasmin activity in human platelets, *Am. J. Physiol.*, 216, 508, 1969.
73. **Ganguly, P.**, A low molecular weight antiplasmin of human blood platelets, *Clin. Chim. Acta*, 39, 466, 1972.
74. **Mui, P. T., James, H. L., and Ganguly, P.**, Isolation and properties of a low molecular weight antiplasmin of human blood platelets and serum, *Br. J. Haematol.*, 29, 627, 1975.
75. **Fritz, H., Tschesche, H., Greene, L. J., and Truscheit, E., Eds.**, *Proteinase Inhibitors*, Springer-Verlag, Berlin, 1974.
76. **Vogel, R., Trautschold, I., and Werle, E.**, *Natural Proteinase Inhibitors*, Academic Press, New York, 1968.
77. **Kraut, H., Frey, E. K., and Bauer, E.**, Ueber ein neues Kreislaufhormon, *Z. Physiol. Chem.*, 175, 97, 1928.
78. **Kunitz, M. and Northrop, J. H.**, Isolation from beef pancreas of crystalline trypsinogen, trypsin, trypsin inhibitor, and inhibitor-trypsin compound, *J. Gen. Physiol.*, 19, 991, 1936.
79. **Kassell, B., Radicevic, M., Berlow, S., Peanasky, R. J., and Laskowski, M., Sr.**, The basic trypsin inhibitor of bovine pancreas. I. An improved method of preparation and amino acid composition, *J. Biol. Chem.*, 238, 3274, 1963.
80. **Avineri-Goldman, R., Snir, I., Blauer, G., and Rigbi, M.**, Studies on the basic trypsin inhibitor of bovine pancreas and its interaction with trypsin, *Arch. Biochem. Biophys.*, 121, 107, 1967.
81. **Fritz, H., Gebhardt, M., Fink, E., Schramm, W., and Werle, E.**, Verwendung wasserunloslicher Enzymharze mit polyanionischer und polyamphoterer Harzmatrix zur Isolierung von Proteaseinhibitoren, *Z. Physiol. Chem.*, 350, 129, 1969.
82. **Werle, E. and Kaufmann-Boetsch, B.**, On the esterase effects of kallikrein and trypsin and their inhibition by kallikrein- and trypsin inhibitors, *Z. Physiol. Chem.*, 319, 52, 1960.
83. **Chauvet, J., Nouvel, G., and Acher, R.**, Structure primaire d'un inhibiteur pancreatique de la trypsine (inhibiteur de Kunitz et Northrop). II. Caracterisation des peptides resultant de l'hydrolyse trypsique, *Biochim. Biophys. Acta*, 115, 130, 1966.
84. **Kassel, B., Radicevic, V., Ansfield, M. J., and Laskowski, M.**, The basic trypsin inhibitor of bovine pancreas. IV. The linear sequence of the 58 amino acids, *Biochem. Biophys. Res. Commun.*, 18, 255, 1965.
85. **Anderer, F. A. and Hörnle, S.**, The disulfide linkages in kallikrein inactivator of bovine lung, *J. Biol. Chem.*, 241, 1568, 1966.
86. **Lazdunski, M., Vincent, J. P., Schweitz, H., Peron-Renner, M., and Pudles, J.**, Mechanism of association of trypsin (or chymotrypsin) with the pancreatic trypsin inhibitors (Kunitz and Kazal). Kinetics and thermodynamics of the interaction, in *Proteinase Inhibitors*, Fritz, H., Tschesche, H., Greene, L. J., and Truscheit, E., Eds., Springer-Verlag, Berlin, 1974, 420.
87. **Rühlman, A., Schwager, P., Kukla, D., Bartels, K., and Hubner, R.**, Structure of the complex formed by bovine trypsin and bovine pancreatic trypsin inhibitor. Refinement of the crystal structure analysis, in *Proteinase Inhibitors*, Fritz, H., Tschesche, H., Greene, L. J., and Truscheit, E., Eds., Springer-Verlag, Berlin, 1974, 497.
88. **Verstraete, M., Ed.**, Report on aprotinin: Trasylol, in *Hemostatic Drugs. A Critical Appraisal*, Martinus Nijhoff, The Hague, The Netherlands, 1977, 108.
89. **Trapnell, J. E., Rigby, C. C., and Talbot, C. H.**, A controlled trial of Trasylol in the treatment of acute pancreatitis, *Br. J. Surg.*, 61, 177, 1974.
90. **McMichan, J. C.**, Post Traumatic Syndrome, Ph.D. thesis, Monash University, Melbourne, Australia, 1976.
91. **Astrup, T. and Sterndorff, I.**, Plasminogen activator in urine and urinary trypsin inhibitor, *Scand. J. Clin. Lab. Invest.*, 7, 239, 1955.

92. **Shulman, N. R.**, Proteolytic inhibitor with anticoagulant activity separated from human urine and plasma, *J. Biol. Chem.*, 213, 655, 1955.
93. **Proksch, G. J., Lane, J., and Nordschow, C. D.**, Interrelation of the urinary trypsin inhibitor to human plasma, *Clin. Biochem.*, 6, 200, 1973.
94. **Hochstrasser, K., Feuth, H., and Hochgesand, K.**, Proteinase inhibitors of the respiratory tract: studies on the structural relationship between acid-stable inhibitors present in the respiratory tract, plasma and urine, in *Proteinase Inhibitors,* Fritz, H., Tschesche, H., Greene, L. J., and Truscheit, E., Eds., Springer-Verlag, Berlin, 1974, 111.
95. **Colowick, S. P. and Kaplan, N. O., Eds. in Chief**, *Methods in Enzymology,* Vol. 45 (Part B), Lorand, L., Ed., Academic Press, New York, 1976.
96. **Umezawa, H.**, Structures and activities of protease inhibitors of microbial origin, in *Methods in Enzymology,* Vol. 45 (Part B), Lorand, L., Ed., Academic Press, New York, 1976, 678.
97. **Hozumi, M., Ogawa, M., Sugimura, T., Takeuchi, T., and Umezawa, H.**, Inhibition of tumorigenesis in mouse skin by leupeptin, a protease inhibitor from *Actinomycetes, Cancer Res.*, 32, 1725, 1972.
98. **Birk, Y.**, Trypsin and chymotrypsin inhibitors from soybeans, in *Methods in Enzymology,* Vol. 45 (Part B), Lorand, L., Ed., Academic Press, New York, 1976, 700.
99. **Kowalski, D., Leary, T. R., McKee, R. E., Sealock, R. W., Wang, D., and Laskowski, M., Jr.**, Replacements, insertions and modifications of amino-acid residues in the reactive site of soybean trypsin inhibitor (Kunitz), in *Proteinase Inhibitors,* Fritz, H., Tschesche, H., Greene, L. J., and Truscheit, E., Eds., Springer-Verlag, Berlin, 1974, 311.
100. **Janin, J., Sweet, R. M., and Blow, D. M.**, The mode of action of soybean trypsin inhibitor as revealed by crystal structure analysis of the complex with porcine trypsin, in *Proteinase Inhibitors,* Fritz, H., Tschesche, H., Greene, L. J., and Truscheit, E., Eds., Springer-Verlag, Berlin, 1974, 513.
101. **Jansen, E. F., Nutting, M. D. F., Jang, R., and Balls, A. K.**, Mode of inhibition of chymotrypsin by diisopropylfluorophosphate: introduction of isopropyl and elimination of fluorine as hydrogen fluoride, *J. Biol. Chem.*, 185, 209, 1950.
102. **Chase, T., Jr. and Shaw, E.**, *p*-Nitrophenyl-*p*′-guanidinobenzoate HCl: a new active site titrant for trypsin, *Biochem. Biophys. Res. Commun.*, 29, 508, 1967.
103. **Shaw, E., Mares-Guia, M., and Cohen, W.**, Evidence for an active-center histidine in trypsin through use of a specific reagent, 1-chloro-3-tosyl-amido-7-amino-2-heptanone, the chloromethyl ketone derived from *N*-alpha-tosyl-L-lysine, *Biochemistry,* 4, 2219, 1965.
104. **Groskopf, W. R., Hsieh, B., Summaria, L., and Robbins, K. C.**, Studies on the active center of human plasmin. The serine and histidine residues, *J. Biol. Chem.*, 244, 359, 1969.
105. **Bachmann, F.**, Development of antibodies against perorally and rectally administered streptokinase in man, *J. Lab. Clin. Med.*, 72, 228, 1968.
106. **Verstraete, M., Vermylen, J., Amery, A., and Vermylen, C.**, Thrombolytic therapy with streptokinase using a standard dosage scheme, *Br. Med. J.*, 1, 454, 1966.
107. **Johnson, A. J. and McCarty, N. R.**, The lysis of artificially induced intravascular clots in man by intravenous infusions of streptokinase, *J. Clin. Invest.*, 38, 1627, 1959.
108. **Hedner, U.**, Inhibitors of the plasminogen activation by urokinase in human serum, in *Thrombosis and Urokinase,* Paoletti, R. and Sherry, S., Eds., Academic Press, London, 1977, 119.
109. **Hedner, U. and Gallimore, M.**, Two human immunochemically distinct low molecular fibrinolytic inhibitors, *Thromb. Haemost.*, 38, 145, 1977.
110. **Gallimore, M. J.**, Inter-α-antiplasmin: its distinction from antiactivator, *Thromb. Res.*, in press.
111. **Harpel, P. C.**, $C\bar{1}$ inactivator, *Methods Enzymol.*, 45, 751, 1976.
112. **Clemmensen, I. and Christensen, F.**, Inhibition of urokinase by complex formation with human α_1-antitrypsin, *Biochim. Biophys. Acta,* 429, 591, 1976.
113. **Ogston, D., Bennet, B., Herbert, R. J., and Douglas, A. S.**, The inhibition of urokinase by alpha 2-macroglobulin, *Clin. Sci.*, 44, 73, 1973.
114. **Abiko, Y. and Iwamoto, M.**, Plasminogen-plasmin system. VII. Potentiation of antifibrinolytic action of a synthetic inhibitor, tranexamic acid, by α_2-macroglobulin antiplasmin, *Biochim. Biophys. Acta,* 214, 411, 1970.
115. **Helle, I.**, Fibrinolysis and coagulation. Effect of calcium and of coagulation on the lysis of fibrin clots, *Scand. J. Haematol. Suppl.*, 4, 1968.
116. **Bennet, N. B.**, Further studies on an inhibitor of plasminogen activation in human serum. Release of the inhibitor during coagulation and thrombus formation, *Thromb. Diath. Haemorrh.*, 23, 553, 1970.
117. **Thorsen, S.**, The inhibition of tissue plasminogen activator and urokinase-induced fibrinolysis by some natural proteinase inhibitors and by plasma and serum from normal and pregnant subjects, *Scand. J. Clin. Lab. Invest.*, 31, 51, 1973.

118. **Fletcher, A. P., Biederman, O., Moore, D., Alkjaersig, N., and Sherry, S.,** Abnormal plasminogen-plasmin system activity (fibrinolysis) in patients with hepatic cirrhosis: its cause and consequences, *J. Clin. Invest.,* 43, 681, 1964.
119. **Tytgat, G., Collen, D., and De Vreker, R. A.,** Investigations on the fibrinolytic system in liver cirrhosis, *Acta Haematol.,* 40, 265, 1968.
120. **Fletcher, A. P., Alkjaersig, N., Sherry, S., Genton, E., Hirsch, J., and Bachmann, F.,** The development of urokinase as a thrombolytic agent. Maintenance of a sustained thrombolytic state in man by its intravenous infusion, *J. Lab. Clin. Med.,* 65, 713, 1965.
121. **Thorsen, S., Brakman, P., and Astrup, T.,** Influence of platelets on fibrinolysis: a critical review, in *Hematologic Reviews,* Vol. 3, Ambrus, J. L., Ed., Marcel Dekker, New York, 1972, 123.
122. **Den Ottolander, G. J. H., Leynse, B., and Cremer-Elfrink, H. M. J.,** Plasmatic and platelet antiplasmins and anti-activators, *Thromb. Diath. Haemorrh.,* 21, 26, 1969.
123. **Murray, J., Crawford, G. P. M., Ogston, D., and Douglas, A. S.,** Studies on an inhibitor of plasminogen activators in human platelets, *Br. J. Haematol.,* 26, 661, 1974.
124. **Moore, S., Pepper, D. S., and Cash, J. D.,** The isolation and characterization of a platelet-specific β-globulin (β-thromboglobulin) and the detection of anti-urokinase and antiplasmin released from thrombin-aggregated washed human platelets, *Biochim. Biophys. Acta,* 379, 360, 1975.
125. **Dubber, A. H. C., McNicol, G. P., Uttley, D., and Douglas, A. S.,** In vitro and in vivo studies with Trasylol, an anticoagulant and a fibrinolytic inhibitor, *Br. J. Haematol.,* 14, 31, 1968.
126. **Bernik, M. B. and Kwaan, H. C.,** Inhibitors of fibrinolysis in human tissues in culture, *Am. J. Physiol.,* 221, 916, 1971.
127. **Kawano, T., Morimoto, K., and Uemura, Y.,** Partial purification and properties of urokinase inhibitor from human placenta, *J. Biochem.,* 67, 333, 1970.
128. **Uszynski, M. and Abildgaard, U.,** Separation and characterization of two fibrinolytic inhibitors from human placenta, *Thromb. Diath. Haemorrh.,* 25, 580, 1971.
129. **Aoki, N. and Kawano, T.,** Inhibition of plasminogen activators by naturally occurring inhibitors in man, *Am. J. Physiol.,* 223, 1334, 1972.
130. **Landmann, N. and Markwardt, F.,** Irreversibele synthetische Inhibitoren der Urokinase, *Experientia,* 26, 145, 1970.
131. **Ong, E. B., Johnson, A. J., and Schoellmann, G.,** Identification of an active site histidine in urokinase, *Biochim. Biophys. Acta,* 429, 252, 1976.
132. **Hijikata, A., Fujimoto, K., Kitaguchi, H., and Okamoto, S.,** Some properties of the plasminogen activator from the pig heart, *Thromb. Res.,* 4, 731, 1974.
133. **Reddy, K. N. N. and Markus, G.,** Mechanism of activation of human plasminogen by streptokinase, *J. Biol. Chem.,* 247, 1683, 1972.
134. **Okamoto, S., Oshiba, S., Mihara, H., and Okamoto, H.,** Synthetic inhibitors of fibrinolysis: in vitro and in vivo mode of action, in Chemistry pharmacology, and clinical applications of proteinase inhibitors, *Ann. N.Y. Acad. Sci.,* 146, 414, 1968.
135. **Verstraete, M., Ed.,** *Haemostatic Drugs : a Critical Appraisal,* Martinus Nijhoff, The Hague, 1977.
136. **Claeys, H. and Vermylen, J.,** Physicochemical and proenzyme properties of NH_2-terminal glutamic acid and NH_2-terminal lysine human plasminogen. Influence of 6-aminohexanoic acid, *Biochim. Biophys. Acta,* 342, 351, 1974.
137. **Wallén, P. and Wiman, B.,** On the generation of intermediate plasminogen and its significance for activation, in *Proteases and Biological Control,* Reich, E., Rifkin, D. B., and Shaw, E., Eds., Cold Spring Harbor Laboratory, Cold Spring Harbor, N.Y., 1975, 291.
138. **Wallén, P.,** Activation of plasminogen with urokinase and tissue activator, in *Thrombosis and Urokinase,* Paoletti, R. and Sherry, S., Eds., Academic Press, London, 1977, 91.
139. **Thorsen, S.,** Human Urokinase and Porcine Tissue Plasminogen Activator, Ph.D. Thesis, University of Copenhagen, 1977.
140. **Sjöholm, I., Wiman, B., and Wallén, P.,** Studies on the conformational changes of plasminogen induced during activation to plasmin and by 6-aminohexanoic acid, *Eur. J. Biochem.,* 39, 471, 1973.
141. **Wiman, B. and Wallén, P.,** Structural relationship between "glutamic acid" and "lysine" forms of human plasminogen and their interaction with NH_2-terminal activation peptide as studied by affinity chromatography, *Eur. J. Biochem.,* 50, 489, 1975.
142. **Thorsen, S., Glas-Greenwalt, P., and Astrup, T.,** Differences in the binding to fibrin of urokinase and tissue plasminogen activator, *Thromb. Diath. Haemorrh.,* 28, 65, 1972.

Chapter 7

ORIGIN OF PLASMINOGEN AND METABOLIC FATE

Robert F. Highsmith

Table of Contents

I. INTRODUCTION

Plasminogen, the inactive zymogen of the fibrinolytic enzyme plasmin, is a plasma protein whose levels in normal plasma are maintained relatively constant at approximately 0.2 mg/mℓ. Despite numerous interesting animal studies, the elucidation of the specific site of production of this substance in the human remains obscure; however, significant insights into the dynamics of its turnover have been achieved under a wide variety of physiological and pathological conditions. In addition, the metabolic turnover properties of purified preparations of plasminogen which vary considerably in amino-terminal residues, isoelectric points, and electrophoretic mobilities have been analyzed. Of particular interest to thrombolytic therapy are the quantitative studies which have now been completed on the metabolic fate of the plasminogen molecule during therapeutic fibrinolysis.

This chapter will be concerned with an evaluation of recent investigations on the synthesis of plasminogen and the metabolic parameters which govern its circulating level. Both human and animal studies will be reviewed only as they relate to this zymogen. The physiological factors regulating plasma fibrinolytic activity, such as plasminogen activator and antiplasmin, will be dealt with in Chapters 2 and 8, respectively.

II. ORIGIN OF PLASMINOGEN

During the past 10 to 15 years, research pertaining to the fibrinolytic zymogen, plasminogen, has centered on the biochemical characterization of this molecule, following its purification from both human and animal plasmas. Since the development of improved isolation and assay techniques, a wide variety of excellent basic studies have now been completed on the mechanism of plasminogen activation by the pharmacological activators, urokinase and streptokinase. However, relatively few physiological investigations have been undertaken to elucidate the anabolic and catabolic pathways for this zymogen. These studies are of great importance, since the activity of the fibrinolytic enzyme system, while partially regulated by circulating plasminogen activator and protease inhibitors, is ultimately limited by the availability of endogenous plasminogen.

The primary site of synthesis of plasminogen has not been firmly established in any species to date. However, several studies have provided indirect evidence which suggests both considerable species variation as well as possible multiple sites of synthesis and/or storage.

Investigations utilizing radioactive isotopes and isolated organ perfusion techniques have supported the view that the liver is the primary locus for the synthesis of nearly all of the plasma proteins. Included in this group are all of the commonly known procoagulants with the exception of Factor VIII, whose additional, extrahepatic source of production has now been well documented.[1] The role of the liver in plasminogen metabolism remains unclear, as evidenced by the complexity of the relationship of the fibrinolytic system as a whole to human liver function. While the normal liver is apparently devoid of fibrinolytic activity,[2] the increased activity seen in cirrhosis has been speculated to occur secondary to cellular destruction and release of plasminogen from damaged liver cells.[3] However, an alternative explanation was offered by Fletcher, et al.,[4] who claimed that the enhanced fibrinolytic activity coincident with cirrhosis was due to an altered clearance mechanism for plasminogen activator. In 1969, Davis and Picoff[5] investigated the possible use of the circulating plasminogen level as an index of liver function. Although they found the proenzyme level was not a useful liver function test in that it did not correlate with any specific hepatic disorder, they consistently noted decreased plasminogen levels in generalized liver disease. These studies suggest a possible role of the liver in plasminogen production; however, the lowered zymogen level could also be interpreted as:

1. Impaired release of stored plasminogen by the liver
2. Production of an inhibitor to plasminogen
3. Increased catabolism of the proenzyme
4. Decreased production of plasminogen in another organ and/or tissue secondary to generalized liver disease

Several other studies suggest that the liver, while intimately involved in plasminogen metabolism in some undefined fashion, is most likely not the primary synthetic site. Using immunofluorescence techniques with a specific antiplasminogen antiserum, Barnhart andRiddle[6] have reported on the cellular localization of plasminogen within the eosinophilic granules of human bone marrow cells. They found no evidence of synthesis or storage of plasminogen in liver, spleen, lymph nodes, or lungs, except that associated with the eosinophils present in these organs. In this carefully controlled study using human marrows and biopsied tissues, the fluorescent antiplasminogen reacted with all types of the eosinophilic cell series, and the zymogen content increased dramatically until maturation had occurred. Mature eosinophils in peripheral blood stained less intensely than the developing granulocytes — an observation which the authors interpreted as evidence for the synthesis of plasminogen in the bone marrow and subsequent transport by and release from the eosinophil into the general circulation. Indirect support for this hypothesis can be found in the observation of a bleeding diathesis, possibly mediated by plasmin, which often occurs in different types of leukemia. Furthermore, in cases of eosinophilic leukemia in which morphologically abnormal granules have been found in this cell type, the most prominent autopsy finding was ventricular mural thrombi.

The studies of Barnhart and Riddle do not appear to corroborate the earlier studies of Miller et al.[7] which failed to demonstrate any α or β globulin synthesis using ^{14}C lysine uptake and functional rat carcasses as an animal model. Since plasminogen is a β globulin and these experimental animals are claimed to possess functional bone marrow tissue, one would expect evidence of some β globulin synthesis under these conditions. However, as noted by Barnhart and Riddle, the nonphysiological status of these experimental animals and their associated stress reactions might have facilitated migration of the newly formed and mature eosinophils into the tissues. In addition, other investigators have noted that approximately 20 hr are required for the maturation of eosinophils by the bone marrow before their release into the peripheral blood. Since the experiments of Miller were completed within 6 hr, it is unlikely that sufficient time had elapsed for the maturation process to be completed, and therefore no β globulin synthesis due to plasminogen production would be detectable. Also, as will be discussed in more detail later, species variation could account for these discrepancies for apparent differences in plasminogen metabolism have been recorded between the rat and other species.[8,9]

It should be emphasized that the immuno-histochemical studies of Barnhart and Riddle were performed primarily on bone marrows and tissue biopsies obtained from patients with a wide variety of clinical disorders. These pathological conditions included acute, subacute, and chronic granulocytic leukemia, Hodgkin's disease, leukocytosis, idiopathic thrombocytopenic purpura, various types of anemia, polycythemia vera, and asthmatics. Although some normal marrows and other tissues were used, one must question whether their findings, which strongly implicate bone marrow and eosinophilic granules as the site of plasminogen synthesis, represent a normal physiological process or a generalized pathological response.

Several other researchers have also reported on the cellular localization of plasminogen. Prokopowicz and Stormorken[10] have demonstrated the presence of the fibrinolytic zymogen in all types of granulocytes and not just in eosinophils. The plasminogen activity as well as the alkaline and acid protease activities of these cell types were dependent on the maturation stage. Their additional finding of a plasminogen activator in these cells confirmed those obtained earlier by Jurgens[11] and by Gans.[12] Lymphocytes were found to be devoid of any detectable proenzyme. Further studies by Prokopowicz have concentrated on the distribution of fibrinolytic activity within the subcellular fractions of human granulocytes.[13] The activity of plasminogen, plasminogen activator, and plasmin obtained on fibrin plates was distributed equally throughout all subfractions. Despite considerable heterogeneity of the fractions, the striking increase in fibrinolytic activity following subfractionation suggested the additional presence of an inhibitor in the granulocyte. This hypothesis was substantiated by analyzing dilution curves of the plasminogen activity of the subfractions which suggested that the inhibitor was primarily an antiactivator. The authors also compared the activity of plasminogen in diluted human plasma with that in corresponding amounts of leukocytes and found that the level of proenzyme in these cells was approximately twice that found in plasma. Although no evidence was presented for the ability of granulocytes to release stored plasminogen, these data may indicate biosynthesis of the zymogen. The observation that plasminogen levels in guinea pig leukocytes decreased rapidly following treatment with an inhibitor of protein synthesis substantiates this conclusion.[14]

Further indirect evidence that plasma plasminogen may be derived from granulocytes can be found in the more recent experiments conducted by Prokopowicz and Niewiarowski in which the physicochemical properties of plasma and granulocyte-derived plasminogens were compared.[15] Plasminogens from both human plasma and granulocytes, purified by DEAE-Sephadex chromatography, were shown to possess similar fibrinolytic, caseinolytic, fibrinogenolytic, and esterolytic activities. The optimum pH for activation of both zymogens was 7.0 to 7.2, and the kinetics of activation by streptokinase and urokinase were quite similar. Also, the plasmins derived from both precursors were similarly inhibited by ε-aminocaproic acid and pancreatic trypsin inhibitor.

Although the above studies strongly suggest that both plasma and granulocyte plasminogens may constitute the same proenzyme, little direct evidence has been presented to substantiate the concept that plasma plasminogen is derived from granulocytes or that these cell types are indeed capable of releasing stored zymogen into the circulation. Furthermore, the presence of plasminogen within the formed elements of the blood is not unique to the granulocyte series, for Sakuragawa[16] has detected significant levels of the fibrinolytic precursor in the hemolysates of red blood cells derived from venous blood and bone marrow. Despite a relatively high concentration of plasminogen within the granulocyte, the total amount present in the cells as compared to that in plasma (approximately 20 mg %) is relatively small and has led other investigators to search for alternative sources of plasminogen production.

Highsmith[9,17] has reported that the kidney is the primary source of plasminogen in the restoration of normal plasma levels following acute depletion of the zymogen in cats. In order to ascertain which organs were involved in the regulation of circulating plasminogen levels, cats were acutely depleted of zymogen by injection of streptokinase, and arterial-venous differences in plasminogen concentration across various organs were determined. No measurable differences were seen for the kidney, liver, spleen, brain, and heart-lung before the injection of activator which suggests that plasminogen metabolism, if occurring in any of these organs, is relatively slow under normal physiological conditions. Following rapid depletion, the plasminogen levels began to increase at 10 hr after the streptokinase injection; reestablishment of the precise preinjection level for each animal was complete by 18 hr. A similar time course of plasminogen restoration after streptokinase injection has been reported for the human.[18] The 10-hr delay before the zymogen levels began increasing suggested synthesis rather than release of stored plasminogen. After the delay, normal values were restored within about 6 to 8 hr. The authors point out that it is unlikely that this could be explained by plasminogen release from granulocytes, for it is highly improbable that enough granulocytes could be produced within this time period to account for the large increase that occurred in circulating plasminogen. These findings, however, do not rule out the participation of bone marrow and the formed elements of the blood in maintaining plasminogen levels required by normal turnover of this zymogen. The finding by Highsmith and Kline[9] of a large, negative arterial-venous difference in plasminogen concentration across the kidney during the restoration phase following acute depletion is most supportive of a major role for the kidney in plasminogen biosynthesis. Furthermore, bilateral nephrectomy blocked the return to normal plasminogen levels which consistently occurred after depletion of intact animals. Although the results of these experiments clearly implicate the kidney as an organ of major importance in plasminogen metabolism, its precise role remains undefined. For instance, the question remains unanswered as to whether the kidney synthesizes the entire plasminogen moiety *de novo* and releases it concurrently with production or, alternatively, that the renal tissue may alter an inactive precursor molecule and release it into the renal vein as a substance with plasminogen activity. It should be noted that the proposed role of the kidney in plasminogen biosynthesis by Highsmith and Kline was derived from experiments using acutely depleted cats, and it remains to be confirmed whether their conclusions are applicable to chronic situations or to the human fibrinolytic system.

Several observations have been made which raise some questions about the role of the kidney in human plasminogen biosynthesis and which also lend support to the existence of considerable species variation in this physiological mechanism. Many investigators have noted that anephric humans maintained on hemodialysis have normal levels of circulating plasminogen. Isacson and Nilsson,[19] in 1969, studied five anephric patients aged 15 to 44 years and found statistically normal plasminogen values in each as compared to normal volunteers. Siefring and Castellino,[8] using lysine-Sepharose® affinity chromatography, have qualitatively determined the level of plasminogen isozymes for anephric plasma vs. normal plasma. These data reveal that the two major forms of plasminogen found in normal human plasma are also present in anephric plasma in approximately equal amounts. It should be noted, however, that both of the above studies were done on patient plasmas which were not obtained until at least 3 months after bilateral nephrectomy was performed and thus would have permitted secondary sources of plasminogen production to become operative. In addition, the results were not expressed as a percentage of prenephrectomy values for each patient, but rather were compared to arbitrary "normal", nonnephrectomized values.

Some further preliminary data have been obtained on the question as to whether the acute animal experiments of Highsmith and Kline have any relevance to normal plasminogen metabolism in the human. These authors reported[20] that in animals which had not received streptokinase, the arterial plasminogen concentration dropped approximately 50% within 2 hr following bilateral nephrectomy. By 10 hr, the concentration of zymogen had returned to control levels. Furthermore, in two patients from whom blood samples were obtained before and after nephrectomy, the plasminogen concentrations also dropped to approximately 50% of their preoperative values within 12 hr and had returned to normal 48 hr later. Although the time course of plasminogen restoration after nephrectomy is somewhat different in the cat and human, their similarity suggests that the cat data may be applicable to the human in regard to a role for the kidney in plasminogen metabolism, but only in situations in which streptokinase was not administered and acute depletion of the zymogen was not provoked.

The more recent findings of Siefring and Castellino[8] suggest that limited *de novo* synthesis of plasminogen may occur in the absence of the kidneys. Their results were obtained by quantitating the rate of incorporation of L-[4,5-^{3}H] leucine into the two major isozymes of rat plasminogen following the injection of labeled amino acid into normal, adrenalectomized, anephric, or sham-operated control rats. The data indicate that the biosynthesis of both isozymes occurs under all of these experimental conditions. However, contrary to their conclusions, the data also clearly show that bilateral nephrectomy reduces the rate of plasminogen synthesis by approximately 65%. The authors did not state what the remaining 35% level after nephrectomy corresponded to in terms of plasma plasminogen concentration. While these findings could be translated as evidence for the kidney being the major source of plasminogen anabolism, Siefring and Castellino elected to interpret them as evidence for *de novo* synthesis of the zymogen in the absence of the kidneys. They base their opinion on a suspicion that the slower rate of plasminogen biosynthesis in nephrectomized rats is probably a result of the decreased cardiac output and systemic shock accompanying this surgical procedure. However, their data do not support this hypothesis, for the rate of leucine incorporation into plasminogen in the sham-operated control rats as well as in the adrenalectomized rats was not significantly different from that obtained in the intact, nontraumatized animal. If the decreased plasminogen synthesis was due to the poor physiological condition of the animal, certainly the rate of incorporation of leucine into plasminogen should have fallen markedly in the surgically operated, intact controls, unless the removal of the kidneys was specifically responsible for the physiological demise of the animal. Although there is no reason a priori to suspect an appreciable decrease in cardiac output under these conditions, one must know the time after nephrectomy at which the leucine incorporation study was initiated in order to evaluate this possible explanation for the decreased plasminogen biosynthesis. Siefring and Castellino did not publish that data in the paper in question, but did provide an alternative explanation for the decreased rate of plasminogen production following nephrectomy. Although the raw data of this critical experiment were not presented, they compared the rate of leucine incorporation into general plasma proteins for normal vs. nephrectomized rats and found that immediately following removal of the kidneys, the rate of protein synthesis was approximately one third of the normal value. Based on this finding, they felt that the apparently decreased rate of plasminogen biosynthesis was most likely artifactual, since the general protein synthetic rate was similarly depressed under these experimental conditions. Apparently, the effect of nephrectomy on depressing generalized protein synthesis must be acute, for they have also reported that 6 months following removal of the kidneys in the human, the anephric plasma plasminogen levels were nearly identical to that found in normal plasma. Likewise, these observations may help to explain why immediately after nephrectomy (12 hr) in the two patients studied, Kline and Highsmith[20] noted a 50% reduction in the circulating zymogen levels. While concluding that none of the circulating plasminogen is produced in the rat kidney, Siefring and Castellino did not study or hypothesize an alternate source of the zymogen in this species.

In summary, it appears that considerable species variation must be operative in regard to the origin(s) of the plasminogen molecule. The findings of Highsmith and Kline in the feline species clearly implicate the kidney as the primary source of plasminogen under conditions of acute, pharmacological depletion of the zymogen. However, using different methodologies, Siefring and Castellino[8] has demonstrated *de novo* biosynthesis of plasminogen in anephric rats, albeit at a slower rate than normal. It would appear that the human kidney may be involved in the synthesis of this molecule, since it has been shown that the plasminogen levels fall immediately after nephrectomy. On the other hand, there must be alternate sources of zymogen production under more chronic conditions, for the structure and content of plasminogen in anephric plasma several months after kidney removal is normal. One might speculate that in the absence of the kidneys, the granulocytic cells of bone marrow may become the dominant source of plasminogen in amounts sufficient to maintain normal levels. This complex story is yet to be resolved and will necessitate further comparative studies of plasminogen production under a wide variety of experimental conditions.

III. PLASMINOGEN: REGULATION OF PLASMA LEVELS

Before considering the catabolic fate of the fibrinolytic zymogen, some additional findings of Highsmith and Kline[17] on the physiological regulation of circulating plasminogen levels will be briefly discussed.

A series of cross-injection experiments in cats were designed to determine the nature of the stimulus which leads to plasminogen production and/or release following acute depletion. Donor plasma was obtained from either intact animals or from those whose plasminogen levels had been depleted for various lengths of time after streptokinase injection. The infusion of normal plasma into normal or into plasminogen-depleted recipients produced no response; however, following the infusion of plasmas obtained from donors which had been depleted for 9 hr, both the normal and the depleted recipients showed a rapid elevation in arterial plasminogen levels. Since the injection of normal plasma produced no response, these results indicate the presence of a substance in the plasma of depleted animals which stimulates the production and/or release of zymogen in the recipients. Thus, it would appear that following acute depletion, plasminogen release is mediated by a blood-borne substance rather than by plasminogen depletion per se, as evidenced by the inability of the plasma from 1- or 3-hr depleted donors to produce such a response in recipients. Apparently, the synthesis and release of this stimulating substance is complete at approximately 5 hr after plasminogen depletion. Furthermore, the data demonstrate that the kidney is intimately involved in this regulatory mechanism, for bilateral nephrectomy of the recipients abolished the response to the injected substance from donor animals. The authors have proposed that in response to acute depletion, a negative feedback control system mediated by a plasma factor results in the restoration of normal circulating plasminogen levels. Although these results have not been confirmed by others, it is interesting to note that Friedman et al.,[21] using a similar cross-injection design in rabbits, have produced evidence suggesting that coagulation factor levels may be regulated by a plasma factor which they termed "coagulopoietin". In previous experiments,[22] they have shown that the vitamin-K dependent clotting proteins, Factors II, VII, IX, and X, may be subject to similar regulatory mechanisms, as evidenced by the elevation of these factors in recipient animals following the injection of plasma from coumadin-treated donors.

From the evidence reviewed above, it appears that the plasma levels of some procoagulants as well as the fibrinolytic precursor, plasminogen, are precisely regulated. In view of their biological importance in the maintenance of a fluid state within the vascular space, it would seem appropriate, if not necessary, that such a physiological mechanism exist. However, it should be noted that the models proposed by Highsmith[17] and by Karpatkin[21] were derived from acute animal experiments, and it remains to be established whether their conclusions are applicable to more chronic situations concerned with normal turnover of the regulated proteins or to the human coagulation and fibrinolytic systems.

IV. PLASMINOGEN: METABOLIC FATE

Considerable information has now been obtained on the metabolic fate of the plasminogen molecule. The investigations utilizing valid metabolic tracers have focused on the kinetics of the synthesis and breakdown of plasminogen in normal subjects, as well as under different experimental and clinical conditions in which abnormal turnover of the zymogen occurs.

A. Normal Plasminogen Metabolism

The level of plasminogen in normal human plasma has been determined by a number of different methods. Although the absolute concentration in plasma is dependent on which assays are used, there appears to be very little, if any, daily fluctuation nor any significant difference between male and female levels. Using a highly specific radioimmunoassay, Rabiner et al.[23] have reported normal values in the human to be 206 ± 36 (SD) $\mu g/m\ell$. This value is in good agreement with other immunological determinations and corresponds to a molar concentration of 2.2×10^{-6} *M*.

Nonimmunological measurements of plasminogen in plasma have given results which differ significantly from the above values. In general, caseinolytic and fibrinolytic assays of plasma plasminogen consistently yield lower values than those obtained by radioimmunoassay or immunodiffusion.[24] These results may indicate that a certain percentage of the zymogen circulates in a biologically inactive form; however, active-site titration of activated plasminogen purified from human plasma does not support this claim. Perhaps a more likely reason for this discrepancy is the existence of substances in plasma which retard the proteolytic activity of activated plasminogen, since the enzymatic assay of plasminogen requires its prior conversion to the active protease, plasmin. In whole plasma, this procedure is complicated by the presence of numerous protease inhibitors, most of which have been shown to possess antiplasmin activity. The pioneering observation by Milstone[25] in 1941 that fibrinolysis by hemolytic streptococcus occurred only with the addition of a "lytic factor" present in the euglobulin component of human plasma paved the way to our current usage of this plasma fraction for the measurement of blood fibrinolytic activity. Indeed, separation of plasminogen from the protease inhibitors by euglobulin fractionation or by other means is required before any measureable biological activity of the activated zymogen can be realized. However, with the advent of monospecific antisera to the human protease inhibitors and more sensitive assays, it has now been established that the frequently used euglobulin preparation is not completely devoid of inhibitor antigen. This observation was made by several authors while investigating new plasminogen assays or while noting the discrepancy between functional and immunological levels of plasminogen in plasma. Evidence by Kluft[26] has demonstrated the presence in euglobulin of considerable amounts of $C1^-$-inactivator and inter-α-trypsin inhibitor — two of the human plasma protease inhibitors which are known to inhibit plasmin in a purified system.[27,28] The increase in fibrinolytic activity of $C1^-$-inactivator-deficient plasma (hereditary angioneurotic edema) as compared to normal suggests that this inhibitor may influence the assayable fibrinolytic activity of this fraction of plasma. Furthermore, Highsmith[29] et al. have demonstrated the physical interaction of $C1^-$-inactivator with activated plasminogen in this plasma component and that more plasmin activity can be obtained from $C1^-$-inactivator-deficient euglobulin than from normal euglobulin, despite the same immunological levels of plasminogen in both samples.

Therefore, it would appear that the primary reason for the discrepancy between immunoreactive and functional levels of plasminogen in plasma is due to the presence of protease inhibitors in that component of plasma which is most frequently utilized in the assessment of blood fibrinolytic activity. Further support for this interpretation lies in the fact that the quantity of plasminogen purified from a specified volume of whole plasma agrees closely with that predicted by immunological assay of the starting material. Consequently, if absolute concentrations of plasminogen in plasma are desired, one should rely on immunological quantitation, for the amount of plasminogen obtained by proteolytic assays of the euglobulin fraction will also be determined in part by the protease inhibitor content of this fraction of plasma.

Following the injection of highly purified radiolabeled plasminogen into normal subjects, the plasma radioactivity declines logarithmically. By fitting such tracer data with a sum of two exponential terms, Collen et al.[30] have calculated various metabolic parameters from these functions using a two-compartment mammillary model. The following results were obtained for plasminogen in 12 healthy male volunteers, age 23 to 63 years; plasma radioactivity half-life of 2.21 ± 0.29 days; fractional catabolic rate constant of 0.55 ± 0.09 of the plasma pool per day; absolute catabolic rate of 4.8 ± 1.2mg/kg/day; and fractional transcapillary efflux rate of 0.38 ± 0.20 of the plasma pool per day. Although very few similar investigations have been done by others, Harker et al.[31] have reported a plasma half-life for plasminogen of 1.62 ± 0.11 days in 20 normal subjects. This value is significantly lower than that reported by Collen, but is most likely due to the use of a nonnative, labeled plasminogen molecule in the studies of Harker. In order to make valid conclusions about the in vivo behavior of any substance in plasma using radiotracer methodology, one must be certain that the labeled compound has the same physicochemical properties as the native endogenous molecule. It would appear that in Harker's studies,[32,33] the apparent use of a partially degraded form of labeled plasminogen with NH_2-terminal lysine rather than the native NH_2-terminal glutamic acid residue could account for the more rapid turnover of the zymogen than that reported by Collen. It has been demonstrated that while NH_2-terminal glutamic acid plasminogen has a half-life of 2.0 to 2.5 days, its partially degraded counterpart with NH_2-terminal lysine or valine has a value of less than 1.0 day.[34]

Another possible reason for the discrepancy in plasminogen half-life values could be explained by a variation in the sialic acid content between the different molecular forms of the zymogen used by the two investigators. It has been shown by Morell et al.[35] that the sialic acid content of glycoproteins may alter the rate at which these molecules are metabolized by the liver. Furthermore, it has been demonstrated that desialylated rabbit plasminogen has a significantly shortened survival time in the plasma of this species.[36] Although the actual sialic acid content of the plasminogens used in the tracer studies of Harker and of Collen were not reported, it appears reasonable that a variation in the content of this moiety could account for the differences in recorded half-lives.

The general catabolic pathways for the plasminogen molecule have been evaluated by studying plasminogen kinetics under pathological conditions, as well as by observing the effects of various agents on these metabolic parameters. However, before examining the breakdown of the zymogen under these nonphysiological conditions, a brief discussion on the metabolism of plasminogen during exercise will be given.

B. Plasminogen Metabolism During Exercise

The increase in euglobulin fibrinolytic activity detectable in postexercise plasma by proteolytic assay has been well documented.[37] Although the mechanism by which this increase occurs after exercise is not well understood, it appears that it is most likely due to an elevation of circulating plasminogen activator levels. During strenuous physical exercise in normal subjects, the plasma radioactivity disappearance rate of plasminogen increases markedly, as manifested by a significant shortening of the half-life for this zymogen.[38] Also of interest is the existence of a parallel increase in the disappearance rate of fibrinogen, but not of prothrombin, under the same experimental conditions of exercise. The fact that the absolute concentrations of plasminogen and fibrinogen, as well as prothrombin, do not change significantly during exercise illustrates the utility of dynamic metabolic studies in detecting changes which would not be realized by static measurements of blood concentrations. Of the many possible explanations, the increased plasminogen and fibrinogen metabolism during exercise is most likely due to specific utilization of these proteins. In fact, one might speculate that the elevation of plasminogen activator levels during exercise results in conversion of plasminogen to plasmin with resultant fibrinogenolysis. Evidence to support this view comes from the finding that exercise has no influence on the metabolism of prothrombin[38] (which is contrary to what one would expect if the increased fibrinogen turnover was due to intravascular coagulation). Also, the finding of significant Aα-chain degradation of fibrinogen in postexercise plasma lends credence to a plasminogen-plasmin-mediated fibrinogenolysis rather than a consumptive decrease in fibrinogen under these conditions. It should be noted, however, that these findings have not been solidly confirmed and may be variable with the particular type of exercise regimen used.

C. Effects of Various Agents on Plasminogen Metabolism

Studies on the effects of various agents on plasminogen turnover have provided insights into the mechanisms by which these compounds influence fibrinolysis. In addition, the use of such agents has assisted in differentiating the various catabolic pathways for plasminogen under normal as well as pathological conditions.

The primary pathway of plasminogen catabolism appears to be by generalized metabolic degradation of the zymogen rather than through activation of the proenzyme to plasmin or by consumption secondary to intravascular coagulation. Supportive evidence for this process is found in the studies on patients with Bechet's syndrome in which a low circulating plasminogen activator level is found. Despite a decreased euglobulin fibrinolytic activity and a prolonged euglobulin clot lysis time, these patients possess a normal plasminogen half-life.[30] Certainly, the rate of plasminogen metabolism as reflected by the half-life would have been significantly altered under these conditions if the primary catabolic pathway was via plasminogen activation. Likewise, attempts have been made to investigate the metabolic effects of inhibiting plasminogen activator in vivo by the administration of Trasylol® (tranexamic acid) to normal subjects. In the presence of tranexamic acid, the turnover rate of plasminogen is increased in a dose-dependent fashion.[30] One would have anticipated a decreased rate of plasminogen metabolism under these conditions if the primary catabolic pathway was through enzyme activation. However, these studies are probably not valid tests of the relative importance of the activation of plasminogen on its turnover rate, for the fibrinolytic inhibitor, tranexamic acid, like ε-aminocaproic acid, is known to induce a conformational change in the plasminogen molecule which most likely would alter its turnover.[39,40] If plasminogen were normally degraded in human plasma by enzymatic activation to plasmin, the subsequent formation of new plasmin-protease inhibitor complexes should be readily detectable. However, experimental data show that while these neoantigenic complexes are indeed present in plasma to which urokinase or streptokinase have been added, they are not present in native human plasma.[41] Therefore, there is little, if any, experimental evidence to support a major role for plasminogen activation in the normal catabolism of this zymogen. Likewise, it appears that under normal conditions, very little of the fibrinolytic zymogen is consumed secondary to in vivo coagulation, for the rate of plasminogen turnover is unchanged during heparin anticoagulation of normal subjects.[30]

Other recent studies[42] indicate that radiolabeled plasminogen may be a useful tool for the quantitation of the consumption of this zymogen for patients in whom fibrinolysis and/or fibrin formation have been induced therapeutically. The administration of streptokinase or urokinase results in the activation of the fibrinolytic system and subsequent depletion of plasminogen. The circulating half-life for the zymogen may be as short as 0.5 day under these conditions. In addition, fibrinogen levels are decreased concomitant with the appearance in plasma of fibrinogen degradation products and high molecular weight complexes of plasmin with the protease inhibitors (primarily α_2-antiplasmin). Although their efficacy remains in doubt, both streptokinase and urokinase are capable of inducing thrombolysis.

The secondary fibrinolytic response to defibrination is well documented and is presumably the mechanism by which the drug reptilase (Defibrase®) is thought to possess similar thrombolytic potential. Although plasminogen consumption and a similar shortening of the half-life of the zymogen occurs following the administration of either reptilase or the exogenous plasminogen activators, the dynamics of plasminogen turnover are different for these two agents. The enhanced disappearance rate of plasminogen following streptokinase infusion is a reflection of the metabolism of plasmin-inhibitor complexes, while that following reptilase infusion is primarily representative of the metabolism and distribution of plasminogen alone.

In conclusion, the normal kinetics of in vivo fibrinolysis and its relationship to the formation and deposition of fibrin within the cardiovascular system have just begun to be appreciated. Metabolic turnover studies done under a wide variety of physiological and pathological conditions have illustrated the utility of such dynamic studies in estimating the degree of ongoing fibrinolysis and fibrinogenolysis. With the availability of purified materials and of reliable tracer methodologies, the advantages which dynamic turnover studies provide over static blood-level measurements are profound. For example, significant in vivo fibrinolysis, as well as ongoing coagulation, can be merely suggested by measuring plasma concentrations of the respective reactants only if their rates of synthesis and degradation are grossly imbalanced. However, turnover studies using labeled tracers which are specifically consumed during the process of coagulation or fibrinolysis are very sensitive to small changes in the degrees of activation of these two systems. In fact, future studies utilizing this dynamic approach hold promise for detecting hypercoagulable and/or hyperfibrinolytic states prior to the overt manifestation of the clinical disorder.

REFERENCES

1. **Veltkamp, J. J., Asfaou, E., van der Torren, K., van der Does, A., van Tilburg, N. H., and Pauwels, E. K.,** Extrahepatic Factor VIII synthesis, *Transplantation,* 18, 56, 1974.
2. **Albrechtsen, O. K.,** The fibrinolytic activity of human tissues, *Br. J. Haematol.,* 3, 284, 1957.

3. **Astrup, T., Rasmussen, J., and Amery, A.**, Fibrinolytic activity of the cirrhotic liver, *Nature (London)*, 185, 619, 1960.
4. **Fletcher, A. P., Biederman, O., Moore, D., Alkjaersig, N., and Sherry, S.**, Abnormal plasminogen-plasmin system activity in patients with hepatic cirrhosis, *J. Clin. Invest.*, 43, 681, 1964.
5. **Davis, R. D. and Picoff, R. C.**, Low plasminogen levels and liver disease, *Am. J. Clin. Pathol.*, 52, 661, 1969.
6. **Barnhart, M. I. and Riddle, J. M.**, Cellular localization of profibrinolysin (plasminogen), *Blood*, 21, 306, 1963.
7. **Miller, L. L., Bly, C. G., and Bale, W. F.**, Plasma and tissue proteins produced by non-hepatic rat organs as studied with lysine-ε-C^{14}, *J. Exp. Med.*, 99, 133, 1954.
8. **Siefring, G. E. and Castellino, F. J.**, *De novo* biosynthesis of plasminogen in the anephric rat, *J. Appl. Physiol.*, 38, 114, 1975.
9. **Highsmith, R. F. and Kline, D. L.**, Kidney: primary source of plasminogen after acute depletion in the cat, *Science*, 174, 141, 1971.
10. **Prokopowicz, J. and Stormorken, H.**, Fibrinolytic activity of leucocytes in smears of bone marrow and peripheral blood, *Scand. J. Haematol.*, 5, 129, 1968.
11. **Jurgens, J.**, Das verhalten des fibrinolytischen systems beider leukämie, *Folia Haematol. (Frankfurt am Main)*, 8, 52, 1963.
12. **Gans, H.**, Fibrinolytic properties of proteases derived from human, dog and rabbit leukocytes, *Thromb. Diath. Haemorrh.*, 10, 379, 1964.
13. **Prokopowicz, J.**, Distribution of fibrinolytic and proteolytic enzymes in subcellular fractions of human granulocytes, *Thromb. Diath. Haemorrh.*, 19, 84, 1968.
14. **Prokopowicz, J., Rejniak, L., and Niewiarowski, S.**, Influence of cytostatic agents on fibrinolytic and proteolytic enzymes and on phagocytosis of guinea pig leucocytes, *Experientia*, 23, 813, 1967.
15. **Prokopowicz, J. and Niewiarowski, S.**, Comparative studies on the properties of human plasma and granulocyte plasminogens, *Bull. Acad. Pol. Sci.*, 16, 261, 1968.
16. **Sakuragawa, N.**, Studies on the fibrinolytic activity of red blood cells, *Acta Haematol. Japon.*, 29, 910, 1966.
17. **Highsmith, R. F. and Kline, D. L.**, Plasminogen restoration by the kidney mediated by a plasma factor, *Am. J. Physiol.*, 225, 1032, 1973.
18. **Fletcher, A. P., Alkjaersig, N., and Sherry, S.**, The maintenance of a sustained thrombolytic state in man. I. Induction and effects, *J. Clin. Invest.*, 38, 1096, 1959.
19. **Isacson, S. and Nilsson, I. M.**, The kidneys and the fibrinolytic activity in the blood, *Thromb. Diath. Haemorrh.*, 22, 211, 1969.
20. **Kline, D. L. and Highsmith, R. F.**, The regulation of blood levels of fibrinolytic enzymes, *Ser. Haematol.*, 6, 513, 1973.
21. **Friedman, E. W., Karpatkin, M., and Karpatkin, S.**, Evidence suggesting the regulation of coagulation factor levels in rabbits by a transferable plasma agent, *Blood*, 48, 949, 1976.
22. **Karpatkin, M. and Karpatkin, S.**, Evidence for a humoral agent capable of raising vitamin-K-dependent coagulation factors in rabbits, *Br. J. Haematol.*, 24, 553, 1973.
23. **Rabiner, S. F., Goldfine, I. D., Hart, A., Summaria, L., and Robbins, K. C.**, Radioimmunoassay of human plasminogen and plasmin, *J. Lab. Clin. Med.*, 74, 265, 1969.
24. **Ganrot, P. O. and Niléhn, J. E.**, Immunochemical determination of human plasminogen, *Clin. Chim. Acta*, 22, 335, 1968.
25. **Milstone, J. H.**, A factor in normal human blood which participates in streptococcal fibrinolysis, *J. Immunol.*, 42, 109, 1941.
26. **Kluft, C.**, Occurrence of C1 inactivator and other proteinase inhibitors in euglobulin fractions and their influence on fibrinolytic activity, *Haemostasis*, 5, 136, 1976.
27. **Ratnoff, O. D., Pensky, J., Ogston, D., and Naff, G. B.**, The inhibition of plasmin, plasma kallikrein, plasma permeability factor, and the C1r subcomponent of the first component of complement by serum C1-esterase inhibitor, *J. Exp. Med.*, 129, 315, 1969.
28. **Steinbuch, M., Audran, R., Reuge, C., and Blatrix, C.**, Etude d'une d-globuline contenant du zinc: la proteine π, in *Protides of the Biological Fluids*, Peeters, H., Ed., Elsevier, Amsterdam, 1966, 185.
29. **Highsmith, R. F., Burnett, C. J., and Weirich, C. J.**, The interaction of $C\bar{1}$-esterase inhibitor and plasmin in human euglobulin, *J. Lab. Clin. Med.*, 93, 459, 1979.
30. **Collen, D., Tytgat, G., Claeys, H., Verstraete, M., and Wallen, P.**, Metabolism of plasminogen in healthy subjects: effect of tranexamic acid, *J. Clin. Invest.*, 51, 1310, 1972.
31. **Harker, L. A., Schmer, G., and Slichter, S. J.**, Plasminogen kinetics in man, in *Proc. 3rd Congr. Int. Soc. Thrombosis and Haemostasis*, Washington, D.C., Abstract volume 294, 1972.
32. **Harker, L. A. and Slichter, S. J.**, Arterial and venous thromboembolism: kinetic characterization and evaluation of therapy, *Thromb. Diath. Haemorrh.*, 31, 188, 1974.

33. **Harker, L. A., Slichter, S. J., Scott, C. R., and Ross, R.,** Homocystinemia. Vascular injury and arterial thrombosis, *N. Engl. J. Med.*, 291, 537, 1974.
34. **Collen, D., Ong, E. B., and Johnson, A. J.,** Human plasminogen: *In vitro* and *in vivo* evidence for the biological integrity of NH_2-terminal glutamic acid plasminogen, *Thromb. Res.*, 7, 515, 1975.
35. **Morell, A. G., Gregoriadis, G., and Scheinberg, H.,** The role of sialic acid in determining the survival of glycoproteins in the circulation, *J. Biol. Chem.*, 246, 1461, 1971.
36. **Siefring, G. E. and Castellino, F. J.,** The role of sialic acid in the determination of distinct properties of isoenzymes of rabbit plasminogen, *J. Biol. Chem.*, 249, 7742, 1974.
37. **Prentice, C. R. M., Hassanein, A. A., McNicol, G. P., and Douglas, A. S.,** Studies on blood coagulation, fibrinolysis and platelet function following exercise in normal and splenectomized people, *Br. J. Haematol.*, 23, 541, 1972.
38. **Collen, D., Semeraro, N., Tricot, J. P., and Vermylen, J.,** Turnover of fibrinogen, plasminogen and prothrombin during exercise in man, *J. Appl. Physiol.*, 42, 865, 1977.
39. **Alkjaersig, N.,** The purification and properties of human plasminogen, *Biochem. J.*, 93, 171, 1964.
40. **Abiko, Y., Iwamoto, M., and Tomikawa, M.,** Plasminogen-plasmin system. V. A stoichiometric equilibrium complex of plasminogen and a synthetic inhibitor, *Biochim. Biophys. Acta*, 185, 424, 1969.
41. **Collen, D.,** Emergence in plasma during activation of the coagulation or fibrinolytic systems of neoantigens, associated with the complexes of thrombin or plasmin with their inhibitors, *Thromb. Res.*, 5, 777, 1974.
42. **Collen, D. and Vermylen, J.,** Metabolism of iodine-labeled plasminogen during streptokinase and reptilase therapy in man, *Thromb. Res.*, 2, 239, 1973.

Chapter 8

PHYSIOLOGY OF FIBRINOLYSIS

Inga Marie Nilsson, Ulla Hedner, and Maurizio Pandolfi

TABLE OF CONTENTS

I. INTRODUCTION

Plasminogen, the inactive precursor of plasmin, exists in the blood and, though in much lower concentration, also in practically all other body fluids. Plasminogen can be activated by an intrinsic and an extrinsic system. Knowledge of the intrinsic (humoral) plasminogen activation pathway is the result of recent studies showing evidence for the occurrence of a Factor XII-dependent pathway, a C3- (Factor XII-independent) dependent pathway,[1] a kininogen-dependent pathway,[2] and a platelet-dependent pathway.[3] The role played by these systems in pathophysiology is still largely unknown (see Chapter 8).

The extrinsic (cellular) fibrinolysis activation pathways have been studied since the early 1930s and are therefore much better understood. Interest in research in fibrinolysis at that time was aroused by Fischer's[4] observation that in vitro cultures of normal and neoplastic cells liquefy the supporting fibrin clot.

Studies using extractive and histochemical methods have revealed a complex pattern of distribution of fibrinolytic activators (plasminogen activators) in the cells of the body. Briefly, tissue plasminogen activator is contained in the endothelium of many vessels (small arteries and veins, some large veins, such as the renal vein and vena cava, and lymphatics) and in several types of epithelium and mesothelium, such as corneal and conjunctival epithelium, pleural mesothelium, uterine and vaginal epithelium, and epithelium of the urinary tract. The subject has recently been reviewed by Pandolfi[5] and Astrup.[6] It is not clear why the endothelium of some vessels is fibrinolytically active, but not that of others. Lack of activity may be due to absence of plasminogen activator in the endothelial cells or coexistence of inhibitors of fibrinolysis.[7] It is noteworthy that fibrinolytic activity may vary in a given structure during life. This applies both to vascular endothelium and epithelium. Thus it has been found that during embryogenesis, fibrinolytic activity in the wall of a vessel may vary with the stage of development of the fetus.[8] In other cells, such as the vaginal epithelium, the fibrinolytic activity varies with the phase of the cycle. It is high in early estrus and disappears in late estrus, a variation apparently under hormonal control.[9] Cellular maturation appears to influence the activity of other cells, such as epithelial cells in the buccal mucosa, whose activity is highest at desquamation.[10] It has also been possible to show that a moderate difference in fibrinolytic activity occurs in homologous vessels according to their location. Thus the fibrinolytic activity of the superficial veins of the arms is clearly higher than that of the corresponding veins of the legs.[11] Recently Nicolaides et al.[12] found the fibrinolytic activity of the vein walls to vary in one and the same limb. Thus the fibrinolytic activity in the wall of the plantar vein was significantly lower than in that of the femoral or popliteal vein.

There is evidence that fibrinolytically active cells continuously release plasminogen activator into the fluids with which they are in contact. The most apparent release is that of the vascular endothelium which is responsible for the maintenance of the spontaneous fibrinolytic activity of the blood. Differences in the fibrinolytic activity of the vessel walls between different regions of the body are reflected by corresponding differences in the spontaneous activity of the blood. Thus the spontaneous fibrinolytic activity of blood collected from the arms is higher than that of blood collected from the legs.[13]

Any form of stress, such as physical exertion or anxiety, stimulates the plasma plasminogen activator activity.[14] Also electroshock[15] and pneumoencephalography[16] raise the fibrinolytic activity in the blood. Infusion of adrenalin,[17,18] salbutamol, isoprenaline,[19,20] nicotinic acid,[21,22] vasopressin or its synthetic analogues, 8-lysine vasopressin (LVP), and 1-desamino-8-D-arginine vasopressin (DDAVP)[23,24] also cause a rapid, brief increase in plasminogen activator activity. Injection of pyrogens stimulates fibrinolysis.[25] Venous occlusion of the limbs[26,27] is followed by a marked increase in the local fibrinolytic activator activity.

The rise in plasminogen activator activity in response to these stimuli has usually been attributed to a release of plasminogen activator from the endothelial cells. The mechanism controlling the release is not properly understood, but two main hypotheses have been put forward, namely adrenoceptor stimulation and a change in vascular motility.

Systemic release of catecholamine is a common response to several of the above-mentioned stimuli. Yet the rise in plasminogen activator activity following infusion of catecholamines is at most partially prevented[28,29] by adrenergic β-blockers. Cash[30] and Gader et al.[29] have studied the fibrinolytic response to different adrenergic-receptor agonists and polyadrenergic-receptor agonists in association with specific blockers. They believe that the catecholamine-mediated plasminogen activator response is related to three different receptor sites. According to Cash,[14] the adrenergic receptors involved in the release of plasminogen activator are not mediated by the known receptors and are not related to β-adrenergic receptors.

There are, however, a number of situations where the plasminogen activator rises rapidly, although adrenoceptor stimulation is unlikely or can be excluded. Such situations are infusion of nicotinic acid, vasopressin and its synthetic analogues, and venous occlusion. Effective β-blockade does not prevent the increase in fibrinolytic activity in these situations.[24,31,32] It has been postulated that change in vascular motility — either decreasing or increasing the calibers of the vessels — is the basis of plasminogen activator release in such situations.[33] This also holds for venous stasis, the trapped blood producing a passive distension of the venous vascular tree.[34] However, many potent vasoactive drugs, such as histamine,[35] serotonin,[36] theophylline and cyclic AMP,[37] have no effect on plasminogen activator in vivo. In addition, DDAVP, which has no vasoactive properties, raises the fibrinolytic activity substantially.[24] Markwardt and Klöcking[38] have shown that the pattern of response in vivo is different from that in isolated perfused organs. They ascribed the plasminogen activator release in man to a complex interaction between the vessel wall on one hand and central nervous influences, regulation processes within different organs, and reactions with blood components on the other.

A question that has been discussed is whether an artificially induced rise in plasminogen activator activity is due not to a release of plasminogen activator from the vessel walls, but to some activation process in the plasma. As Factor XII is the common initiator of the kinin-forming, fibrinolytic, and intrinsic clotting systems, it has been suggested that activation of Factor XII starts the sequence of reactions resulting in the activation and seeming rise of plasminogen activator activity. However, no evidence is available in support of this possibility, Nilsson and Robertson[27] found that after venous occlusion, Factor XII-deficient individuals developed the same fibrinolytic activity as normal individuals. Adrenalin infusion raises the plasminogen activator activity, but has no effect on Factor XII.[20]

II. METHODS FOR MEASURING FIBRINOLYTIC ACTIVITY

It is clear from the preceding section that assessment of the fibrinolytic activity in the body and tissues should preferably be based on:

1. The spontaneous fibrinolytic activity of blood.
2. The fibrinolytic response to stimuli known to stimulate the release of activators

from the vessel walls into the blood stream (plasminogen activator release assays).

3. The plasminogen activator content of vessel walls.

A. Methods for Measuring the Spontaneous Fibrinolytic Activity of the Blood

The fibrinolytic activity of the blood is the composite effect of fibrinolytic activators and inhibitors. To obtain a more specific measure of the fibrinolytic activators, various methods have been devised in which the inhibitory effect is claimed to have been eliminated or diminished by dilution of the plasma, denaturation (treatment with chloroform or acetone), or by fractionation of the plasma (euglobulin precipitation)[41]. The inhibitor activity is not completely eliminated by such procedures.[39,40] The tests and determinations most widely used for measuring the fibrinolytic activator activity in blood are

1. Euglobulin clot lysis test
2. Diluted blood clot lysis time
3. Fibrin plate method

1. Euglobulin Clot Lysis Test (ELT)

The euglobulin fraction is prepared by diluting plasma with distilled water and by then acidifying the solution with acetic acid or carbon dioxide. The euglobulin fraction contains the plasminogen, plasmin, fibrinogen, and plasminogen activators, while most of the fibrinolytic inhibitors remain in the supernatant. The euglobulin fraction is dissolved in buffer and coagulated with thrombin, and the time necessary for the clot to dissolve is noted.

Some factors influence the method. Kluft and Brakman[40] have shown that the amounts of inhibitors coprecipitated with the euglobulin fraction vary with the pH and dilution of the plasma. They found that C1-inactivator was precipitated in considerable amounts (up to 80 to 100%) in the euglobulin fraction, especially at low pH and low ionic strength. Only traces of α_1-antitrypsin and α_2-macroglobulin were found. It is therefore recommended to use plasma diluted 1:10 to secure an appropriate ionic strength and a pH 5.9 to 6.0 for precipitation of euglobulin in order to avoid coprecipitation of C1-inactivator.

Fibrinolytic activators are labile. The test must be processed within 2 hr of collection of the blood.[42] The result of a test may vary with the anticoagulant used.[43] Euglobulin clots from oxalated plasma and heparinized plasma lyse less readily than euglobulin clots from citrated plasma. A standardized procedure is therefore absolutely necessary. Such methods have been described by Conard,[42] Kluft and Brakman,[40] and Nilsson and Olow.[44] The euglobulin clot lysis time is normally 3 to 20 hr.

If fibrinolysis is severe, the dissolution time will be short (at most 30 min). EACA and heparin are not precipitated in the euglobulin fraction.[42] The test can therefore be used in patients receiving heparin treatment.

By careful reading of long lysis times (with an automatic lysis recorder), it is possible to detect any abnormally low fibrinolytic activity.[45]

Since the lysis time varies inversely with the fibrinolytic activity,[46] the results can also be expressed as units of activity calculated according to the method of McNicol et al.[47] in which the reciprocal of a lysis time of 300 min is taken as unity.

2. Diluted Blood Lysis Time

To assess fibrinolytic activator, Fearnley and co-workers[48] devised a dilution method for determining the lysis time of clots prepared from blood or plasma diluted 1:10 in phosphate buffer at pH 7.4 and clotted with thrombin. The method usually gives lysis times three times as long as the euglobulin clot lysis test.

The diluted blood lysis time technique has been used mainly for estimating the normal variation of blood fibrinolytic activity and for following up patients receiving drugs to raise or lower the fibrinolytic activity of their blood. The long incubation time implies a considerable source of error (growth of bacteria, unsatisfactory observation, etc.).

3. Fibrin Plate Method

The fibrin plate method is a sensitive and accurate tool for measuring fibrinolytic activity. It can measure plasminogen activator activity and plasmin activity together or separately. A measured amount of test material, such as plasma, euglobulin fraction, or other body fluids or tissue extracts, is deposited onto the surface of a uniform layer of fibrin. A plasminogen-rich fibrin substrate is used for measuring plasminogen activator activity, but a plasminogen-free substrate is used for plasmin. A plasminogen-free fibrin plate can be prepared by heat inactivation of the plasminogen[49] or with the use of fibrinogen treated with bentonite to adsorb the plasminogen.[50] On incubation of the plates at 37°C, active agents, if any, produce circular areas of lysis in the fibrin plate. Comparison with the lysed areas produced by a standard preparation of tissue activator or urokinase will give a measure of the fibrinolytic activity of a given sample.

Fibrin plate methods have been described by Astrup and Müllertz,[51] Brakman,[52] Nilsson and Olow,[44] and Haverkate and Brakman.[53] The precision of the fibrin plate method is high. The S.D. is 13% for values above 50 mm.[2,54] The lower limit of detection of the method is extremely low, e.g., 0.3 ng (10^{-14} mol of trypsin).[53]

B. Plasminogen Activator Release Assays

The capacity of an individual to release plasminogen activator (his fibrinolytic capacity) can be assessed with the aid of various stimuli, such as exercise, injection of nicotinic acid, adrenalin, vasopressin, and venous occlusion of the limbs, known to enhance the release of plasminogen activators into the blood stream. Some persons respond weakly or not at all to such stimuli.[14,55,56] They are called poor responders.

1. Nicotinic Acid

The high percentage of poor responders among volunteers and the long period of nonresponsiveness after such an injection makes the use of nicotinic acid (i.v.) unsuitable as a routine method for assessing the fibrinolytic capacity.[22]

2. Exercise and Adrenalin

Exercise and adrenalin have been used particularly by Cash and co-workers.[57-60] The stimuli have been standardized, and reproducible results have been obtained. There is a close correlation between the response to exercise and that to adrenalin (i.v.). These stimuli can detect habitually poor responders, but these methods are not suitable for most patients.

3. Venous Occlusion

At the Coagulation Laboratory in Malmö, we have estimated for some years the fibrinolytic capacity in a given person from the local response of the fibrinolytic activity to venous occlusion of the arms.[55,61] It is a rather simple method without any side effects and therefore suitable for routine clinical use. In this method, venous occlusion is produced by placing a sphygmomanometer cuff around each upper arm and inflating it to a pressure midway between the systolic and diastolic blood pressure for 20 min. Blood samples for determination of the fibrinolytic activity of resuspended euglobulin precipitate on fibrin plates are obtained before application and just before deflation of the cuff. The mean increase in the fibrinolytic activity in the samples from each arm is taken as a measure of the fibrinolytic capacity.

Several workers use the venous cuff test, but apply venous occlusion for only 5, 10, or 15 min.[62-64] As shown by Aberg and Nilsson,[56] it is possible to identify poor responders by shortening the period of occlusion, but then the method is less sensitive.

4. *Vasopressin and DDAVP in Plasminogen Activator Release*

Aberg and Nilsson[56] studied the fibrinolytic response to vasopressin and to venous occlusion in healthy volunteers and patients with thrombotic disease. A close correlation was found between the fibrinolytic response to vasopressin and that to venous occlusion. However, vasopressin is not suitable for release assays because of its effects, namely vasoconstriction and abdominal cramps.

DDAVP (1-desamino-8-D-arginine) is a synthetic derivative of vasopressin. It produces a striking increase in the antidiuretic-pressor ratio of activities, but has no vasoactive properties and no side effects on the intestines.[65] Mannucci et al.[24] have shown that DDAVP enhances the fibrinolytic activity of the blood still more than does vasopressin. Aberg and Nilsson[66] therefore studied DDAVP for its possible use in release assays. DDAVP in a dose of 0.4 μg / kg bodyweight was given by i.v. infusion for 30 min to 30 normal patients and to 42 patients with thrombotic disease. The response to venous occlusion was also tested. Of the 42 patients with thrombosis, 25 were poor responders to DDAVP. A total of 16 of these patients responded poorly also to venous occlusion. DDAVP may, perhaps, prove useful in the evaluation of plasminogen activator release in clinical studies. The fact that the fibrinolytic response is not only local but a systemic response might be regarded as an advantage.

C. Plasminogen Activator Content of Vessel Walls

The histochemical film technique for demonstrating fibrinolytic activity in tissue was described by Todd.[67] Pandolfi et al.[68,69] have developed the histochemical method to allow quantitative determination of the fibrinolytic activity in the vessel wall, usually in biopsy specimens of superficial hand veins. A frozen section of the vessel is incubated in contact with a plasminogen-rich fibrin film. During incubation, the plasminogen activator present in the section converts the plasminogen contained in the adjacent fibrin to plasmin with local lysis as a result. Staining reveals fibrinolysis at the sites of active structures of the section as white gaps in the fibrin film. By incubating sections for different periods and evaluating the size of the lysed zones, it is possible to quantitate the activity. The activity is expressed in arbitrary units ranging from 0 to 12 (normal range 6 to 10).

III. FIBRINOLYSIS IN VARIOUS PHYSIOLOGICAL CONDITIONS

A. Sex, Age, and Race

Cash[70] found the spontaneous fibrinolytic activity to be somewhat higher in women than in men, a finding that could not be corroborated by Hamilton et al.[71] Robertson et al.[72] found the fibrinolytic response of the arms to venous occlusion not to vary with sex between the ages of 18 and 50, but to be significantly stronger in women at higher ages.

Some workers have found the fibrinolytic activity of the blood not to vary with age,[71,73-75] while others have found it to increase.[72,76,77]

The fibrinolytic activity is higher in black African males than in white European males.[78,79] The fibrinolytic activity is also higher in people living at high altitudes.[80]

B. Diurnal Variation

The fibrinolytic activity tends to be low in the morning and to increase during the daytime to reach its highest level between 5 and 8 p.m.[48,81-84] According to Fearnley et al.,[48] the diurnal pattern of fibrinolysis is not appreciably affected by physical activity.

C. Fibrinolytic Activity in Arterial and Venous Blood

The fibrinolytic activity in arterial blood is somewhat lower than that in venous blood[85,86] which has been ascribed to a higher level of plasminogen activator in the veins. Almer et al.[87] compared the plasminogen activator activity in biopsy specimens of the temporal artery and of a superficial dorsal hand vein. They found no noteworthy difference between the activator content of the veins and that of the arteries.

D. Pregnancy

The spontaneous fibrinolytic activity in the blood decreases during pregnancy and is barely detectable at term.[88-91] During labor the fibrinolytic activity is still very low, as measured with clot lysis assays or on fibrin plates, but returns to nonpregnancy values immediately after delivery. According to most authors, this decline in fibrinolytic activity during pregnancy is due to deficiency of an activator of fibrinolysis. Åstedt et al.[92-95] studied the response of the fibrinolytic activity to venous occlusion during pregnancy and at the same time determined the plasminogen activator activity in the vein walls with the histochemical method of Pandolfi et al.[69] During pregnancy the fibrinolytic activity after venous occlusion successively decreased and was often barely demonstrable at term. The plasminogen activator activity in the vein walls also decreased, but only slightly. Cash[14] has also shown that the response to exercise is decreased in pregnancy. Taken together these findings indicate that the low fibrinolytic activity during pregnancy is due, above all, to inhibition of the release of fibrinolytic activators from the vessel walls. Åstedt[95] produced evidence indicating that the decline of the fibrinolytic activity during pregnancy is due to some direct or indirect effect of placental hormones, particularly progestagens and estrogens, on the synthesis and release of fibrinolytic activators in the vessel wall. Patients with retention of the placenta thus have low fibrinolytic activity until the delivery of the placenta.

E. Hormones

The fibrinolytic activity of the blood can also be influenced by hormones. Åstedt[96] found that an estrogenic compound, ethinylestradiol, in a dose of 250 μg a day for 10 days significantly decreased the plasminogen activator content of the vein wall, while the spontaneous fibrinolytic activity of blood and the local fibrinolytic response to venous occlusion tended to increase. Åstedt assumed that ethinylestradiol inhibits the synthesis of activators or stimulates their release to a rate exceeding that of their production. This assumption was strengthened by the observation by Sobrero et al.[97] that combined oral contraceptives raised the spontaneous fibrinolytic activity, even when they contained little progestagen. It is noteworthy that the natural estrogenic hormone, 17-β-estradiol, has no effect on the plasminogen activator content.[98] Progestagen preparations[99] have been found to have no effect on the plasminogen activator content of the vessel wall, but have been reported to decrease the spontaneous fibrinolytic activity.[100]

Extensive investigation of the effect of anabolic steroids on fibrinolysis has shown that such steroids can produce long-term stimulation of fibrinolysis and then both stimulate synthesis of plasminogen activator in the vessel wall and enhance spontaneous fibrinolysis and the release of activators from the vessels.[101-103]

F. Exercise

Biggs and co-workers[104] were the first to show that exercise increased systemic plasma fibrinolytic activity. Several workers have since confirmed this observation.[57,70,83,84,105-111] They also pointed out that such an increase is only brief. It is not associated with any decrease of plasminogen or fibrinogen, appearance of free plasmin, or increase in fibrinogen/fibrin degradation products. Most workers have found that the increase in fibrinolytic activity varies with the intensity and duration of the exercise and the time of day it is performed. Short periods of intense exercise caused marked increases, while less strenuous exercise required a longer time to produce similar increases. The increase during prolonged, gentle exercise is small and comparable to that seen in the resting diurnal variation.[84,109,111] The increase in fibrinolysis seen after exercise appears to be similar to that seen in other stress situations and after infusion of adrenalin. However, it is now established that fibrinolysis following exercise cannot be prevented by β-adrenergic blockers and that there is no correlation between adrenalin levels and euglobulin lysis times.[28,107,109] This contrasts with the increase in Factor VIII seen after exercise which is preventable by β-adrenergic blockers. The increased perfusion of muscle capillaries and veins in association with physical activity has been thought to lead to an increased release or availability of plasminogen activator from the endothelial cells.

What is the significance of the increase stimulated by exercise? As pointed out earlier, only very strenuous exercise will increase fibrinolysis and even then for only a short time. Moderate exercise such as walking does not cause any significant increase in fibrinolysis. Exercise is associated not only with increased fibrinolysis, but also with an increase in Factor VIII. It is quite possible that in such situations a higher level of plasminogen activator is important for maintaining a satisfactory hemostatic balance.

G. Effect of Drinking and Certain Food Products

Fearnley and co-workers[112] found that beer and wine lowered the fibrinolytic activity in the blood, while whisky, gin, and absolute alcohol did not. They felt that some fermentation product other than ethyl alcohol was responsible for this change. Nilsson et al.[113] also found that consumption of wine and beer, but not of ethyl alcohol, lowered the fibrinolytic activity of the blood, as measured on fibrin plates. The minimal amount necessary to inhibit the fibrinolytic activity was 100 mℓ of red wine or 1000 mℓ of beer. The inhibiting effect of red wine persisted after removal of the alcohol by boiling. Grapes, grape juice, and carbohydrate meals had no effect on the fibrinolytic activity. In vitro experiments showed that wine and beer contained a principle that inhibited fibrinolytic activators. This principle was purified from grape pulp and found to consist of pectin with a molecular weight of about 10,000 and a degree of esterification of 29%. The failure of grapes to produce antiactivator effect in vivo was explained by the fact that the pectin was combined with other constituents in the pulp and that the active pectin is not released unless extracted by boiling or by the fermentation procedure involved in wine preparation. Apple pectin, citrus pectin, beet pectins, and pectin extracts from carrots possessed no inhibitory activity, while pectins from bilberries and black currants did.

In any investigation of the fibrinolytic activity in health and in disease attention must be given to dietary and drinking habits.

H. Smoking

Opinions differ on the effect of smoking on the fibrinolytic activity of the blood.

Thus Pozner and Billimoria[114] found heavy smoking to shorten the euglobulin lysis times, while Kaur and Sharma[115] and Dalderup et al.[116] found the spontaneous fibrinolytic activity, as measured with the dilute blood clot lysis times, to be lower in smokers than in nonsmokers. Janzon and Nilsson[117] compared the spontaneous fibrinolytic activity and fibrinolytic activity after venous occlusion in randomly selected heavy smokers and nonsmokers, all men, of uniform age. The smokers were examined after a 12-hr abstention. No difference was found between the smokers and nonsmokers. In those smokers who refrained from smoking for 8 to 9 weeks, the fibrinolytic activity did not differ from that initially recorded. Smoking of six cigarettes within a short time resulted in a shorter euglobulin clot lysis time. This was ascribed to the combined effect of nicotine and carbon monoxide.

Smoking thus seems not to have any significant effect on the fibrinolytic activity.

I. Alimentary Lipemia

Whether animal or vegetable dietary fat reduces the fibrinolytic activity of the blood is still debatable, but at present most authors agree that there is little unequivocal evidence that it does.[118-121] Lee et al.[122] found the fibrinolytic activity of the blood to be higher in a group using a very low-fat diet than in one using a high-fat diet. However, as the groups differed in ethnic origin, it is not possible to attribute this difference to diet alone. Menon[123] thus showed that after a 4-year stay in the U.K., Nigerian students still had a much higher fibrinolytic activity than British students using the same diet. Cronberg and Nilsson[124] found that infusion of a fat emulsion, Intralipid® (consisting of soya bean fat emulsified with egg yolk lecithin), had no effect on the fibrinolytic activity of the blood. Korsan-Bengtsen and Holm[125] studied the effect of free fatty acids on plasma fibrinolytic activity. The free fatty acid concentration was raised by infusion of noradrenalin. The fibrinolytic activity did not vary with fluctuation of the free fatty acid concentration.

Menon[126] found that fasting raised the fibrinolytic activity. This was obviously not due to the lipemia as such, but to the increase in adrenalin caused by the fasting.

Thus, it has not yet been shown that alimentary lipemia following intake of meals rich in animal or vegetable fat has any significant influence on the fibrinolytic activity of the blood.

J. Primary Carbohydrate-Induced Hypertriglyceridemia (PCH)

In PCH the fibrinolytic activity of the blood is significantly decreased.[127,128] Spöttl et al.[129] found the response to venous occlusion to be abnormally weak. Similar findings have also been reported by Almêr.[130] A very high proportion of poor responders to exercise has been demonstrated in patients with Type IV hyperlipoproteinemia.[131]

K. Obesity

The fibrinolytic activity in blood, as measured by dilute blood clot lysis time or euglobulin clot lysis time, tends to be low in obesity.[132-137] It has also been shown that obese subjects respond to exercise with a small rise in plasminogen activator activity.[134] Almêr[130] has shown that the response to venous occlusion decreased with increasing overweight. Almêr[130] and Almêr and Janzon[138] also found that the plasminogen activator activity of the vessel walls is significantly more often low in obesity (total of 315 subjects). This is incompatible with the reports by Grace and Goldrick,[139] who found no correlation between the degree of overweight and activator activity of s.c. tissue in seven obese and seven lean subjects. It has clearly been shown that this decrease in fibrinolytic activity is independent of the blood lipid levels.[130] Neither triglycerides nor chylomicrons inhibit the activation of plasminogen.[140]

The mechanism responsible for the low fibrinolytic activity in obesity is not known. It has been ascribed to functional and morphological changes in small vessels.[130] In obesity changes occur in the microcirculation with loss of normal vascular tone and a general dilatation of the smallest veins.[141] The impairment of the circulatory flow in the terminal vessels leads to hypoxia which might reduce the synthesis and release of plasminogen activator in the endothelium.

IV. FIBRINOLYSIS IN VARIOUS PATHOLOGICAL CONDITIONS

The vascular endothelium contains not only fibrinolytic activators, but also other substances of importance for maintenance of the hemostatic balance. These substances occur in the vascular endothelium and are therefore readily available for interaction with clotting and fibrinolytic factors of the blood. Thus, any injury to the vascular endothelium may result in a release of both fibrinolytic and coagulant agents.

A. Surgical Trauma and Shock

Surgery raises the fibrinolytic activity in the circulating blood.[142-144] The increase is highest during the actual operation.[144-147] The activity measured immediately after the operation is subnormal[146-148] and remains so for 3 to 11 days.[149] The fibrinolytic activity in the vessel wall during and after surgery has been studied by Aberg and Nilsson,[150] using both the histochemical method of Pandolfi[5] and the venous occlusion test.[13] Both the vessel wall activity, assayed histochemically, and the response to venous occlusion decreased significantly on the third day after operation in 22 patients operated upon because of rectal carcinoma. The decrease in the fibrinolytic response after venous occlusion was found to be correlated with the order of the surgical trauma[146,150] and has been explained by a more marked exhaustion of the endothelial fibrinolytic activators during major surgery.[146] A low fibrinolytic activity of the vessel wall is associated with an increased tendency to deep venous thrombosis.[151] In the material of Aberg and Nilsson,[150] all the patients who developed postoperative deep venous thrombosis had a decreased fibrinolytic activity in the vessel wall on the first postoperative day, compared with 60% of the remaining patients. These findings thus suggest an association between a low fibrinolytic activity in the vessel walls and development of postoperative venous thrombosis.[148,150]

The increase in the fibrinolytic activity observed in the blood during surgery has been tentatively ascribed to tissue injury resulting in an excessive release of plasminogen activators from the damaged endothelial cells into the circulation.[152] Other probable causal factors are hypoxia and anoxia.[153,154] The same mechanism is involved in various forms of shock. However, endothelial damage also stimulates a release of coagulant agents.[155] The hemostatic disturbances seen in shock therefore include signs of activation of the fibrinolytic as well as of the coagulation system, i.e., pathological proteolysis. Also proteolytic enzymes from disintegrating leukocytes probably contribute to such pathological proteolysis.[156] However, the hemostatic disorders observed in shock are only secondary phenomena, for which reason treatment should aim at controlling the primary disease.

B. Liver Disorders

The most striking disorders seen in liver diseases are those due to deficient synthesis of coagulation factors. Thus, low levels of vitamin-K-dependent clotting factors are seen in all forms of liver disease.[157,158] The fibrinolytic activity in the blood is often increased in liver cirrhosis.[159,160] This increase is ascribed to impaired hepatic clearing of plasminogen activator.[161] Also the α_2-antiplasmin and plasminogen levels are low.[162,163] The prolonged thrombin time commonly seen in liver cirrhosis[164] has been attributed to hypofibrinogenemia, an increase in physiological antithrombins, or to acquired dysfibrinogenemia.[165] Recently defective fibrin polymerization has also been demonstrated[166,167] and attributed to severe primary hepatocellular dysfunction.

In biliary obstruction, the fibrinolytic activity is decreased,[168] presumably owing to the changes in lipid metabolism occurring in cholestasis.

C. Arteriosclerosis and Diabetes Mellitus

The thrombogenic theory of arteriosclerosis published in 1844 by Rokitansky and later reviewed by Duguid in 1949[169] stimulated investigation of the question whether there is any relationship between arteriosclerosis and suppression of systemic fibrinolysis. However, the results of such studies are conflicting. Some workers have found decreased fibrinolytic activity in ischemic heart disease,[132,170,171] whereas others have been able to find this decrease in arterial blood, but not in venous blood,[86] and still others have not found any significant difference at all.[172,173] It is known that the incidence of coronary disease is low in liver cirrhosis in which fibrinolysis is increased.[174] The fibrinolytic activity has been reported to be low in intermittent claudication[175] and in patients with various signs of arteriosclerosis.[176]

In diabetes mellitus (DM), a disease often associated with arteriosclerosis, the results are less discordant. Most researchers have found the fibrinolytic activity to be decreased in DM.[132,171,177,178] Moser and Hajjar[179] and Cash and McGill,[59] who used the euglobulin clot lysis time, found no such suppression, and Lassman et al.[180] found the activity to be, if anything, increased in experimental diabetes. Diabetics react poorly to stimuli known to enhance fibrinolysis, such as exercise[59] and venous occlusion,[177] though no decrease in response to adrenalin has been observed by Tanser.[181] Almer and Nilsson[177] also found the level of the plasminogen activator in the vessel wall to be low in DM. Furthermore, the level of fibrinolytic inhibitors, such as α_2-macroglobulin and inhibitors of plasminogen activation, has been found to be high.[177] No correlation has been found between the severity of microcirculatory damage such as diabetic retinopathy and any of the changes in fibrinolysis.[182]

Fluctuation of the blood glucose level and the type of therapy used presumably affect the fibrinolytic activity in DM. As clearly shown by Hedlin,[183] exogenous or endogenous insulin enhances the fibrinolytic activity of the blood. However, such an enhancement is not direct, but the results of the action of hormones such as adrenalin released to control hyperglycemia. Thus, injection of insulin is not followed by any increase in fibrinolytic activity before the blood glucose has fallen to 30 to 60%; on the other hand, administration of glucose, as in the glucose tolerance tests, stimulates fibrinolysis when the blood glucose level has been normalized by the action of endogenous insulin.

As for antidiabetic drugs, Fearnley et al.[184] found that sulfonylurea and phenformin increase the blood fibrinolytic activity, an effect which cannot be ascribed by hypoglycemia. However, such an increase lasts for only a few months. The fibrinolytic properties of phenformin have recently been confirmed by Banerjee et al.[185] In a series of 221 diabetics, Almer[188] found a low spontaneous blood fibrinolytic activity in those treated with chloropropamide, while many of those treated with sulfonylurea had a low fibrinolytic activity of the vessel wall. Assessment of these findings is complicated by the fact that adiposity per se is often associated with a low fibrinolytic activity, and as is well known, adiposity is overrepresented in a diabetic population.

D. Thrombotic Disease

A low fibrinolytic activity in the vessel wall has been found to be associated with an increased tendency to develop deep venous thrombosis (DVT).[151,186]

Thus, in 70% of a series of 289 patients with severe thromboembolic disease, the fibrinolytic defence was impaired, i.e., a decreased fibrinolytic activity in the vessel walls and/or a defective release of the activator into the circulation.[151]

Phenformin combined with ethylestrenol stimulates the release of the fibrinolytic activity in the vessel walls in patients with a defective fibrinolytic defence system associated with recurrent DVT. The frequency of DVT episodes tended to fall[187] with the normalization of the fibrinolytic system. Also ethylestrenol alone has been found to have a similar effect.[103]

V. CONCLUDING REMARKS

This review may warrant a few concluding remarks:

1. Of the different fibrinolytic systems found in the organism, the extrinsic system seems to have the best documented physiopathological relevance.
2. Tissue (vessel wall) fibrinolytic activity varies widely in various districts of the body. Its pattern of distribution is constant and variations, when they occur, are moderate. To produce changes of tissue fibrinolysis, prolonged stimuli are necessary, such as the long-term treatment with phenformin and anabolizing hormones which increase the activity or chronic conditions (diabetes mellitus, obesity, and pregnancy) which are followed by a depressed fibrinolytic activity. In other cases, a depressed fibrinolytic activity in the vessel walls appears to be primary and possibly plays a role in thrombogenesis.
3. Blood fibrinolytic activity (unlike tissues) is subject to wide variations, both in the same individual and in different subjects. Thus, blood fibrinolytic activity shows diurnal variation and may readily be enhanced by various stimuli, both physiological (venous stasis and physical exercise) and pharmacological (injection of adrenalin and nicotinic acid). Blood fibrinolysis may be influenced also by alimentary habits. Interindividual variations of blood fibrinolysis often reflect similar variations of fibrinolysis in the vessel walls. Thus, a depressed blood spontaneous and stimulated fibrinolytic activity is usually observed in patients with pregnancy, venous thrombosis, obesity, and DM, where the fibrinolytic activity of the vascular walls is low.

REFERENCES

1. **Schreiber, A. D. and Austen, K. F.**, Hageman factor-independent fibrinolytic pathway, *Clin. Exp. Immunol.*, 17, 587, 1974.
2. **Wuepper, K. D., Miller, D. R., and Lacombe, M. J.**, Flaujaec trait: deficiency of kininogen in man, *Fed. Proc. Fed. Am. Soc. Exp. Biol.*, 34, 859, 1975.
3. **Taylor, F. B., Jr.**, A new approach to the study of hypercoagulability. A discussion of the mechanism and application of a coagulolysis assay which measures both coagulative and fibrinolytic activities, *Thromb. Diath. Haemorrh. Suppl.*, 54, 223, 1973.
4. **Fischer, A.**, *Gewebezuchtung. Handbuch der Biologie der Gewebezellen In Vitro,* Müller and Steinicke, Munich, 1930.
5. **Pandolfi, M.**, Histochemistry and assay of plasminogen activator(s), *Eur. J. Clin. Biol. Res.*, 17, 254, 1972.
6. **Astrup, T.**, Cell-induced fibrinolysis. A fundamental process, in *Proteases and Biological Control,* Vol. 2, Reich, E. et al., Eds., Cold Spring Harbor: Laboratory, Cold Spring Harbor, N.Y., 1975, 343.

7. **Noordhoek-Hegt, V.**, Localization and distribution of fibrinolysis inhibition in the walls of human arteries and veins, *Thromb. Res.*, 10, 121, 1977.
8. **Pandolfi, M.**, Localization of fibrinolytic activity in the developing rat eye, *Arch. Ophthalmol.*, 78, 512, 1967.
9. **Henriksen, J. and Astrup, T.**, Fibrinolytically active rat vaginal epithelial cells, *J. Pathol. Bacteriol.*, 93, 706, 1967.
10. **Wünschmann-Henderson, B. and Astrup, T.**, Relation of fibrinolytic activity in human oral epithelial cells to cellular maturation: the influence of smoking, *J. Pathol.*, 108, 293, 1972.
11. **Pandolfi, M., Nilsson, I. M., Robertson, B., and Isacson, S.**, Fibrinolytic activity of human veins, *Lancet*, 2, 127, 1967.
12. **Nicolaides, A. N., Clark, C. T., Thomas, R. O., and Lewis, J. D.**, Fibrinolytic activator in the endothelium of the veins of the lower limb, *Br. J. Surg.*, 63, 881, 1976.
13. **Robertson, B., Pandolfi, M., and Nilsson, I. M.**, Response of local fibrinolytic activity to venous occlusion of arms and legs in healthy volunteers, *Acta Chir. Scand.*, 138, 437, 1972.
14. **Cash, J. D.**, Neurohumoral pathways associated with the release of plasminogen activator in man, in *Progress in Chemical Fibrinolysis and Thrombolysis*, Vol. 1, Davidson, J. F., Samama, M. M., and Desnoyers, P. C., Eds., Raven Press, New York, 1975, 97.
15. **Pina-Cabral, J. M. and Rodrigues, C.**, Blood catecholamine levels, factor VIII and fibrinolysis after therapeutic electroshock, *Br. J. Haematol.*, 27, 371, 1974.
16. **Schneck, S. A. and von Kaulla, K. N.**, Fibrinolysis and the nervous system, *Neurology*, 11, 959, 1961.
17. **Biggs, R., Macfarlane, R. G., and Pilling, J.**, Observations on fibrinolysis. Experimental activity produced by exercise or adrenaline, *Lancet*, 1, 402, 1947.
18. **Ingram, G. I. C.**, Increase in antihaemophilic globulin activity following infusion of adrenaline, *J. Physiol. (London)*, 156, 217, 1961.
19. **Gader, A. M. A., Clarkson, A. R., and Cash, J. D.**, The plasminogen activator and coagulation Factor VIII response to adrenaline, noradrenaline, isoprenaline and salbutamol in man, *Thromb. Res.*, 2, 9, 1973.
20. **Ingram, G. I. C., Jones, R. V., Hershgold, E. J., Denson, K. W. E., and Perkins, J. R.**, Factor-VIII activity and antigen, platelet count and biochemical changes after adrenoceptor stimulation, *Br. J. Haematol.*, 35, 81, 1977.
21. **Weiner, M., Redisch, W., and Steele, M. J.**, Occurrence of fibrinolytic activity following administration of nicotinic acid, *Proc. Soc. Exp. Biol. Med.*, 98, 755, 1958.
22. **Robertson, B.**, Effect of nicotinic acid on fibrinolytic activity in health, in thrombotic disease and in liver cirrhosis, *Acta Chir. Scand.*, 137, 643, 1971.
23. **Gader, A. M. A., Da Costa, J., and Cash, J. D.**, A new vasopressin analogue and fibrinolysis, *Lancet*, 2, 1417, 1973.
24. **Mannucci, P. M., Åberg, M., Nilsson, I. M., and Robertson, B.**, Mechanism of plasminogen activator and factor VIII increase after vasoactive drugs, *Br. J. Haematol.*, 30, 81, 1975.
25. **Meneghini, P.**, La shock-vaccino terapia nelle cura di un caso di trombosi traumatica della vena cava inferiore, *Arch. E. Maragliano Patol. Clin.*, 4, 771, 1949.
26. **Clarke, R. L., Orandi, A., and Cliffton, E. E.**, Induction of fibrinolysis by venous obstruction, *Angiology*, 11, 367, 1960.
27. **Nilsson, I. M. and Robertson, B.**, Effect of venous occlusion on coagulation and fibrinolytic components in normal subjects, *Thromb. Diath. Haemorrh.*, 20, 397, 1968.
28. **Cash, J. D., Woodfield, D. G., and Allan, A. G. E.**, Adrenergic mechanism in the systemic plasminogen activator response to adrenaline in man, *Br. J. Haematol.*, 18, 487, 1970.
29. **Gader, A. M. A., Da Costa, J., and Cash, D. J.**, The effect of propranolol, alprenolol and practolol on the fibrinolytic and factor VIII response to adrenaline and salbutamol in man, *Thromb. Res.*, 4, 25, 1974.
30. **Cash, J.**, Physiological aspects of fibrinolytis, in *Synthetic Fibrinolytic Thrombolytic Agents*, von Kaulla, K. N. and Davidson, J. F., Eds., Charles C Thomas, Springfield, Ill., 1975, 5.
31. **Ponari, O., Civardi, E., Megha, A., Pini, M., Poti, R., and Dettori, A. G.**, Effect of alpha- and beta-blocking drugs on the clotting and fibrinolytic response to venous stasis in man, *Br. J. Haematol.*, 24, 463, 1973.
32. **Butler, M. J., Smith, M., Irving, M. H., Gordon, Y. B., Ratky, S. M., Rivers, J. W. P., and Hawkey, C.**, The influence of beta-adrenergic blockade upon baseline blood coagulation and fibrinolytic activity and upon the responses to venous occlusion, *Thromb. Diath. Haemorrh.*, 34, 169, 1975.
33. **Holemans, R., Mann, L. S., and Cope, C.**, Fibrinolytic activity of renal venous and arterial blood, *Am. J. Med. Sci.*, 254, 330, 1967.
34. **Nilsson, I. M. and Pandolfi, M.**, Fibrinolytic response of the vascular wall, *Thromb. Diath. Haemorrh. Suppl.*, 40, 231, 1970.

35. **Weiner, M., de Crinis, K., Redisch, W., and Steele, M. J.,** Influence of some vasoactive drugs on fibrinolytic activity, *Circulation,* 19, 845, 1959.
36. **Thomson, W. B., Green, J., and Evans, I. L.,** The effect of some physiological stimuli on fibrinolytic activity in man measured by the heparin fractionation method, *J. Clin. Pathol.,* 17, 341, 1964.
37. **Mannucci, P. M. and Barbi, G. L.,** Effect of cyclic AMP and related drugs on plasminogen activator, *Eur. J. Clin. Invest.,* 3 (Abstr.), 253, 1973.
38. **Markwardt, F. and Klöcking, H. P.,** Studies on the release of plasminogen activator, *Thromb. Res.,* 8, 217, 1976.
39. **Lauritsen, O. S.,** Inhibition of plasminogen activation and plasmin activity after euglobulin precipitation and acidification of plasma, *Scand. J. Clin. Invest.,* 23, 121, 1969.
40. **Kluft, C. and Brakman, P.,** The effect of flufenamate on euglobulin fibrinolysis: involvement of Cl-inactivator, in *Progress in Chemical Fibrinolysis and Thrombolysis,* Vol. 1, Davidson, J. F., Samama, M. M., and Desnoyers, P. C., Eds., Raven Press, New York, 1975, 375.
41. **Milstone, H.,** A factor in normal human blood which precipitates in streptococcal fibrinolysis, *J. Immunol.,* 42, 109, 1941.
42. **Conard, J.,** Plasma plasminogen activator — clot lysis assay techniques, in *Progress in Chemical Fibrinolysis and Thrombolysis,* Vol. 2, Davidson, J. F., Samama, M. M., and Desnoyers, P. C., Eds., Raven Press, New York, 1976, 15.
43. **Blix, S.,** Studies on the fibrinolytic system in the euglobulin fraction of human plasma. A. A methodological study. B. Application of the methods, *Scand. J. Clin. Lab. Invest. Suppl.,* 13, 58, 1961.
44. **Nilsson, I. M. and Olow, B.,** Fibrinolysis induced by streptokinase in man, *Acta Chir. Scand.,* 123, 247, 1962.
45. **Preston, F. E.,** Automated euglobulin clot lysis time, in *Progress in Chemical Fibrinolysis and Thrombolysis,* Vol. 2, Davidson, J. F., Samama, M. M., and Desnoyers, P. C., Eds., Raven Press, New York, 1976, 25.
46. **Sherry, S. and Alkjaersig, N.,** A study of the fibrinolytic enzyme of human plasma, *Thromb. Diath. Haemorrh.,* 1, 264, 1957.
47. **McNicol, G. P., Gale, S. B., and Douglas, A. S.,** In-vitro and in-vivo studies of a preparation of urokinase, *Br. Med. J.,* 1, 909, 1963.
48. **Fearnley, G. R., Balmforth, G., and Fearnley, E.,** Evidence of a diurnal fibrinolytic rhythm; with a simple method of measuring natural fibrinolysis, *Clin. Sci.,* 16, 645, 1957.
49. **Lassen, M.,** Heat denaturation of plasminogen in the fibrin plate method, *Acta Physiol. Scand.,* 27, 371, 1952.
50. **Brakman, P.,** Bovine fibrinogen without detectable plasminogen, *Anal. Biochem.,* 11, 149, 1965.
51. **Astrup, T. and Müllertz, S.,** The fibrin plate method for estimating fibrinolytic activity, *Arch. Biochem.,* 40, 346, 1952.
52. **Brakman, P.,** *Fibrinolysis. A Standardized Fibrin Plate Method, and a Fibrinolytic Assay of Plasminogen,* Scheltema & Holkema, Amsterdam, 1967.
53. **Haverkate, F. and Brakman, P.,** Fibrin plate assay, in *Progress in Chemical Fibrinolysis and Thrombolysis,* Vol. 1, Davidson, J. F., Samama, M. M., and Desnoyers, P. C., Eds., Raven Press, New York, 1975, 151.
54. **Robertson, B. R., Pandolfi, M., and Nilsson, I. M.,** "Fibrinolytic capacity" of healthy volunteers as estimated from effect of venous occlusion of arms, *Acta Chir. Scand.,* 138, 429, 1972.
55. **Nilsson, I. M.,** Methods for assessment of fibrinolytic activator activity, in *Synthetic Fibrinolytic Thrombolytic Agents,* von Kaulla, K. N. and Davidson, J. F., Eds., Charles C Thomas, Springfield, Ill., 1975, 20.
56. **Åberg, M. and Nilsson, I. M.,** Fibrinolytic response to venous occlusion and vasopressin in health and thrombotic disease, in *Progress in Chemical Fibrinolysis and Thrombolysis,* Vol. 1, Davidson, J. F., Samama, M. M., and Desnoyers, P. C., Eds., Raven Press, New York, 1975, 121.
57. **Cash, J. D. and Allan, A. G. E.,** Fibrinolytic response to moderate exercise and intravenous adrenaline in the same subjects, *Br. J. Haematol.,* 13, 376, 1967.
58. **Cash, J. D. and Woodfield, D. G.,** Fibrinolytic response to moderate, exhaustive and prolonged exercise in normal subjects, *Nature (London),* 215, 628, 1967.
59. **Cash, J. D. and McGill, R. C.,** Fibrinolytic response to moderate exercise in young male diabetics and nondiabetics, *J. Clin. Pathol.,* 22, 32, 1969.
60. **Cash, J. D., Woodfield, D. G., and Allan, A. G. E.,** Adrenergic mechanisms in the systemic plasminogen activator response to adrenaline in man, *Br. J. Haematol.,* 18, 487, 1970.
61. **Nilsson, I. M. and Pandolfi, M.,** Assay of fibrinolytic activity of the vessel wall, in *Progress in Chemical Fibrinolysis and Thrombolysis,* Vol. 2, Davidson, J. F., Samama, M. M., and Desnoyers, P. C., Eds., Raven Press, New York, 1976, 1.
62. **Amery, A., Vermylen, J., Maes, H., and Verstraete, M.,** Enhancing the fibrinolytic activity in human blood by occlusion of blood by occlusion of blood vessels, *Thromb. Diath. Haemorrh.,* 7, 70, 1962.

63. **Iatridis, S. G., Iatridis, P. G., and Ferguson, J. H.,** The role of HF (factor XII) in the pathogenesis of the thrombolytic state induced by venous occlusion, *Thromb. Diath. Haemorrh.*, 16, 207, 1966.
64. **Davidson, J. F., Walker, I. D., and McCallum, H. I.,** Study of the mechanism of action of anabolic steroids on fibrinolysis, in *Progress in Chemical Fibrinolysis and Thrombolysis*, Vol. 1, Davidson, J. F., Samama, M. M., and Desnoyers, P. C., Eds., Raven Press, New York, 1975, 311.
65. **Andersson, K.-E., Arner, B., Hedner, P., and Mulder, J. L.,** Effects of 8-lysine-vasopressin and synthetic analogues on release of ACTH, *Acta Endocrinol. (Copenhagen)*, 69, 640, 1972.
66. **Åberg, M. and Nilsson, I. M.,** Plasminogen activator release after venous occlusion and infusion of DDAVP, *6th Int. Congr. Thrombosis and Haemostasis, 12th Congr. World Fed. Hemophilia*, Philadelphia, 1977, 298 (Abstr.).
67. **Todd, A. S.,** The histological localization of fibrinolysin activator, *J. Pathol. Bacteriol.*, 78, 281, 1959.
68. **Pandolfi, M., Isacson, S., and Nilsson, I. M.,** Low fibrinolytic activity in the walls of veins in patients with thrombosis, *Acta Med. Scand.*, 186, 1, 1969.
69. **Pandolfi, M., Bjernstad, A., and Nilsson, I. M.,** Technical remarks on the microscopical demonstration of tissue plasminogen activator, *Thromb. Diath. Haemorrh.*, 27, 88, 1972.
70. **Cash, J. D.,** Effect of moderate exercise on the fibrinolytic system in normal young men and women, *Br. Med. J.*, 2, 502, 1966.
71. **Hamilton, P. J., Dawson, A. A., Ogston, D., and Douglas, A. S.,** The effect of age on the fibrinolytic enzyme system, *J. Clin. Pathol.*, 27, 326, 1974.
72. **Robertson, B., Pandolfi, M., and Nilsson, I. M.,** "Fibrinolytic capacity" in healthy volunteers at different ages as studied by standardized venous occlusion of arms and legs, *Acta Med. Scand.*, 191, 199, 1972.
73. **Sawyer, D. W., Fletcher, A. P., Alkjaersig, N., and Sherry, S.,** Studies on the thrombolytic activity of human plasma, *J. Clin. Invest.*, 39, 426, 1960.
74. **Fearnley, G. R., Chakrabarti, R., and Avis, P. R. D.,** Blood fibrinolytic activity in diabetes mellitus and its bearing on ischaemic heart disease and obesity, *Br. Med. J.*, 1, 921, 1963.
75. **Nilsson, I. M.,** Blood coagulation studies in the aged, in *Age With a Future*, Proc. 6th Int. Congr. Gerontology, Copenhagen, Munksgaard, Copenhagen, 1964, 629.
76. **Swan, H. T.,** Fibrinolysis related to age in men, *Br. J. Haematol.*, 9, 311, 1963.
77. **Hume, R.,** The relationship to age and cerebral vascular accidents of fibrin and fibrinolytic activity, *J. Clin. Pathol.*, 14, 167, 1961.
78. **Walker, W. R.,** Fibrinolytic activity of whole blood from South African Bantu and white subjects, *Am. J. Clin. Nutr.*, 9, 461, 1961.
79. **Ferguson, J. C., Mackay, N., and McNicol, G. P.,** Effect of feeding fat on fibrinolysis, stypven time, and platelet aggregation in Africans, Asians and Europeans, *J. Clin. Pathol.*, 23, 580, 1970.
80. **Chochan, I. S., Singh, I., and Balakrihsnan, K.,** Fibrinolytic activity at high altitude and sodium acetate buffer, *Thromb. Diath., Haemorrh.*, 32, 65, 1974.
81. **Moser, K. M.,** The compleat fibrinolyticist: a study in septophrenia, *Fed. Proc. Fed. Am. Soc. Exp. Biol.*, 25, 94, 1966.
82. **Mann, R. D.,** Effect of age, sex, and diurnal variation on the human fibrinolytic system, *J. Clin. Pathol.*, 20, 223, 1967.
83. **Menon, I. S., Burke, F., and Dewar, H. A.,** Effect of strenuous and graded exercise on fibrinolytic activity, *Lancet*, 1, 700, 1967.
84. **Rosing, D. R., Brakman, P., Redwood, D. R., Goldstein, R. E., Beiser, G. D., and Epstein, S. E.,** Blood fibrinolytic activity in man. Diurnal variation and the response to varying intensities of exercise, *Circ. Res.*, 27, 171, 1970.
85. **Fearnley, G. R. and Ferguson, J.,** Arteriovenous difference in natural fibrinolysis, *Lancet*, 2, 1040, 1957.
86. **Naimi, S., Goldstein, R., and Proger, S.,** Studies of coagulation and fibrinolysis of the arterial and venous blood in normal subjects and patients with atherosclerosis, *Circulation*, 27, 904, 1963.
87. **Almer, L.-O., Pandolfi, M., and Åberg, M.,** The plasminogen activator activity of arteries and veins in diabetes mellitus, *Thromb. Res.*, 6, 177, 1975.
88. **Nilsson, I. M. and Kullander, S.,** Coagulation and fibrinolytic studies during pregnancy, *Acta Obstet. Gynecol. Scand.*, 47, 286, 1967.
89. **Brakman, P.,** The fibrinolytic system in human blood during pregnancy, *Am. J. Obstet. Gynecol.*, 94, 14, 1966.
90. **Bonnar, J., McNicol, G. P., and Douglas, A. S.,** Fibrinolytic enzyme system and pregnancy, *Br. Med. J.*, 3, 387, 1969.
91. **Bonnar, J., McNicol, G. P., and Douglas, A. S.,** Coagulation and fibrinolytic mechanisms during and after childbirth, *Br. Med. J.*, 2, 200, 1970.

92. **Åstedt, B., Isacson, S., Nilsson, I. M., and Pandolfi, M.,** Fibrinolytic activity of veins during pregnancy, *Acta Obstet. Gynecol. Scand.,* 49, 171, 1970.
93. **Åstedt, B.,** Fibrinolytic activity during labour, *Acta Obstet. Gynecol. Scand.,* 51, 171, 1972.
94. **Åstedt, B.,** Fibrinolytic activity of veins in the puerperium, *Acta Obstet. Gynecol. Scand.,* 51, 325, 1972.
95. **Åstedt, B.,** Demonstration of significance of placenta in depression of fibrinolytic activity during pregnancy, *J. Obstet. Gynaecol. Br. Commonw.,* 79, 205, 1972.
96. **Åstedt, B.,** Low fibrinolytic activity of veins during treatment with ethinyloestradiol, *Acta Obstet. Gynecol. Scand.,* 50, 279, 1971.
97. **Sobrero, A. J., Brakman, P., and Astrup, T.,** Effects on blood fibrinolysis of an oral contraceptive low in progestin (Ovulen), *Am. J. Obstet. Gynecol.,* 110, 122, 1971.
98. **Åstedt, B. and Jeppsson, S.,** 17-β-oestradiol and the fibrinolytic activity of vein walls, *J. Obstet. Gynaecol. Br. Commonw.,* 81, 719, 1974.
99. **Åstedt, B., Jeppsson, S., and Pandolfi, M.,** Fibrinolytic activity of veins during use of depot medroxyprogesterone acetate as a contraceptive, *Fertil. Steril.,* 23, 489, 1972.
100. **Brakman, P., Sobrero, A. J., and Astrup, T.,** Effects of different systemic contraceptives on blood fibrinolysis, *Am. J. Obstet. Gynecol.,* 106, 187, 1970.
101. **Fearnley, G. R., Chakrabarti, R., and Evans, J.,** Fibrinolytic and defibrinating effect of phenformin plus ethyloestrenol in vivo, *Lancet,* 1, 910, 1969.
102. **Davidson, J. F., Lochhead, M., McDonald, G. A., and McNicol, G. P.,** Fibrinolytic enhancement by stanozolol: a double blind trial, *Br. J. Haematol.,* 22, 543, 1972.
103. **Hedner, U., Nilsson, I. M., and Isacson, S.,** Effect of ethyloestrenol in the vessel wall, *Br. Med. J.,* 2, 729, 1976.
104. **Biggs, R., MacFarlane, R. G., and Pilling, J.,** Observations on fibrinolysis, *Lancet,* 1, 402, 1947.
105. **Sherry, S., Lindemeyer, R. I., Fletcher, A. P., and Alkjaersig, N.,** Studies on enhanced fibrinolytic activity in man, *J. Clin. Invest.,* 38, 810, 1959.
106. **Iatridis, S. G. and Ferguson, J. H.,** Effect of physical exercise on blood clotting and fibrinolysis, *J. Appl. Physiol.,* 18, (Suppl. 2), 337, 1963.
107. **Cohen, R. J., Epstein, S. E., Cohen, L. S., and Dennis, L. H.,** Alterations of fibrinolysis and blood coagulation induced by exercise, and the role of beta-adrenergic-receptor stimulation, *Lancet,* 2, 1264, 1968.
108. **Karp, J. E. and Bell, W. R.,** Fibrinogen-fibrin degradation products and fibrinolysis following exercise in humans, *Am. J. Physiol.,* 227, 1212, 1974.
109. **Hawkey, C. M., Britton, B. J., Wood, W. G., Peele, M., and Irving, M. H.,** Changes in blood catecholamine levels and blood coagulation and fibrinolytic activity in response to graded exercise in man, *Br. J. Haematol.,* 29, 377, 1975.
110. **Britton, B. J., Wood, W. G., Smith, M., Hawkey, C., and Irving, M. H.,** The effect of beta adrenergic blockade upon exercise-induced changes in blood coagulation and fibrinolysis, *Thromb. Haemostas.,* 35, 396, 1976.
111. **Davis, G. L., Abildgaard, C. F., Bernayer, E. M., and Britton, M.,** Fibrinolytic and hemostatic changes during and after maximal exercise in males, *J. Appl. Physiol.,* 40, 287, 1976.
112. **Fearnley, G. R., Ferguson, J., Chakrabarti, R., and Vincent, C. T.,** Effect of beer on blood fibrinolytic activity, *Lancet,* 1, 184, 1960.
113. **Nilsson, I. M., Bjorkman, S. E., von Studnitz, W., and Hallén, A.,** Antifibrinolytic activity of certain pectins, *Thromb. Diath. Haemorrh.,* 6, 177, 1961.
114. **Pozner, H. and Billimoria, J. D.,** Effect of smoking on blood-clotting and lipid and lipoprotein levels, *Lancet,* 1, 1318, 1970.
115. **Kaur, S. and Sharma, K. S.,** Fibrinolytic activity and its variation in normal healthy subjects, *Indian J. Physiol. Pharmacol.,* 14, 137, 1970.
116. **Dalderup, L. M., Zwartz, J. A., Keller, G. H. M., Schouten, F., and van Haard, W. B.,** Serum lipids, typing, fibrinolysis, and smoking, *Br. Med. J.,* 3, 223, 1970.
117. **Janzon, L. and Nilsson, I. M.,** Smoking and fibrinolysis, *Circulation,* 51, 1120, 1975.
118. **Ogston, D. and Fullerton, H. W.,** Effect of alimentary lipaemia on plasma fibrinolytic activity, *Br. Med. J.,* 2, 1288, 1962.
119. **Merskey, C. and Marcus, A. J.,** Lipids, blood coagulation and fibrinolysis, *Annu. Rev. Med.,* 14, 323, 1963.
120. **Howell, M.,** Effects of plasma lipids on fibrinolysis, *Br. Med. Bull.,* 20, 200, 1964.
121. **Nilsson, I. M.,** The Development of Thrombosis, Thule Int. Symp. Stroke, 1966, *Nordiska Bokhandelns Förlag,* Stockholm, 1967, 101.
122. **Lee, K. T., Kim, D. N., [illegible], and Thomas, W. A.,** Geographic pathology of atherosclerosis and thrombosis, *J. Atheroscler. Res.,* 6, 203, 1966.

123. **Menon, I. S.**, Fibrinolytic activity in the blood of Nigerian students after four years' residence in the United Kingdom, *Lab. Pract.*, 16, 574, 1967.
124. **Cronberg, S. and Nilsson, I. M.**, Coagulation studies after administration of a fat emulsion, Intralipid®, *Thromb. Diath. Haemorrh.*, 18, 664, 1967.
125. **Korsan-Bengtsen, K. and Holm, T.**, Free fatty acids (FFA) — blood clotting, fibrinolysis and platelet function, *Scand. J. Haematol.*, 13, 65, 1974.
126. **Menon, I. S.**, Fasting and non-fasting fibrinolytic activity, *Lab. Pract.*, 16, 469, 1967.
127. **Sweet, B., Rifkind, B. M., and McNicol, G. P.**, The relationship between blood lipids and the fibrinolytic enzyme system, *J. Atheroscler. Res.*, 6, 359, 1966.
128. **Blatny, J., Kojecky, Z., and Fischerova, E.**, Hyperlipemie essentialle et fibrinolyse, *Nouv. Rev. Fr. Hematol.*, 8, 259, 1968.
129. **Spöttl, F., Holzknecht, F., and Braunsteiner, H.**, Enhancement of the fibrinolytic activity by venous occlusion in patients with primary "carbohydrate-induced" hypertriglyceridemia, *Acta Haematol.*, 51, 154, 1969.
130. **Almér, L.-O.**, Effect of obesity on endogenous fibrinolytic activity in diabetes mellitus, *J. Med.* (Westbury, N.Y.), 6, 351, 1975.
131. **Epstein, S. E., Rosing, D. R., Brakman, P., Redwood, D. R., and Astrup, T.**, Impaired fibrinolytic response to exercise in patients with type-IV hyperlipoproteinemia, *Lancet*, 2, 631, 1963.
132. **Fearnley, G. R., Chakrabarti, R., and Avis, P. R. D.**, Blood fibrinolytic activity in diabetes mellitus and its bearing on ischaemic heart disease and obesity, *Br. Med. J.*, 1, 921, 1963.
133. **Shaw, D. A. and MacNaughton, D.**, Relationship between blood fibrinolytic activity and body fatness, *Lancet*, 1, 352, 1963.
134. **Ogston, D. and McAndrew, G. M.**, Fibrinolysis in obesity, *Lancet*, 2, 1205, 1964.
135. **Bennett, N., Ogston, C., McAndrew, G., and Ogston, D.**, Studies on the fibrinolytic enzyme system in obesity, *J. Clin. Pathol.*, 19, 241, 1966.
136. **Grace, C. S. and Goldrick, R. B.**, Fibrinolysis and body build, *J. Atherscler. Res.*, 8, 705, 1968.
137. **Warlow, C. P., McNeill, A., Ogston, D., and Douglas, A. S.**, Platelet adhesiveness, coagulation, and fibrinolytic activity in obesity, *J. Clin. Pathol.*, 25, 484, 1972.
138. **Almér, L.-O. and Janzon, L.**, Low vascular fibrinolytic activity in obesity, *Thromb. Res.*, 6, 171, 1975.
139. **Grace, C. S. and Goldrick, R. B.**, Tissue fibrinolytic activity in obesity, *Aust. J. Exp. Biol. Med. Sci.*, 47, 397, 1969.
140. **Spöttl, F., Holzknecht, F., and Braunsteiner, H.**, Inhibitors of the plasminogen activation in patients with primary "carbohydrate-induced" hypertriglyceridemia, *J. Atheroscler. Res.*, 8, 821, 1968.
141. **Romani, J.-D., Bonnet-Bontier, M., Got, O., and Bernheim, R.**, Manifestations angiopathiques chez les diabethiques et chez les obese. Etude comparative de leurs caracteres et de leur frequence, *Presse Med.*, 77, 669, 1969.
142. **Macfarlane, R. G.**, Fibrinolysis following operation, *Lancet*, 1, 10, 1937.
143. **Macfarlane, R. G. and Biggs, R.**, Observations on fibrinolysis: spontaneous activity associated with surgical operation, trauma, etc., *Lancet*, 2, 862, 1946.
144. **Andersson, L., Nilsson, I. M., and Olow, B.**, Fibrinolytic activity in man during surgery, *Thromb. Diath. Haemorrh.*, 7, 391, 1962.
145. **MacIntyre, I. M. C., Webber, R. G., Crispin, J. R., Jones, D. R. B., Wood, J. K., Allan, N. C., Prescott, R. J., and Ruckley, C. V.**, Plasma fibrinolysis and postoperative deep vein thrombosis, *Br. J. Surg.*, 63, 694, 1976.
146. **Griffiths, N. J., Woodford, M., and Irving, M. H.**, Alteration in fibrinolytic capacity after operation, *Lancet*, 2, 635, 1977.
147. **Olow, B.**, Postoperative changes in the coagulation factors and the fibrinolytic system, *Scand. J. Clin. Lab. Invest.*, 16 (Suppl. 78), 30, 1964.
148. **Knight, M. T. N., Dawson, R., and Melrose, D. G.**, Fibrinolytic response to surgery. Labile and stabile patterns and their relevance to post-operative deep venous thrombosis, *Lancet*, 2, 370, 1977.
149. **Britton, B. J., Hawkey, C., Wood, W. G., and Peele, M.**, Stress — a significant in venous thrombosis? *Br. J. Surg.*, 61, 814, 1974.
150. **Åberg, M. and Nilsson, I. M.**, Fibrinolytic activity of the vein wall after surgery, *Br. J. Surg.*, in press.
151. **Isacson, S. and Nilsson, I. M.**, Defective fibrinolysis in blood and vein walls in recurrent "idiopathic" venous thrombosis, *Acta Chir. Scand.*, 138, 313, 1972.
152. **Kwaan, H. C.**, Disorders of fibrinolysis, *Med. Clin. North Am.*, 56, 163, 1972.
153. **Tagnon, H. J., Levenson, S. M., Davidson, C. S., and Taylor, F. H. L.**, The occurrence of fibrinolysis in shock, with observations on the prothrombin time and the plasma fibrinogen during hemorrhagic shock, *Am. J. Med. Sci.*, 211, 88, 1946.

154. **Kwaan, H. C. and McFadzean, A. J. S.**, On plasma fibrinolytic activity induced by ischemia, *Clin. Sci.*, 15, 245, 1956.
155. **Hardaway, R. M., Dixon, R. S., Foster, E. F., Karabin, B. L., Scifres, F. D., and Meyers, T.**, The effect of hemorrhagic shock on disseminated intravascular coagulation, *Ann. Surg.*, 184, 43, 1976.
156. **Schmidt, W., Egbring, R., and Havemann, K.**, Effect of elastase-like and chymotrypsin-like neutral proteases from human granulocytes on isolated clotting factors, *Thromb. Res.*, 6, 315, 1975.
157. **Owren, P. A.**, The diagnostic and prognostic significance of plasma prothrombin and factor V levels in parenchymatous hepatitis and obstructive jaundice, *Scand. J. Clin. Lab. Invest.*, 1, 131, 1949.
158. **Losowsky, M. S., Simmons, A. V., and Miloszewski, K.**, Coagulation abnormalities in liver disease, *Postgrad. Med.*, 53, 147, 1973.
159. **DeNicola, P. and Soardi, F.**, Fibrinolysis in liver diseases. Study of 109 cases by means of the fibrin plate method, *Thromb. Diath. Haemorrh.*, 2, 290, 1958.
160. **Grossi, C. E., Moreno, A. H., and Rousselot, L. M.**, Studies on spontaneous fibrinolytic activity in patients with cirrhosis of the liver and its inhibition by epsilon amino caproic acid, *Ann. Surg.*, 153, 383, 1961.
161. **Tytgat, G., Collen, D., de Vreker, R., and Verstraete, M.**, Investigations on the fibrinolytic system in liver cirrhosis, *Acta Haematol.*, 40, 265, 1968.
162. **Brakman, P., Mohler, E. R., and Astrup, T.**, Blood fibrinolysis in liver disease, *Haemostasis*, 2, 209, 1973/74.
163. **Teger-Nilsson, A.-C., Gyzander, E., Hedner, U., Myrvold, H., Noppa, H., Olsson, R., and Wallmo, L.**, Protein Inhibitors of Fibrinolysis, 3rd Int. Conf. Synthetic Fibrinolytic Thrombolytic Agents, Glasgow, September 28-30, 1976, (Abstract no. 26).
164. **Jim, R. T. S.**, A study of the plasma thrombin time, *J. Lab. Clin. Med.*, 50, 45, 1957.
165. **Von Felten, A., Straub, P. W., and Frick, P. G.**, Dysfibrinogenemia in a patient with primary hepatoma. First observation of an acquired abnormality of fibrin monomer aggregation, *N. Engl. J. Med.*, 280, 405, 1969.
166. **Green, G., Thomson, J. M., Dymock, I. W., and Poller, L.**, Abnormal fibrin polymerization in liver disease, *Br. J. Haematol.*, 34, 427, 1976.
167. **Dettori, A. G., Ponari, O., Civardi, E., Megha, A., Pini, M., and Poti, R.**, Impaired fibrin formation in advanced cirrhosis, *Haemostasis*, 6, 137, 1977.
168. **Jedrychowski, A., Hillenbrand, P., Ajdukiewicz, A. B., Parbhoo, S. P., and Sherlock, S.**, Fibrinolysis in cholestatic jaundice, *Br. Med. J.*, 1, 640, 1973.
169. **Duguid, J. B.**, Pathogenesis of atherosclerosis, *Lancet*, 2, 925, 1949.
170. **Chakrabarti, R., Hocking, E. D., and Fearnley, G. R.**, Fibrinolytic activity and coronary-artery disease, *Lancet*, 1, 987, 1968.
171. **Badawi, H., E.-Sawi, M., Mikhail, M., Nomeir, A. M., and Tewfik, S.**, Platelet, coagulation and fibrinolysis in diabetic and non-diabetic patients with quiescent coronary heart disease, *Angiology*, 21, 511, 1970.
172. **Shaper, A. G., Jones, K. W., Kyobe, J., and Jones, M.**, Fibrinolysis in relation to body fatness, serum lipids and coronary heart disease in African and Asian men in Uganda, *J. Atheroscler. Res.*, 6, 313, 1966.
173. **Gormsen, J. and Laursen, B.**, Studies on pharmacological enhancement of blood fibrinolytic activity, *Angiology*, 21, 546, 1970.
174. **Howell, W. L. and Manion, W. C.**, The low incidence of myocardial infarction in patients with portal cirrhosis of the liver. A review of 639 cases of cirrhosis of the liver from 17,731 autopsies, *Am. Heart J.*, 60, 341, 1960.
175. **Nestel, P. J.**, Fibrinolytic activity of the blood in intermittent claudication, *Lancet*, 2, 373, 1959.
176. **Peabody, R. A., Tsapogas, M. J., Wu, K. T., Deveraj, K. T., Allastair, M., and Eckert, C.**, Altered endogenous fibrinolysis and biochemical factors in atherosclerosis, *Arch. Surg.* (Chicago), 109, 309, 1974.
177. **Almér, L.-O. and Nilsson, I. M.**, On fibrinolysis in diabetes mellitus, *Acta Med. Scand.*, 198, 101, 1975.
178. **Bogie, W., George, J., and Crane, C. W.**, Fibrinolytic activity in treatment of diabetes, *Lancet*, 2, 312, 1976.
179. **Moser, K. M. and Hajjar, G. C.**, Age and disease-related alterations in fibrinogen-euglobulin (fibrinolytic) behavior, *Am. J. Med. Sci.*, 251, 536, 1966.
180. **Lassman, H. B., Wilkens, H. J., and Black, N.**, Biochemical pharmacology of the fibrinolysin system of the rat. I. The effect of alloxan-induced hyperglycemia, *J. Pharmacol. Exp. Ther.*, 189, 317, 1974.
181. **Tanser, A. R.**, Fibrinolytic response of diabetics and nondiabetics to adrenaline, *J. Clin. Pathol.*, 20, 231, 1967.
182. **Almér, L.-O. and Pandolfi, M.**, Fibrinolysis and diabetic retinopathy, *Diabetes*, 25, 807, 1976.
183. **Hedlin, A.**, Insulin and blood fibrinolytic activity, *Thromb. Diath. Haemorrh.*, 29, 293, 1973.

184. **Fearnley, G. R., Chakrabarti, R., and Vincent, C. R.,** Effect of the sulphonylureas on fibrinolysis, *Lancet*, 2, 622, 1960.

185. **Banerjee, R. N., Kumar, V., Rao, S. R., Gralni, A. L., Arya, M., and Bardhan, J.,** Antifibrin action of phenformin, *Diabetologia*, 11, 105, 1975.

186. **Nilsson, I. M.,** Coagulation, fibrinolysis and venous thrombosis, *Triangle (Engl. Ed.,)*, 16, 19, 1977.

187. **Nilsson, I. M., Hedner, U., and Isacson, S.,** Phenformin and ethyloestrenol in recurrent venous thrombosis, *Acta Med. Scand.*, 198, 107, 1975.

188. **Almér, L.-O.,** personal communication.

Chapter 9

A FAR-REACHING PROGRAM: RAPID, SAFE, AND PREDICTABLE THROMBOLYSIS IN MAN

M. Verstraete

TABLE OF CONTENTS

I. INTRODUCTION

The possibility of restoring the patency of vessels obstructed by thrombi is an old dream shared by many investigators. Trypsin, the first protease used for this purpose, was found to be too toxic, and so the surgical approach of thrombectomy remained unchallenged for many years, particularly after the introduction of Fogarty's catheter, better synthetic grafts, and autologous venous or umbilical bypasses. However, surgical skill is mainly limited to arteries and is hampered by the smallness of arterial size and by poor distal run-off.

In the meantime, considerable progress has been made in our understanding of the fibrinolytic system and the biochemistry of thrombolytic agents of human (plasmin and urokinase), animal (porcine plasmin), or microbial (streptokinase and brinase) origin. Nevertheless, regardless of the thrombolytic agent used, two major problems have still not been circumvented: (1) the slow dissolution of a thrombus which in an arterial segment may occur too late to avoid irreversible tissue damage and (2) the small surface available for biochemical interchange which in an occluding thrombus is restricted to the area directly exposed to the circulating blood. In addition, the complex organization of a thrombus also impedes its lysis, as does the presence in the circulating blood of antibodies or inhibitors to the agent used.

II. THE RESTRICTED ACTION OF PLASMIN ON FIBRIN IN PHYSIOLOGICAL FIBRINOLYSIS

Any plasmin generated in vivo is very rapidly neutralized by a fast-acting antiplasmin present in large excess in plasma, the plasmin and its inhibitor forming a 1:1 stoichiometric complex devoid of enzymatic activity. Plasmin bound to fibrin is only slowly inactivated by antiplasmin. The two interactions are mediated by the lysine binding sites in the plasmin molecule, and the plasmin-antiplasmin complex does not seem to dissociate in the presence of fibrin. The molecular model for physiological fibrinolysis recently proposed by Wiman and Collen seems therefore a plausible hypothesis. When fibrin is formed, a small amount of plasminogen is specifically bound to it through its lysine binding site(s). Plasminogen activator present in the blood or released from the vascular endothelium is adsorbed on the fibrin surface and efficiently activates the adsorbed plasminogen. The plasmin so formed has its lysine binding site(s) occupied in complex formation with fibrin and is also involved in fibrin degradation by way of its active site and therefore reacts very slowly with antiplasmin. In contrast, plasmin which is released from digested fibrin is rapidly and irreversibly neutralized by antiplasmin in the circulation.

III. THROMBOLYTIC AGENTS IN CLINICAL USE

Although the low physiological levels of the endogeneous fibrinolytic activity in shed blood can be augmented by synthetic agents, the resulting effect is weak and slow acting and has never been shown to dissolve major arterial or venous thrombi. Clinical experience with thrombolytic agents is so far limited mainly to streptokinase, urokinase, and (to a minor extent) brinase.

A. Urokinase

Urokinase (UK) is a trypsin-like enzyme consisting of a single polypeptide chain. There are two forms of urokinase: S_1, the more active, has a molecular weight of 34,500 ± 2,000 and a specific activity of 218,000 IU/mg protein; the values for the S_2

form are a molecular weight of 54,000, with a specific activity of 93,500 IU/mg protein.[2] The S_1 form probably represents a breakdown product of urokinase which arises as a result of the purification procedure (autocatalytic cleavage or uropepsin activity?); its amino acid sequence is very similar to the B-chains of thrombin and plasmin. The Asp–His–Ser–triad, common to all serine proteases, is responsible for their catalytic activity and can be irreversibly inhibited by DFP. Both forms of urokinase split a single Arg–Val bond in Glu- and in Lys-plasminogen.[3,4] It was recently suggested that the S_1 preparation may lyse two peptide bonds in Glu–Plg.[5] The S_1 form activates Glu–Plg two to five times more slowly than does S_2, whereas the kinetics for Lys–plasminogen are the same for the two urokinase forms.[6]

Urokinase is freely soluble in water, is not destroyed by alcohol or acetone, and is very stable, withstanding temperatures up to 50°C and pH values between 1 and 10. In urine, the enzyme is rapidly inactivated at acid pH, presumably by the enzyme uropepsin. Urokinase has antigenic characteristics different from those of the plasma activator, and it is therefore likely that urokinase is secreted by the kidney rather than being the excreted form of plasma activator.

Normal urine contains about 6 IU/mℓ or a few micrograms of pure enzyme protein per milliliter; a total of 2,300 ℓ of urine are required to produce 29 mg of highly purified urokinase (specific activity 35,000 CTA units per milligram protein).* At present, considerable quantities of urokinase are harvested from human embryonic kidney cell cultures, as first described by Bernik et al.[7] Since it is derived from human tissues, urokinase is not antigenic; it does not cause allergic reactions. A disadvantage is that a thromboplastic contamination of the best preparations causes a variable degree of transient hypercoagulation, and when the product is used in low doses, platelet aggregation may be induced.

Less than 25% of radiolabeled urokinase remains in the circulation 15 min after injection, and most radioactivity appears in the liver and bladder within 15 min. The estimated half-life is 10 to 15 min.

B. Streptokinase

Streptokinase (SK) is a nonenzymatic protein with a molecular weight of 47,000. It is a catabolic byproduct of a strain of β-hemolytic streptococci (Lancefield Group C) and is antigenic in man. The molecule consists of a single peptide chain without stabilizing disulfide bridges. One unit of streptokinase equals about 0.01 μg protein. The commercial preparations of streptokinase are at present purified to such a high degree that serious pyrogenic or allergic side effects are rare and minor. Unlike urokinase, streptokinase is not a direct activator of plasminogen. Streptokinase forms a 1:1 complex with plasminogen, exposing an active catalytic site on the latter molecule which gives an activator property to the whole complex. The plasminogen in the complex is converted to plasmin, and this streptokinase-plasmin complex also has activator properties. Further, plasmin is then formed mainly from noncomplexed plasminogen by cleavage of a single arginyl–valine bond.

C. Brinase

The mold *Aspergillus oryzae* produces a proteolytic agent, Protease I or brinase. Unlike the activators, brinase has a direct fibrinolytic activity. There are naturally occurring inhibitors against brinase in blood and body tissues, and they are mainly

* The activity of urokinase is expressed in CTA (Committee on Thrombolytic Agents) units or in International Units (IU). One IU is equivalent to 1 CTA unit and corresponds to the activity of 1.41 Meq of the international reference preparation; 1 IU = 0.074 Guest-Celander units, 0.740 Ploug units, 0.286 NOVO units, 1.429 Remmert and Cohen units, and 1.200 Sgouris units.

found in the α-2-macroglobulin and α_1-antitrypsin fractions.[8] It has been shown that the α_2-macroglobulin/enzyme complex retains part of its proteolytic effect; this explains why a thrombolytic effect could be obtained in animal experiments, even when the enzyme was given in amounts not exceeding the inhibitor capacity of the plasma.[9]

IV. DISCUSSION OF DIFFERENT APPROACHES TO THE USE OF STREPTOKINASE

Although it has been 20 years since streptokinase was shown quite convincingly to lyse thrombi in the human circulation,[10] the search still continues for a more effective dose regimen with a lesser bleeding hazard. The conventional scheme of SK administration consists of a loading dose, followed by continuous maintenance for one or several days. The procedure and rationale for continuous infusion of SK are summarized below, and recent modifications of this conventional scheme are discussed.

A. Continuous Infusion of Streptokinase

The initial loading dose of streptokinase is administered to overcome the antistreptokinase antibody level which varies among individuals and must be titrated in vitro to calculate the individual antibody neutralizing dose. However, a standard initial dose of 600,000 units SK is large enough for the majority of patients; even 300,000 units SK would be sufficient to neutralize inhibitors and antibodies in 95% of the adult population.[11] Furthermore, the reaction between SK and its antibodies is apparently rather slow, which means that complex formation between SK and plasminogen proceeds parallel to the antibody reaction.

The titrated or standard loading dose of SK is administered i.v. over a period of 10 to 30 min, followed by a maintenance dose of 100,000 IU hourly for the next 24 to 72 hr. This scheme results in a brisk increase of plasmin which causes a sharp fall in fibrinogen, a rise in FDPs, and a rapid depletion of plasminogen, followed by the maintenance of a low plasminogen level (between 5 to 10% of the normal value). Such a low plasminogen level is desirable, as any newly synthesized plasminogen will, in the presence of an excess of SK, form an activator, leaving few free plasminogen molecules available to be activated to plasmin in the circulation. Further degradation of circulating fibrinogen can thus be avoided.[12] Complete depletion of the plasminogen level may, however, reduce the thrombolytic potential, and in case of rethrombosis, the new thrombus would be poor in plasminogen and thus resistant to lysis.

B. Intermittent Administration of Streptokinase

There is reasonable evidence that the plasmin(ogen)-SK-complex is adsorbed onto the fibrin surface, where it can exert its effect without being significantly influenced by circulating antiplasmin. Intermittent administration of SK could therefore provide a repeated pulse of plasmin generated in the thrombus. If the SK infusions are given at 24-hr intervals, newly synthesized plasma plasminogen will restore the plasminogen levels, and after each SK injection, a high but brief circulating activator (plasminogen-SK complex) level could enrich the thrombus with this complex, resulting in an increased lysis rate.

We used the following dosage scheme in nine patients with chronic obliterative arterial disease and in eight patients with deep venous thrombosis.[13] After 25 mg prednisolone had been given i.v., an initial dose of 600,000 IU SK was administered over a 30-min period. At 24-hr intervals during the next 3 days, injections of 250,000 IU SK were given over a 5-min period. Immediately after the first administration of 600,000 units SK, the plasminogen level fell to about 17% of the starting value and remained at this level for the first 3 hr, but had returned to a level of 50% 23 hr after each pulsing dose of SK. The synthesis rate of plasminogen is not affected when an SK injection is repeated at 24-hr intervals for 3 days. The level of plasmin-antiplasmin complex dropped gradually during the first few hours and had become negligible after 24 hr. By this time, the concentration of free antiplasmin had again risen to approximately 60% of the preinfusion value. Plasmin activity was found to be high 1 hr after each administration of SK but was barely detectable after 24 hr. The fibrinogen level fell to a minimum of 20% of its original value during the first 3 hr after infusion and had risen to 50% 24 hr later. It fell again to between 25 and 40% following each subsequent SK injection. The thrombin time reached a peak value 2 hr after administration of the initial dose and was still about three times the starting value 24 hr later. Daily injections of 250,000 units of SK resulted in a sustained prolongation of the thrombin time which was at least twice the original value, even 24 hr after the SK injection. The fibrinogen degradation products reached their highest concentration 2 hr after administration of the initial dose (1668 $\mu g/m\ell$); this level was still 291 $\mu g/m\ell$ a day later, but tended to decrease gradually, notwithstanding the daily injections of 250,000 units of SK.

Our trial did not primarily aim to evaluate the clinical effectiveness of this administration scheme of SK. Of the nine patients with chronic obliterative arterial disease, only four claimed to have a decrease in rest pain, but arterial pulses reappeared or distal pressure at ankles increased in only two of them. The clinical signs improved in four of the five patients with extended superficial phlebitis, but in none of the three with nonrecent deep venous thrombosis. Using the same schedule of intermittent infusion of SK in 15 patients, Kakkar et al.[14] failed to observe complete clearing in repeated phlebograms of recent thrombotic femoral or iliac vein occlusions, whereas Ziemski et al.[15] obtained complete phlebographic clearance of recent thrombi in tibial or popliteal veins in all six of their patients. These three trials were conducted with the same dosage scheme of intermittent SK administration. As early as 1968, Heikinheimo recommended the intermittent administration of SK (loading dose 500,000 units over 60 min), followed by 250,000 units over 4 hr whenever the fibrinogen level rose above 80 mg% in plasma; the clinical results were satisfactory.[16,17] Another administration scheme consists of a loading dose of SK followed by a daily maintenance dose of 100,000 units per hour for 16 hr. This schedule was applied for no more than 6 days in 62 patients with an occlusion of limb arteries of no longer than 2 months duration; 22 had arteriographically confirmed thrombolysis.[18]

C. Infusion of an Equimolar Streptokinase-Plasminogen Complex

Streptokinase has by itself neither protease nor esterase activity.[19] When SK and human plasminogen (Plg) are mixed, a 1:1 stoichiometric complex (SK-Plg) is formed, and an active serine hydrolytic center is exposed; this complex can activate plasminogen.[20,21] It was reported that the SK-Plg complex has no activity on heated fibrin plates and does not react with antisera against human plasminogen, the latter experiment suggesting that the antigenic nature of the SK-Plg complex is different from that of plasminogen.[22] The failure of the SK-Plg complex to inhibit the hemagglutination of SK-coated cells indicates that the human antibody does not recognize the SK-Plg complex, even though one third by weight of the complex is SK.[23]

Administration of SK in man is associated with an immediate and a late immunological problem. As a result of previous streptococcal infections, patients have high affinity antibodies to streptokinase which must be saturated before infused SK can be effective. The late problem is the boosting effect of the SK infusion on the production of antibodies, which impedes both the continuation of the treatment for more than 5 days and renewed treatment within 4 to 6 months. Because the SK molecule present in the SK-Plg complex contains fewer accessible antigenic determinants than the intact molecule,[22] a systemic thrombolytic state might be obtained with a much lower dose of SK, and immediate side reactions would be less frequent. It is also possible that the immunogenicity of SK with antigenic sites masked by complex formation would be lower than that of the unbound SK.

We have tested these two hypotheses in man.[13] Two preparations of a 1:1 stoichiometric streptokinase-plasminogen complex were tested, the first in five patients (24-hr infusion) and the second one in four patients (6-hr infusion) with chronic obliterative arteriosclerotic disease in whom arterial surgery was considered to be neither feasible nor desirable. The dramatic increase seen in the anti-SK titer within 1 week of the administration of the first preparation of SK-Plg complex can be explained by the presence of residual free SK or SK fragments. It is known that heat inactivated plasminogen binds SK and forms a complex which is devoid of activator activity,[22,23] but that SK molecules are released after injection and act as an antigen and immunogen.

For this reason, we used another preparation of SK-Plg complex, prepared using unheated plasminogen obtained from hepatitis-free donors. Thorough precautions were taken to ensure that the final preparation contained no unbound SK as measured by assays on human and bovine fibrin plates and by polyacrylamide gel electrophoresis. Although this second preparation of SK-Plg complex contained no unbound streptokinase, an enhanced level of antibodies against SK was also found in all four patients treated with this preparation.

The results described above do not support the hypothesis that complex formation between SK and plasminogen prior to parenteral administration would abolish its antigenicity and immunogenicity.

The clinical efficacy of an equimolar streptokinase-plasminogen complex was studied by Martin et al.[24] In eight patients with occlusion or stenosis of the iliac or femoral artery, a loading dose of activator was followed by a continuous infusion of 100,000 units of activator per hour for 48 hr. A moderate decrease of plasminogen concentration and a measurable plasmin activity were found during the whole course of activator infusion; neither activator nor streptokinase quantities were measurable. Of the eight cases treated, complete thrombolysis was obtained in four, and the remaining four had widening of their stenoses. Whether this preparation was immunogenic is not stated in the report.

D. Intermittent Streptokinase-Plasminogen Administration

A total of 26 patients with extensive deep venous thrombosis were given 600,000 IU SK daily, followed by 90 mg of Glu-plasminogen for 5 days. Complete lysis was obtained in 27% and partial lysis in 23% of the patients.[14] These results compare poorly with the results obtained with Lys-plasminogen administered before SK infusion.

E. Intermittent Plasminogen-Streptokinase Administration

In purified systems, it has been shown[25] that the native form of plasminogen (with NH_2-terminal glutamic acid) has a weak affinity for fibrin, whereas partially degraded plasminogen (with NH_2-terminal lysine) formed by autocatalytic digestion has a stronger affinity. Approximately 4% of native and 8% of partially degraded plasminogen is specifically adsorbed to the fibrin in a whole plasma system.[26] Several groups have reported that the plasminogen content of thrombi formed in the circulation is small,[27-29] but can increase when the thrombi are placed in an artificial circulatory system.[30,31] It was therefore tempting to enrich the circulation of thrombotic patients with human Lys-plasminogen which has a higher affinity for fibrin. Kakkar et al.[14,32]

have given to 29 consecutive patients with a recent deep vein thrombosis either 90 or 120 mg of a preparation that was mainly Lys-plasminogen of placental origin over a period of 4 to 6 hr, followed by 600,000 IU SK over 30 min. The same treatment was repeated every 24 hr for the next 4 days. Phlebographically confirmed complete lysis was observed in 60% and partial lysis in 23%, and in 17% thrombi remained unchanged. The mean plasminogen levels remained between 20 to 40% of the starting value; the fibrinogen level dropped to approximately half the pretreatment level, but gradually decreased further to 1 mg/mℓ, while the plasma concentration of FDP also dropped over the same period.[14]

Phlebographically confirmed complete lysis was observed in 55% of patients treated every 24 hr with plasminogen and streptokinase administered in sequence. In contrast, thrombi remained virtually unchanged by phlebographic measurement in 12 out of 15 other patients (nonrandomized) receiving daily the same amount of SK, but no plasminogen. The thrombi were estimated to be of the same age and extent in the two treatment groups.[33]

F. Infusion of Porcine Plasmin Followed by Streptokinase

Porcine plasmin has a slow and often partial thrombolytic effect in man.[34] Duckert et al.[35] initiated thrombolytic treatment with an infusion of 30 units of plasmin per kilogram body weight over 90 min, followed by roughly the same dose over 6 to 10 hr and continued by only 10,000 IU SK per hour for 4 to 5 days. An intense fibrinolytic effect was noted, but with a higher bleeding incidence than with conventional SK treatment. Complete or partial lysis of venous thrombi was confirmed by phlebography in 71.5% of the patients.[36]

G. Initial Fibrinogen Removal Followed by Streptokinase

Besides fibrin in the thrombus, several substrates compete for interaction with plasmin generated in the circulation. One is fibrinogen, and its degradation products inhibit the aggregation of platelets and fibrin polymerization and thus give rise to an impaired hemostasis. Removal of fibrinogen from the circulation with the use of thrombin-like enzymes, such as Defibrase, Botropase, or Arvin, prior to SK administration would circumvent these problems.

Thrombin-like enzymes exclusively liberate fibrinopeptide A from the fibrinogen molecule, thus leading to circulating des-A fibrin monomer which complexes with fibrinogen to yield a soluble fibrin monomer complex. This complex can be readily converted to a fibrin clot by thrombin or give rise to paracoagulation and cryofibrinogenemia. Whereas the action of thrombin is limited by its adsorption to the fibrin clot and neutralization by circulating antithrombin, this is not the case with the above-mentioned viper enzymes which remain unimpeded in the blood stream and have therefore a more prolonged action than thrombin. After 24 to 48 hr of treatment with a purified extract of viper venom, the FDP of plasma are so decreased (about 20 ± 10 μ/mℓ) that they probably have no clinical significance.[37] The same authors went further and complemented the defibrinogenating treatment with a thrombolysis induced by SK (initial dose of 250,000 IU followed by 100,000 units per hour or 10,000 units per hour). Surprisingly, the euglobulin lysis times were highest when the lowest SK dose was given. The authors reported that the patients seemed to have fewer hemorrhagic complications while on this combined drug schedule than on conventional SK therapy. The clinical effectiveness of this combined treatment must still be demonstrated.[38]

V. DISCUSSION OF DIFFERENT APPROACHES TO THE USE OF UROKINASE

A. Continuous Infusion of Urokinase

The dosage regimen for urokinase is still being investigated. In the U.S., a maintenance dose of 5000 to 7000 IU/kg/hr has mainly been given, while in France a moderate dose of 1500 to 3000 IU/kg/hr was used. In Japan a very low dose of 100 to 1000 IU/kg/day is recommended. This difficult problem was recently reinvestigated by Samama et al.[39] A standard primary dose of 150,000 IU was given in 30 men, followed by an hourly dose of 1000, 2000, or 2500 IU/kg for 15 hr. The lowest dose did not induce a fibrinolytic state or induced one of low intensity; the highest dose of 2500 IU/kg/hr was consistently associated with an intense fibrinolytic activity. Fletcher et al.[40] also confirmed that a maintenance dose of 2400 to 3000 units per kilogram produces a substantial increase of plasma fibrinolytic activity.

Most clinical trials were conducted with an initial dose of 4400 units per kilogram of body weight given i.v. over 10 to 30 min, followed by a maintenance dose of 4000 units per kilogram of body weight per hour for 12 to 72 hr. This dose was shown to be thrombolytic and provided satisfactory clinical results. It is, however, possible that a lower and more economical drug dosage would also be adequate. Monitoring of this treatment with laboratory tests is not essential.

B. Plasminogen-Urokinase Infusion

Human plasminogen (95% Lys-plasminogen) has been given in doses ranging from 90 to 150 microkatals units (50 to 75 mg plasminogen) 6 hr before administration of a maintenance dose of 112,500 units urokinase per hour for 24 hr in patients with a recent major pulmonary embolism. The clinical results obtained with this sequential treatment were found to be superior to earlier results obtained with urokinase infusion without plasminogen.[41]

VI. CLINICAL USE OF STREPTOKINASE OR UROKINASE

A vast amount of literature has now accumulated on the use of streptokinase and to a minor extent of urokinase in a variety of clinical situations. As so often happens, many reports are uncontrolled trials or are limited to a small number of patients. Although favorable results were obtained in some conditions, well-designed clinical trials are the only reasonable basis for delineating the clinical indications of any drug, including thrombolytic agents. Reliable information and consistent good results allow the recommendation of thrombolytic agents in only a few indications.

A. Recent Deep Venous Thrombosis

An ideal therapy of established deep venous thrombosis would restore vascular patency, eliminate the risk of pulmonary embolism and later rethrombosis, and preserve the valve function, thereby avoiding the postphlebitic syndrome: a chronically swollen limb prone to stasis ulceration.

During treatment with streptokinase, a partial or complete clearance of the occluded vein is obtained in 65 to 80% of the cases, compared with 10 to 25% in heparin-treated patients.[42] In general, venous thrombi are less susceptible to lysis when more than 4 days old; however, in the trial conducted by Duckert et al.,[43] five of ten deep-vein occlusions of 10- to 15-day duration reopened after streptokinase treatment and so did the occlusions in one of seven patients with symptoms dating from 22 to 56 days. This is not an argument for postponing thrombolytic treatment once the diagnosis is made, but does encourage the study of patients with nonrecent deep vein thrombosis to see whether a relatively late reopening of the veins with streptokinase can really prevent chronic venous insufficiency.

In general, proximal veins are more readily reopened with streptokinase than distal veins, but one has to bear in mind that the highest occlusions are usually more recent, since the patient seeks medical help sooner; partial calf vein thrombosis may remain clinically silent for a lengthy period.

Rethrombosis of a lysed thrombus does occur in spite of anticoagulation, and little is known about its frequency. Rethrombosis occurred only once in the 93 patients admitted to the trial of Duckert et al.[43] in which the control phlebograms were taken at a mean of 5.8 days after the beginning of streptokinase treatment. Another study revealed that the patients with complete thrombus regression immediately after thrombolytic treatment also had normal phlebograms at a follow-up 6 to 50 (mean 21) months later.[44] It now appears that the risk of rethrombosis is considerably less after thrombolysis than after thrombectomy.

Whether streptokinase treatment can restore the venous function of the leg and reduce the incidence of the late sequellae or postthrombotic syndrome has only been studied in a few trials. In the trial of Kakkar et al.,[45] venous valve function judged by ascending functional cinephlebography was normal 6 to 12 months after thrombolytic treatment in those patients in whom the diagnosis was made within 26 hr and the thrombus rapidly and completely dissolved. In another follow-up study performed on average 21 months after thrombolytic treatment, a normal phlebogram as well as plethysmographic findings (venous reserve volume and maximal venous-emptying capacity) confirmed the normal valve function in those patients who had good initial results.[44] Widmer[46] published the results of a 4.8-year follow-up of 67 patients who had a partial or complete clearing of the occluded vein after thrombolytic treatment and of 78 patients in whom the initial treatment was not effective as shown by phlebography. All patients had been on oral anticoagulation for the first 6 months after acute treatment. Leg ulcers did not occur in the group with successful thrombolysis, but did occur in 11% of the patients in whom venous patency could not be restored initially. Leg edema assessed by circumference measurements was significantly less in the group successfully treated by thrombolysis. Thus, the normal valvular function in most patients without phlebographically-detectable thrombotic remnants after thrombolysis contrasts with the valvular destruction observed after venous thrombectomies and constitutes an important argument in favor of thrombolytic therapy in acute deep venous thrombosis causing clinical symptoms in younger patients.

During thrombolytic treatment of deep venous thrombosis, pulmonary embolism has always been a hazard to be feared. It is likely that small lysed fragments of the thrombus do embolize, but are rapidly dissolved in the lung circulation by the systemic fibrinolytic system, reducing the severity of the associated hemodynamic disturbances. The incidence of reported nonfatal pulmonary embolism during thrombolytic treatment of deep vein thrombosis varies considerably, a fact which is also partly due to the sensitivity of the various diagnostic methods used.[47] In the trial of Duckert et al.,[43] comprising 187 patients with acute or subacute deep vein thrombosis treated either with streptokinase or heparin, the incidence of nonfatal pulmonary embolism was not greater during thrombolytic treatment (7.5%) than during heparinization (12%). A randomized trial comparing a treatment schedule of 24 hr of heparin, streptokinase, or urokinase in acute deep vein thrombosis revealed the superiority of the latter two agents to heparin; the effectiveness of urokinase or streptokinase appeared to be similar.[48]

From the evidence so far available, streptokinase or urokinase are probably best reserved for patients with extensive recent thrombi involving calf and more proximal veins which cause clinical symptoms, provided these clinical features have not been present for longer than 72 hr. In patients with recent occlusive iliofemoral thrombosis, venous thrombectomy or thrombolytic therapy may be used. Both forms of treatment are less effective when older thrombi are involved; thrombectomy is more often associated with rethrombosis than is thrombolytic therapy. The present trend is definitely in favor of streptokinase treatment, but other factors, particularly contraindications and surgical skill, will determine which of the two forms of treatment should be used in a given medical center.

In general, streptokinase or urokinase are given for up to 3 or 4 days and are followed by anticoagulants, preferably heparin, for 5 to 7 days, which are discontinued once oral anticoagulation has reached the desired level. Treatment with coumarin drugs is continued for at least 4 but preferably 6 months. Patients with recurrent deep venous thrombosis should perhaps be kept indefinitely on oral anticoagulants unless fibrinolytic stimulants, such as the anabolic steroid ethyloestranol and/or antiaggregating drugs, prove to be satisfactory for secondary prevention.

Since deep venous thrombosis is not infrequent before and after childbirth, it is important to know that streptokinase passes the placental barrier only slightly and can be given during pregnancy without increasing the fibrinolytic activity in the fetus. This treatment should, however, be avoided during the first 18 weeks of pregnancy, until the trophoblast is firmly attached to the uterus. No adverse effects in the babies have been reported.[49] Thrombolytic treatment should not be started earlier than 10 days postpartum.

B. Acute Pulmonary Embolism

The aims of an effective treatment of fresh and massive pulmonary embolism are to reduce mortality, decrease the period of incapacity, and improve the long-term effective pulmonary function.

Pulmonary embolism which is associated with considerable morbidity and mortality is most often a complication of a silent peripheral-vein thrombosis. In patients with massive pulmonary embolism resulting in acute right heart failure and shock, mortality is almost 75% in the first 2 hr, thus before any treatment can be given.

For treatment purposes, pulmonary embolism may be classified in four different categories:

1. The emboli may be so massive as to occlude the bifurcation of the pulmonary artery and be immediately fatal, no form of treatment being of value.
2. The emboli may be large enough to occlude two thirds or more of the main branches of the pulmonary artery and cause acute right heart failure with shock, dyspnea, progressive deterioration, and usually death.
3. The emboli may cause collapse followed by partial recovery, but residual hemodynamic problems.
4. The emboli may be small, causing segmental infarctions in the peripheral lung circulation, and may even remain clinically silent until repeated embolism obliterates so much of the vascular bed that pulmonary hypertension and cor pulmonale appear.

Reports of clinical trials in which urokinase or streptokinase have been compared with heparin in patients with severe pulmonary embolism (Categories 2 and 3) have been reviewed.[50,51] All studies indicated that recent pulmonary emboli dissolved much more readily with these thrombolytic agents than with heparin. The National Heart and Lung Institute cooperative trial of urokinase and streptokinase in acute pulmonary embolism is the largest, best documented, and most comprehensive study to date on this subject. The results of the first phase of this trial[52, 53] are based on 160 patients with recent (less than 12 hr) massive pulmonary embolism (significant filling defects or obstruction of at least two arteries). All patients were treated with heparin during diagnostic evaluation, and 82 were randomly allocated to further treatment with urokinase and 78 to heparin treatment. Furthermore, all patients who received a 12-hr infusion.of urokinase were given heparin for 5 days after urokinase was discontinued. No difference in short-term mortality (14 days) was obtained between the two treatment groups. It appeared that 24 hr after initiation of thrombolysis, the urokinase-treated patients had a significantly greater resolution rate of pulmonary emboli than the heparin-treated patients, as judged by arteriography, hemodynamics, and lung scanning; right heart function improved more rapidly than when heparin was given. Serial lung scanning revealed that these differences in embolus resolution rates decreased after 14 days. Pulmonary embolism recurred in 17% of the urokinase patients, compared with 23% of the heparin patients. There were episodes of bleeding in 45% of the urokinase patients, compared with 27% of the heparin patients. Urokinase had a greater effect on the criteria used to judge the resolution of lung emboli in patients with massive embolism.

In the second phase of the same trial,[54] a 12-hr infusion of urokinase was compared with a 24-hr infusion of urokinase or streptokinase treatment in 167 patients; 12 of these patients were in shock. There were no significant differences in mortality, resolution rate of emboli, or the mean changes in right heart hemodynamic parameters after 24 hr between the three treatment groups. A total of 24 hr of urokinase treatment resulted in a greater improvement of the lung scans than did streptokinase treatment, and this difference reached a level of significance in massive pulmonary embolism. Drug-related morbidity was minimal. However, lung scans repeated up to 6 months after the acute event showed no differences between patients treated with thrombolytic agents or with heparin.

Thrombolysis with streptokinase or urokinase appears to be the current treatment of choice for most patients with acute massive life-threatening pulmonary embolism (Categories 2 and 3), who have survived the initial episode and are stabilized with supportive measures, but whose immediate course is precarious. Even if only partial lysis is obtained, it will increase the patient's reserve and furthermore may lyse fresh deep vein thrombi, reducing the incidence of recurrent embolism. However, the decision to be taken by the physician in the presence of an individual patient with a very severe lung embolism, shock, and an immediate risk of dying, is whether to mobilize the heart surgeon and the pump team. According to the Peter Bent Brigham group, patients surviving more than an hour or so after massive infarction comprise a prognostically better group in whom the chance of surviving embolectomy is smaller than the probability of survival without surgery.[55] However, it is likely that surgical skill will improve for this type of emergency. Eventually the physician in charge will have to assess the limitations of the thrombolytic and surgical treatments which are available at the hour of his decision making on behalf of a patient with massive pulmonary embolism.

C. Acute Myocardial Infarction

One way to improve the function of the myocardium is to increase the oxygenation to areas of injury near the infarct. On theoretical grounds, thrombolytic agents could be useful for this purpose. Indeed, lysis or prevention of microthrombi would improve the circulation in the area of infarction; a decrease in the viscosity of the blood may favorably affect the coronary circulation, and if a fibrin occlusion of a coronary artery is present, prevention of its distal propagation or timely restoration of arterial continuity would reduce the ultimate size of the myocardial necrosis. These postulated effects of thrombolytic agents should, by salvaging muscle cells and augmenting myocardial function in ischemic areas, increase cardiac output.

Up to now, ten controlled clinical trials with fibrinolytic drugs in recent myocardial infarction have been presented.[56] All were essentially mortality-type trials in which the mortality in the treated group was compared to the mortality in the control group. The study design of the trials was different in many respects, such as upper age limit of the patients included, age of infarction, randomization procedure, treatment schedules, etc. The mortality statistics in five out of six trials with streptokinase which can be regarded as adequately designed reveal a trend to reduced mortality in patients treated with streptokinase, as compared to the controls which is statistically significant only in three trials. One large-scale urokinase trial showed no positive effect of the treatment.[57] It must be concluded that the usefulness of streptokinase in patients with recent myocardial infarction is not established, but that there is a trend to a reduction of mortality which cannot be overlooked.

D. Recent Arterial Occlusions of Limb Arteries

Clinical experience with streptokinase in the treatment of recent occlusion of peripheral arteries is largely confined to occlusions of the lower limbs. Central to the selection of thrombolytic drugs as a mode of treatment of acute peripheral artery occlusion is, of course, not only the question of how frequently such treatment will ultimately produce an arteriographically satisfactory result, but also two other important questions: how long is thrombolytic treatment required to produce thrombolysis and increased blood flow and is the limb likely to remain viable during this time?

The partial or complete angiographic clearance rate of arterial occlusions is about 70% if streptokinase treatment is started within the first 12 hr of acute onset of symptoms and 63% if started between 12 and 42 hr.[58] Thrombolysis is obtained at an average time of 39 hr when the thrombolytic treatment is started within the first 19 hr, but the mean lysis time is 62 hr when streptokinase is started later.[59] While it is likely that an increase of limb blood flow was obtained considerably earlier than these figures suggest, it must be emphasized that even when thrombolytic therapy is successful in opening an occluded artery in an atherosclerotic limb, substantial delays in the effect of treatment must be anticipated.

Since the introduction of Fogarty's balloon catheter and the Dotter procedure, surgery is likely to be more successful and more reliable. The choice of treatment depends on several factors, such as age, extent and site of the occlusion, the degree of pretreatment ischemia, and the general condition of the patient.[58] In our center, the Fogarty catheter is used in patients with acute thrombosis in large atheromatotic arteries, particularly if there is evidence to suggest impending irreversible damage to the limb. Thrombolytic treatment with streptokinase is initiated only if the thrombotic occlusion is located in an artery too distally located for the surgical approach or when this almost local form of surgery is contraindicated or has failed.

E. Chronic Arterial Occlusion of Limb Arteries

Several investigators have used thrombolytic therapy when either the age of the arterial occlusion was unknown or the clinical history suggested that acute occlusion had occurred several months (up to 6) previously and have shown a 20% success rate.[60, 61] In a recent report, Martin[62] presented the results of streptokinase treatment in 435 chronic arterial occlusions. In 225 chronic occlusions of the popliteal-superficia femoral artery, patency was obtained in 8.9%; the corresponding clearing rate for 169 chronic occlusions of the common or external iliac arteries was 18.9%, and in 41 chronic occlusions of the abdominal aorta with or without concomitant bilateral iliac occlusion, it was 24.3%.

As only unorganized thrombi can lyse, these surprising results suggest that in some cases organization of thrombi may be delayed, possibly because the atherosclerotic lesions form a mechanical barrier for the ingrowth of fibroblasts involved in thrombus organization.

F. Retinal Artery or Vein Occlusion

Circulatory disturbances in the retinal arteries are caused by hypertension, atherosclerosis, inflammation, or thromboemboli; an occlusion of the retinal artery almost invariably damages the vision severely. Thrombolytic treatment is therefore not always indicated. In general, neither anticoagulants nor thrombolytic drugs have been shown to prevent further deterioration in retinal function.

Central retinal vein occlusion has a poor prognosis, but occasionally resolves spontaneously, but not necessarily with improved vision.[63] Two of three recent controlled trials comparing anticoagulants with thrombolytic drugs suggest that chances of improvement or return of vision in central retinal vein occlusion is greater, even up to 1 month after onset of symptoms, with thrombolytic agents used correctly.[64-66]

G. Occluded Arteriovenous Shunts

Arteriovenous external cannulae in patients on long-term hemodialysis occasionally occlude. When clots cannot be removed by irrigation with heparinized saline, streptokinase or urokinase is injected into either or both ends of the cannula; this results in rapid clearance in nearly all cases.

H. Miscellaneous Conditions

Streptokinase and urokinase have been used to clear acute thrombotic obstructions of heart valve prostheses, to dissolve clots in the peritoneal cavity obstructing outflow during peritoneal dialysis, and in severe angina pectoris. As very limited information is available on these and other situations where thromboembolism is a contributing factor, no valid statement can be made on the relative merits of the thrombolytic agent used.

The chance that thrombolytic agents could be useful in cerebral thromboembolism are meager, as the results of therapy also depend on the length of viability of the ischemic brain.[40] Moreover, the risk of hemorrhage within the reperfused infarcted area has prevented the extensive use of thrombolytic agents in this indication.

VII. CLINICAL EXPERIENCE WITH BRINASE

The i.v. infusion of brinase in amounts not exceeding the inhibitor capacity of plasma has been reported to relieve symptoms and increase the blood pressure in the legs of patients with chronic, severe obstructive arterial disease.[67-69] These three open studies do not include a simultaneously followed control group and are therefore open to criticism. Fitzgerald et al.[70] have recently followed 18 patients with stable intermittent claudication for at least 6 months. After an observation period of 3 months during which oral anticoagulants were started, the patients were allocated by randomization to six infusions over 2 weeks of either brinase (100 mg per infusion) or saline. After the last infusion, a significant improvement both of peripheral systolic blood pressures and Doppler ultrasound scanning were observed in the brinase-treated patients. This study does not reveal long-term results. We have performed a randomized single-blind trial with repeated (9 in 19 days) i.v. infusions of 100 mg brinase in 70 patients with severe chronic limb ischemia (Stage III or IV), who were candidates for lumbar sympathectomy or amputation. After the last infusion, a significant increase in calf and ankle pressure index was found in the brinase-treated patients only. After 6 months of follow-up, the proposed surgical procedure was avoided in a significantly higher number of brinase-treated patients ($p = 0.01$); this figure was not significantly higher when 10 patients with Burger's disease were omitted from the analysis. Patients treated with a combination of brinase and coumarins had a better clinical outcome than patients receiving either of them separately.[71]

REFERENCES

1. **Wiman, B. and Collen, D.**, Molecular mechanism of physiological fibrinolysis, *Nature (London)*, 272, 549, 1978.
2. **White, W. F., Barlow, G. H., and Mozen, M. M.**, The isolation and characterization of plasminogen activators (urokinase) from human urine, *Biochemistry*, 5, 2160, 1966.
3. **Summaria, L., Arzadon, L., Bernabe, P., and Robbins, K. C.**, The activation of plasminogen to plasmin by urokinase in the presence of the plasmin inhibitor trasylol. The preparation of plasmin with the same NH_2-terminal heavy (A) chain sequence as the parent zymogen, *J. Biol. Chem.*, 250, 3988, 1975.
4. **Summaria, L., Boreisha, I. G., Arzadon, L., and Robbins, K. C.**, Activation of human Glu-plasminogen to Glu-plasmin by urokinase in presence of plasmin inhibitor, *J. Biol. Chem.*, 252, 3945, 1977.
5. **Lormeau, J., Goulay, J., Vairel, E. G., and Choay, J.**, The action of urokinase on plasminogen, *Thromb. Haemostasis*, 38, 257, 1977.
6. **Lormeau, J. C., Goulay, J., Vairel, E. G., and Choay, J.**, A comment on the activities of high and low molecular weight urokinases, in *Fibrinolysis Current Fundamental and Clinical Concepts*, Gaffney, P. and Balkuv-Ulutin, G., Eds., Academic Press, London, 1978, 77.
7. **Bernik, M. B. and Kwaan, H. C.**, Origin of fibrinolytic activity in cultures of human kidney, *J. Lab. Clin. Med.* 70, 650, 1967.
8. **Kiessling, H. and Svensson, R.**, Influence of an enzyme from *Aspergillus oryzae*, Protease 1, on some components of the fibrinolytic system, *Acta Chem. Scand.*, 24, 569, 1970.
9. **Bergkvist, R. and Svard, P. O.**, Studies on the thrombolytic effect of a protease from *Aspergillus oryzae*, *Acta Physiol. Scand.*, 60, 363, 1964.
10. **Johnson, A. J. and McCarty, W. R.**, The lysis of artificially induced intravascular clots in man by intravenous infusions of streptokinase, *J. Clin. Invest.*, 38, 1627, 1959.
11. **Verstraete, M., Vermylen, J., Amery, A., and Vermylen, C.**, Thrombolytic therapy with streptokinase using a standard dosage scheme, *Br. Med. J.*, 1, 454, 1966.
12. **Verstraete, M., Vermylen, J., and Donati, M. B.**, The effect of streptokinase infusion on chronic occlusions and stenosis, *Ann. Intern. Med.*, 74, 377, 1971.
13. **Verstraete, M., Vermylen, J., Holleman, W., and Barlow, G. H.**, Biological effects of the administration of an equimolar streptokinase-plasminogen complex in man, *Thromb. Res.*, 11, 227, 1977.
14. **Kakkar, V. V., Sagar, S., Scully, M. F., and Lane, D. A.**, Intermittent plasminogen-streptokinase treatment of deep vein thrombosis, *Aktuel. Probl. Angiologie*, 37, 142, 1978.
15. **Ziemski, J. M., Marchlewski, S., Meissner A. J., Rudowski, W., Kolakowsky, L., Lopaciuk, S., and Latallo, Z. S.**, Clinical effects of intermittent streptokinase therapy in deep vein thrombosis, *Aktn. Probl. Angiologie*, 37, 187, 1978.
16. **Heikinheimo, R.**, Fibrinolysis by "minidosage", *Curr. Ther. Res. Clin. Exp.*, 10, 382, 1968.
17. **Heikinheimo, R. and Ruosteenoja, R.**, Further experience with "minidosage" in fibrinolytic treatment, *Curr. Ther. Res. Clin. Exp.*, 13, 444, 1971.
18. **Fiessinger, J. N., Aiach, M., Brunet, G., Cormier, J. M., Leclerc, M., and Housset, E.**, Intermittent treatment with streptokinase in arterial disease of the limbs, *Vas. Surg.*, 2, 384, 1978.
19. **Takada, A., Takada, Y., and Ambrus, L.**, Proactivators in the fibrinolytic system, *Thromb. Diath. Haemorrh. Suppl.*, 47, 37, 1971.

20. **McClintock, D. K. and Bell, P. H.**, The mechanism of activation of human plasminogen by streptokinase, *Biochem. Biophys. Res. Commun.,* 43, 694, 1971.
21. **Reddy, K. N. N. and Markus, G.**, Mechanism of activation of human plasminogen by streptokinase, *J. Biol. Chem.,* 247, 1683, 1972.
22. **Barlow, G. H., Devine, E., and Finley, R.**, Immunochemical and biochemical comparison of streptokinase and the streptokinase-plasminogen complex, *Res. Comm. Chem. Pathol. Pharmacol.,* 10, 465, 1975.
23. **Barlow, G. H., Finley, R., and Castellino, F. J.**, Immunological comparison of native streptokinase with streptokinase fragments, *Thrombos. Res.,* 8, 237, 1976.
24. **Martin, M. and Heimburger, N.**, Clinical and laboratory findings in the course of activator (equimolar SK-plg complex) infusion, *Aktuel. Probl. Angiologie,* 37, 169, 1978.
25. **Thorsen, S.**, Differences in the binding to fibrin of native plasminogen and plasminogen modified by proteolytic degradation. Influence of amino carboxylic acids, *Biochim. Biophys. Acta,* 393, 55, 1975.
26. **Rakoczi, I., Wiman, B., and Collen, D.**, On the biological significance of the specific interaction between fibrin, plasminogen and antiplasmin, *Biochim. Biophys. Acta,* 540, 295, 1978.
27. **Hedner, U., Nilsson, I. M., and Robertson, B.**, Determination of plasminogen in clots and thrombi, *Thromb. Diath. Haemorrh.,* 16, 38, 1966.
28. **Ogston, C. M., Ogston, D., Fullerton, H. W., and Robertson, H. W.**, Observations on the lysis of artificial thrombi by urokinase, *Thromb. Diath. Haemorrh.,* 19, 107, 1968.
29. **Gottiob, R. and Blumel, G.**, Uber den Nachweis der Plasminogen-verarmung in retrahierten Vollblutgerinnseln uber deren Bedeutung fur die Lysierbarheit mit Streptokinase, *Thromb. Diath. Haemorrh.,* 15, 570, 1966.
30. **Scully, M. F., Strachan, C. J. L., and Kakkar, V. V.**, Binding of iodinated proteins to forming and preformed thrombi, *Biochem. Soc. Trans.,* 1, 1204, 1973.
31. **Strachan, C. J. L., Scully, M. F., and Kakkar, V. V.**, The behavior of isotopic labelled blood proteins in thrombosis, *Thromb. Res.,* 4, 303, 1974.
32. **Kakkar, V. V.**, Fibrinolytic treatment of venous thrombosis, *Thromb. Diath. Haemorrh. Suppl.,* 59, 227, 1974.
33. **Scully, M. F., Lane, D. A., Sagar, S., Thomas, D. P., and Kakkar, V. V.**, Intermittent plasminogen-streptokinase treatment of deep vein thrombosis, *Thromb. Haemostas.,* 37, 162, 1977.
34. **Storm, O., Ollendorff, P., Drawsen, E., and Tang, P.**, Acute deep vein thrombosis treated with porcine plasmin, *Thromb. Diath. Haemorrh.,* 32, 468, 1974.
35. **Duckert, F., Walter, M., Marbet, G. A., Six, P., Nyman, D., Madar, G., DaSilva, M. A., Widmer, L. K., Schmitt, H. E., and Vokal, J.**, Results of a combined streptokinase-plasmin therapy in deep vein thrombosis, *Aktuel. Probl. Angiologie,* 37, 175, 1978.
36. **Marbet, G. A., Walter, M., Six, P., Nyman, D., Rüst, O., Biland, L., Duckert, F., Madar, G., DaSilva, M. A., Widmer, L. K., Schmitt, H. E., and Vokal, J.**, in *Blutgerinnung und Antikoagulantien,* Neuhaus, K. and Duckert, F., Eds., Schattauer Verlag, Stuttgart, 1977, 87.
37. **Latallo, Z. S., Lopaciuk, S., and Meissner, J.**, A combined treatment with Defibrase and streptokinase, *Aktuel. Probl. Angiologie,* 26, 181, 1975.
38. **Forbes, C. D., Barbenell, J., and Prentice, C. R. M.**, Treatment of thrombosis by sequential therapy with ancrod followed by streptokinase. Clinical pharmacology and rheology, *Haemostasis,* 5, 348, 1976.
39. **Samama, M. and Conard, J.**, Biological results during urokinase therapy at different doses, in *Thrombosis and Urokinase,* Paoletti, R. and Sherry, S., Eds., Academic Press, London, 1977, 243.
40. **Fletcher, A. P., Alkjaersig, N., Lewis, M., Tulevski, V., Davies, A., Brooks, J. E., Hardin, W. B., Landau, W. M., and Raichle, M. E.**, A pilot study of urokinase therapy in cerebral infarction, *Stroke,* 7, 135, 1976.
41. **Brochier, M., Planiol, T., Griguer, P., Raynaud, Ph., Fauchier, J. P., Charbonnier, B., Latour, F., and Pellois, A.**, Interet du traitement sequentiel lysyl-plasminogene-urokinase et therapeutique thrombolytique, *Coeur Med. Interne,* 16, 513, 1977.
42. **Kakkar, V. V.**, Fibrinolytic treatment of venous thrombosis, *Thromb. Diath. Haemorrh. Suppl.,* 59, 227, 1974.
43. **Duckert, F., Muller, G., Nyman, D., Benz, A., Prisender, S., Madar, G., DaSilva, M. A., Widmer, L. K., and Schmitt, H. E.**, Treatment of deep vein thrombosis with streptokinase, *Br. Med. J.,* 1, 479, 1975.
44. **Johansson, E., Ericson, K., and Zetterquist, S.**, Streptokinase treatment of deep vein thrombosis of the lower extremity, *Acta Med. Scand.,* 199, 89, 1976.
45. **Kakkar, V. V., Flanc, C., Howe, C. T., O'Shea, M. J., and Flute, P. T.**, Treatment of deep vein thrombosis. A trial of heparin, streptokinase and arvin, *Br. Med. J.,* 1, 806, 1969.

46. **Widmer, M. Th., Madar, G., and Widmer, L. K.,** Incidence of post-thrombotic syndrome. Follow-up on 99 patients with a deep venous thrombosis and thrombolytic or heparin treatment, *Aktuel. Probl. Angiologie,* 37, 191, 1978.
47. **Hess, H.,** Zur Streptokinase-Therapie akuter Verschlusse von Gliedmassengefässen, *Thromb. Diath. Haemorrh. Suppl.,* 32, 275, 1969.
48. **Sharma, G. V. R. K., O'Connell, D. J., Belko, J. S., and Sasahara, A. A.,** Thrombolytic therapy in deep vein thrombosis, in *Thrombosis and Urokinase,* Paoletti, R. and Sherry, S., Eds., Academic Press, London, 1977, 181.
49. **Ludwig, H.,** Results of streptokinase therapy in deep venous thrombosis during pregnancy, *Postgrad. Med. J.,* 49 (Suppl. 5), 65, 1973.
50. **Brogden, R. N., Speight, T. M., and Avery, G. S.,** Streptokinase: a review of its clinical pharmacology, mechanism of action and therapeutic uses, *Drugs,* 5, 357, 1973.
51. **Ly, B., Arnesen, H., Eie, H., and Hol, R.,** A controlled clinical trial of streptokinase and heparin in the treatment of major pulmonary embolism, *Acta Med. Scand.,* 203, 465, 1978.
52. The urokinase pulmonary embolism trial. A cooperative study. Phase I results, *JAMA,* 214, 2163, 1970.
53. The urokinase pulmonary embolism trial. A national cooperative study: *Circulation,* 47, Suppl. 11, 1973.
54. The urokinase-streptokinase embolism trial. A national cooperative study. Phase II results, *JAMA,* 229, 1606, 1974.
55. **Alpert, J. S., Smith, R. E., Ockene, I. S., Askenazi, J., Dexter, L., and Dalen, J. E.,** Treatment of massive pulmonary embolism: the role of pulmonary embolectomy, *Am. Heart J.,* 89, 413, 1975.
56. **Van de Loo, J. and Verstraete, M.,** Fibrinolytic treatment of acute myocardial infarction: a question still open, *Thromb. Diath. Haemorrh. Suppl.,* 59, 203, 1974.
57. A European Collaborative Study, Controlled trial of urokinase in myocardial infarction, *Lancet,* 2, 624, 1975.
58. **Amery, A., Deloof, W., Vermylen, J., and Verstraete, M.,** Outcome of recent thromboembolic occlusions of limb arteries treated with streptokinase, *Br. Med. J.,* 11, 639, 1970.
59. **Schmutzler, R. and Koller, F.,** Thrombolytische therapie, in *Recent Advances in Blood Coagulation,* Poller, L., Ed., Churchill, London, 1969, 299.
60. **Schoop, W., Martin, M., and Zeitler, E.,** Beseitigung after Arterienverschlüsse durch intravenose Streptokinase-Infusion, *Dtsch. Med. Wochenschr.,* 93, 2321, 1968.
61. **Schoop, W., Levy, H., and Zeitler, E.,** Late results of thrombolytic therapy of chronic arterial occlusion, *Ger. Med.,* 1, 66, 1971.
62. **Martin, M.,** Application of streptokinase treatment in chronic arterial occlusions, *Aktuel. Probl. Angiologie,* 37, 180, 1978.
63. **Drance, S. M.,** An ophthalmologist's approach to fibrinolytis, *Angiology,* 12, 149, 1961.
64. **Den Ottolander, G. J. H. and Craandijk, A.,** Treatment of thrombosis of the central retinal vein with streptokinase, *Thromb. Diath. Haemorrh.,* 20, 415, 1968.
65. **Kohner, E. M., Pettit, J. E., Hamilton, A. M., Bulpih, C. J., and Dollery, C. T.,** Streptokinase in central retinal vein occlusion: a controlled clinical trial, *Br. Med. J.,* 1, 550, 1976.
66. **Kwaan, H. C., Dobbie, J. G., and Fetkenhour, C. L.,** The use of anticoagulants and thrombolytic agents in occlusive retinal vascular disease, in *Thrombosis and Urokinase,* Paoletti, R., and Sherry, S., Eds., Academic Press, London, 1977, 191.
67. **Fitzgerald, D. E., Frisch, E. P., and Thornes, R. D.,** Thrombolytic therapy with brinase of chronic peripheral arterial disease, *J. Ir. Coll. Physicians Surg.,* 1, 123, 1972.
68. **Fitzgerald, D. E. and Frisch, E. P.,** Relief of chronic peripheral artery obstruction by intravenous brinase, *J. Ir. Med. Assoc.,* 66, 3, 1973.
69. **Lund, F., Ekestrom, S., Frisch, E. P., and Magaard, F.,** Thrombolytic treatment with I.V. brinase of advanced arterial obliterative disease, *Angiology,* 26, 534, 1975.
70. **Fitzgerald, D. E., Frisch, E. P., and Milliken, J. C.,** Relief of chronic arterial obstruction using intravenous brinase — a control trial, *Scand. J. Thorac. Cardiovasc. Surg.,* in press.
71. **Verhaeghe, R., Verstraete, M., Schetz, J., Vanhove, Ph., Suy, R., and Vermylen, J.,** Clinical trial of brinase and anticoagulants as a method of treatment for advanced limb ishcemia, *Eur. J. Clin. Pharmacol.,* 16, 165, 1979.

Chapter 10

MOLECULAR BASIS FOR MEASUREMENT OF CIRCULATING FIBRINOGEN DERIVATIVES*,**

George D. Wilner

TABLE OF CONTENTS

* Supported by USPHS Program Project Grant HL-15486 and Grant HL-22642 from the National Heart and Lung Institute and NIH Career Development Award HL-70447.

** Reprinted from Wilner, G. D., *Prog. Hemostasis Thromb.*, 4, 211, 1978. With permission.

I. INTRODUCTION

Fibrinogen is a relatively large, sparingly soluble glycoprotein whose abundance in plasma reflects its physiologic function as a major component in hemostatic plug formation. In concert with platelet aggregate formation, fibrin generation represents a basic mechanism by which vertebrates maintain normal hemostasis. The demonstration by Mosher[1] that fibrin may covalently bind to proteins produced by fibroblasts suggests that fibrin formation may be critical for normal wound healing as well.

Morphologic examination of human material, as well as studies in experimental animal models, indicate that fibrin forms a major component in venous thrombi but is present to a lesser extent in arterial thrombi[2] (see Figure 1). The course of fibrin clot formation and dissolution in vivo is believed to be associated with the activities of at least three enzymes for which fibrinogen or fibrin represents the primary substrate: thrombin, whose action catalyzes the conversion of fibrinogen to fibrin; Factor XIII, which introduces cross links into the fibrin clot; and plasmin, which digests both fibrinogen and fibrin. The activities of each of these three enzymes are associated with detectable changes in either the chemical or physical properties of fibrinogen, rendering it distinguishable from the native protein. In addition, the action of thrombin or plasmin on fibrinogen results in the release of soluble, specific proteolytic fragments whose quantitation, in theory, may be used as indices of that enzyme's in vivo activity. Advances in the past two decades in our knowledge of the structure of enzyme-altered fibrinogen and its proteolytic fragments, as well as the advent of highly specific and sensitive analytical techniques such as radioimmunoassays and affinity chromatogra-

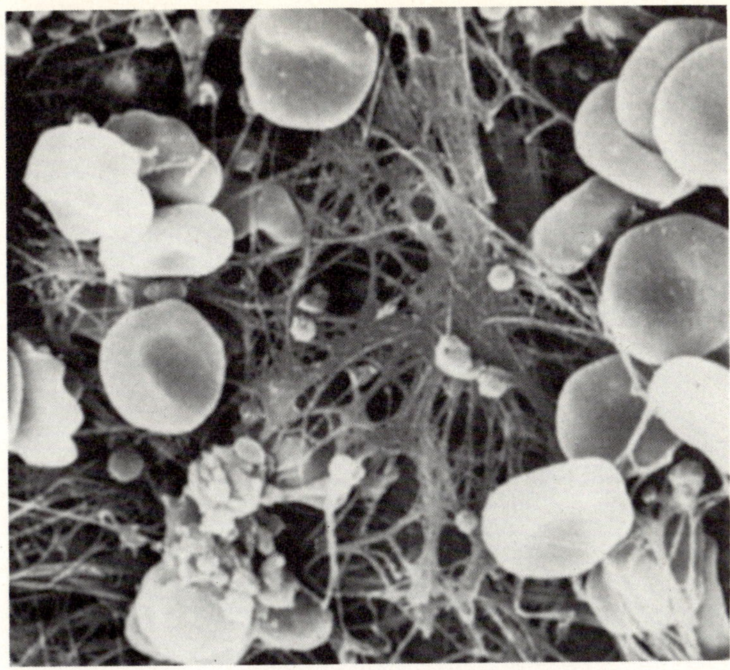

FIGURE 1. Scanning electron micrograph of red thrombus showing erythrocytes and platelet masses trapped in a fibrin meshwork. (Magnification × 2250.) (Courtesy of Dr. D. Fenoglio.)

phy, have made such measurements a reality. The properties of these fragments and the extent to which they represent circulating *de novo* products, which can be quantified as indices of the action of specific coagulant and fibrinolytic enzymes, form the basis for this review.

II. FIBRINOGEN STRUCTURE

The chemical and physical properties of fibrinogen and fibrin have been the subject of intensive investigation by many laboratories, and space permits only a superficial overview of this subject. The reader is referred to recent reviews for further details.[3-6]

Fibrinogen circulates as a dimeric structure whose component halves are linked by three pairs of disulfide bonds.[7] It is generally accepted that the molecular weight of human fibrinogen is 340,000 ± 20,000 daltons and the molecular weights of most mammalian fibrinogens are also in this range.[3]

Currently, much of our knowledge of the organization and structure of the fibrinogen molecule has been derived from studies of changes in electrophoretic mobility of reduced, separated chains of fibrinogen or fibrin that had been subjected to degradation by either enzymatic or chemical means. These techniques, because of their relative simplicity, have been widely used by many investigators and have greatly contributed to our present understanding of this molecule. Predictably, disputes have arisen in the interpretation of these electrophoretic data which will be resolved only when our knowledge of the primary structure of fibrinogen is complete.

Prolonged digestion of fibrinogen by plasmin produces two major families of products, fragments D and E, consisting of remnants of all three component chains of fibrinogen.[8-10] Fragment E, whose primary structure has now been completely deter-

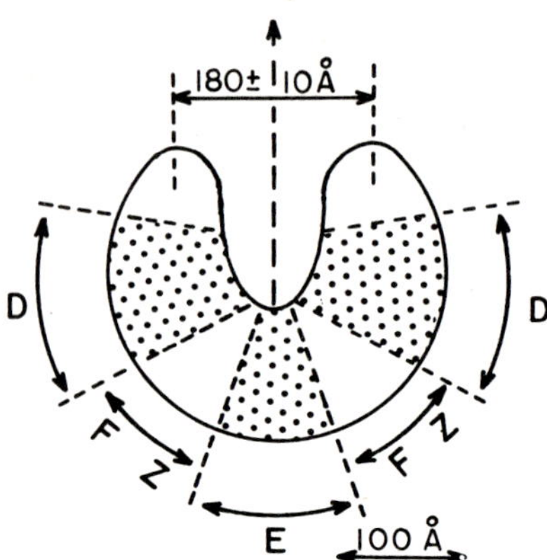

FIGURE 2. Molecular plan of fibrinogen as proposed by Marguerie and Stuhrmann.[28] FZ, zones of increased flexibility, permitting a bent-rod configuration. Proposed localization of plasmic fragments D and E are also shown. (Adapted from Marguerie, G. and Stuhrmann, H. B., *J. Mol. Biol.*, 102, 143, 1976.)

mined,[11] consists of the dimeric amino-terminal region of the fibrinogen molecule, where its 6 chains are covalently linked by 11 pairs of disulfide bonds. Fragment D is a family of monomeric fragments whose molecular weights vary between 85,000 and 100,000 daltons, depending upon the extent to which the γ chain has been degraded.[10,12,13] Although there is universal agreement that fragment D represents remnants of the carboxy-terminal region of the fibrinogen molecule that are covalently bound by at least six to eight disulfide bonds,[5,13,14] the question as to whether early forms of fragment D are in fact dimeric structures remains incompletely resolved.[4,15] The majority of biochemical evidence[10,13,16-24] at present supports the idea that digestion of 1 mol of fibrinogen with plasmin results in the release of 2 mol of fragment D, representing the separate carboxyl-terminal regions of the fibrinogen dimer, and 1 mol of fragment E, representing the dimeric amino-terminal disulfide knot region.

These findings support the hypothesis suggested initially by Nussenzweig and coworkers,[8] later elaborated by Marder,[16] that fibrinogen consists of three domains, which these residual products of plasmin digestion represent. Electron micrographs of dried shadowcast fibrinogen films by Siegel et al.[25] and by Hall and Slayter[26] showed an elongated trinodular structure that could be interpreted as evidence that these plasmin-resistant domains in fibrinogen exist in fact as discreet structural entities. Other studies have questioned whether the nodular-appearing fibrinogen molecules may be related to the techniques used.[27] Recent findings by Marguerie and Stuhrmann[28] with neutron scattering techniques suggest that the hydrated molecule may be a sausage- or spheroid-shaped structure rather than an elongated trinodular molecule, as had been previously assumed (Figure 2).

The plasmin-resistant D and E domains represent functionally distinct regions within the fibrinogen molecule that undergo thermal denaturation independently.[29] Affinity chromatographic studies by Kudryk et al.[30] with techniques developed by Henne and Matthias,[31] suggest that the D and E domains contain specific sites involved in fibrin polymerization, and that the sites within the E domain become available due to the action of thrombin.

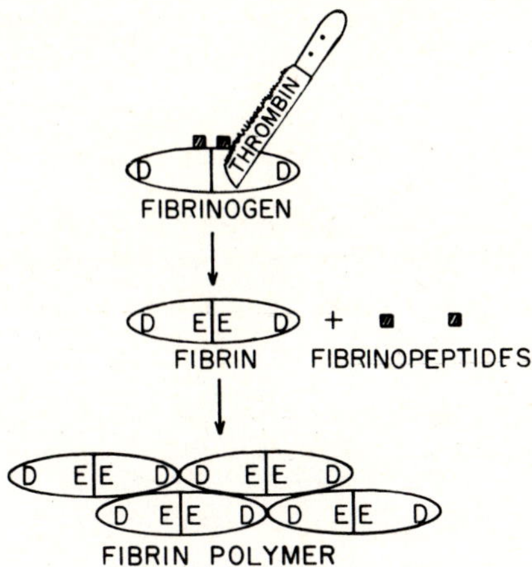

FIGURE 3. Theoretical function of fibrinopeptides as advocated by Blombäck and associates.[5] Fibrinopeptides block polymerizing sites within the E domain of the fibrinogen molecule. Following fibrinopeptide removal by thrombin, unmasked E domain sites react with complementary sites in the D domain, permitting fibrin polymerization to proceed spontaneously.

III. PROPERTIES AND STRUCTURE OF CIRCULATING FIBRINOGEN DERIVATIVES

A. Derivatives Resulting from Thrombin Action

1. Fibrinopeptides A and B

a. Physiologic Properties

Polymerization of fibrinogen is preceded by the limited proteolysis by thrombin of at least one pair of activation peptides from the amino-termini of the Aα chains.[32-34] Removal of these peptides, which are called fibrinopeptides A, after their chain of origin, defines the transformation of fibrinogen to soluble fibrin, i.e., "fibrin monomer". The principal function of this peptide appears to be to mask a specific polymerization site within the E domain of the fibrinogen molecule[5] (see Figure 3). The precise location of the polymerization site that is protected by fibrinopeptide A has not been completely resolved. Affinity chromatographic studies by Kudryk et al.[35] with the mutated fibrinogen Detroit (Aα 19 → Ser)[36] suggest that the polymerization site is critically affected by the region of the fibrinogen molecule where this mutation occurs.

In addition to releasing fibrinopeptide A, thrombin will cleave a second pair of activation peptides from the amino-termini of the Bβ chain at a much slower rate.[37-46] Removal of these peptides, called fibrinopeptides B, may not be required for fibrin polymerization under physiologic conditions.[32-34] However, Shainoff and Dardik[41,281] have demonstrated that selective removal of fibrinopeptide B under conditions in which fibrinopeptide A is intact will coagulate fibrinogen at temperatures below 14°C. These findings suggest the existence of a second, lower affinity polymerizing site that is protected by fibrinopeptide B. By means of selective plasmin digestion, this second polymerizing site has been localized to the Bβ chain. As Laurent and Blombäck[42] have shown, activation of this lower affinity polymerizing site by fibrinopeptide B removal results in the formation of a more dense fibrin polymer network than when only fibrinopeptide A has been removed (Figure 4).

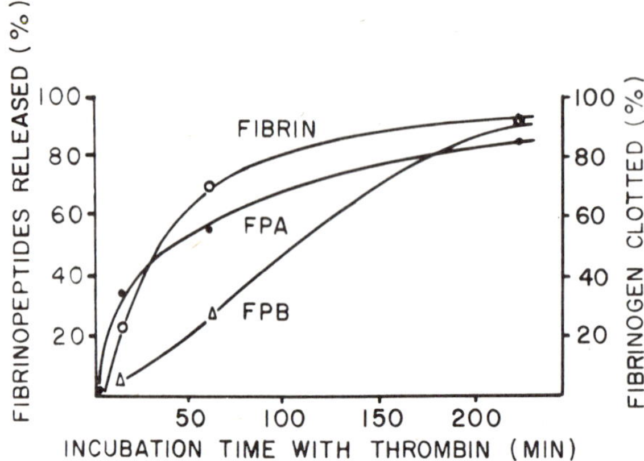

FIGURE 4. Kinetics of fibrinopeptide A (FPA) and fibrinopeptide B (FPB) release following addition of thrombin to solutions of bovine fibrinogen. Correlation of fibrin formation with fibrinopeptide release is also shown. (Adapted from Blombäck, B. and Vestermark, A., *Ark. Kemi,* 12, 173, 1958.)

In addition to their functioning as reversible protecting groups, there is some suggestion that the fibrinopeptides themselves, particularly fibrinopeptide B, may possess other diverse physiologic functions. The observed effects include potentiation of bradykinin-induced smooth muscle contraction[43,44] and vasoconstriction, presumably due to the direct stimulation of vascular smooth muscle cells.[45-47] With a purified reagent system, Osbahr and Custodio[48] demonstrated that relatively large quantities of bovine fibrinopeptide B (10^{-4} to 10^{-8} *M*) produced a 12-fold acceleration in the rate of superprecipitation of rabbit myosin B, which was associated with a doubling in the rate of ATP hydrolysis. The authors offered these data as chemical evidence of a relationship between fibrinopeptide B and smooth muscle contraction, although the precise nature of the relationship is unclear. The physiologic relevance of these observations on the muscle-stimulating effects of fibrinopeptides is difficult to assess because of the relatively large quantities of fibrinopeptides required for their production.

Fibrinopeptide B has also been reported by Kay et al.[49] to possess chemotactic activity for neutrophils and monocytes. Ittyerah et al.[50] studied the effects of clot supernatant, prepared by clotting purified rat fibrinogen, on fibrinogen synthesis in rats. They were unable to confirm earlier observations by Kropatkin and Izak[51] that fibrinogen synthesis could be stimulated by prior administration of clot supernatant to experimental animals, presumably due to fibrinopeptides.

Fibrinopeptides in relatively high concentrations are capable of competitively inhibiting the reaction of thrombin with fibrinogen. This phenomenon was first described by Bettelheim,[37] who observed prolongation of the recalcification time of human plasma following addition of a mixture of fibrinopeptides A and B. More detailed studies by Blomback et al.[44] with synthetic peptide analogs demonstrated that the site on fibrinopeptide A recognized by thrombin involves the carboxy-terminal arginine and a phenylalanine residue located eight residues from the amino-terminal. The spacing between Phe and Arg is apparently critical for thrombin inhibitory activity. The site on fibrinopeptide A recognized by thrombin contributes in only a minor way to the specificity of thrombin action on fibrinogen. Studies by Hageman and Scheraga[52] and by Hogg and Blomback[53] demonstrate that the critical thrombin recognition site on human fibrinogen Aα chains appears to be located in the region Aα 17 to 51.

b. Chemical Properties

Mammalian fibrinopeptides are small, largely hydrophilic peptides 9 to 21 residues in length.[34] The primary structures for most mammalian and some nonmammalian fibrinopeptides[54] have been determined. Mammalian fibrinopeptides, particularly the B peptides, show extraordinary variability in primary structure, even in peptides from closely related species.[34] These homologies and differences in fibrinopeptide structure have been used by Blomback and Doolittle,[55-56] Doolittle et al.,[57] and more recently by Balestrieri et al.[58] to probe phylogenetic relationships between various species. In addition, variants of fibrinopeptide structure are normally present within individuals of certain species. As examples, a minority of human A peptide molecules lack amino-terminal alanine (AY), and the serine residues in others are phosphorylated (AP).[59] Furthermore, a significant portion of canine fibrinopeptide B molecules possess tyrosine-O-sulfate residues, as well as phosphoserine.[3,34] Tyrosine-O-sulfate residues have been found in other mammalian B peptides as well as in B peptides from several nonmammalian vertebrates.[3,54]

The physicochemical properties of fibrinopeptides have received relatively little attention. Huseby[60] studied the circular dichroic spectral characteristics of a variety of mammalian A and B fibrinopeptides. His studies indicate that a definite small area of ordered structure exists in the relatively hydrophobic portion of the carboxy-terminal half of the fibrinopeptide molecule. Despite differences in amino acid sequence, this finding was a constant feature of all of fibrinopeptides studies. These data are consistant with the hypothesis of Blomback et al.[5] that the COOH-terminal half of the fibrinopeptide molecule contains a site recognized by thrombin, and this would help to explain the lack of species specificity in thrombin-fibrinogen reactions.[61]

c. Isolation and Purification

The most frequently used method for isolating fibrinopeptides has been cation-exchange chromatography of fibrin clot supernatant, using conditions and procedures similar to those described by Blomback and Vestermark.[38] Modifications of this method have been described.[62]

Because the structure of fibrinopeptides is known and they are small in size, solid-phase peptide synthesis[63] has become an important alternative method for their preparation. This method is of particular importance for immunologic and physiologic studies in which relatively large quantities of fibrinopeptides are required or tyrosyl analogs of fibrinopeptides are needed that may be conveniently radiolabeled. Synthesis of human fibrinopeptides A and B, as well as homologs and analogs of these peptides, has been carried out by several laboratories.[49,64-71] Canine fibrinopeptide A, its amino tyrosyl analog,[72] and guinea pig fibrinopeptide A[73] have also been synthesized. A synthetic analog of fibrinopeptide A, N-benzoyl-L-phenyl-alanyl-L-valyl-L-arginine-P-nitro-anilide hydrochloride, appears to be useful as a chromogenic substrate for quantitating the amidolytic activity of several enzymes.[74]

d. Kinetics of Fibrinopeptide Release

The observation that fibrinopeptide A release proceeds much more rapidly than the release of fibrinopeptide B as a result of thrombin action on bovine fibrinogen was first made by Bettelheim,[37] who used qualitative electrophoretic techniques. Quantitative studies on the release of fibrinopeptides from bovine fibrinogen were first carried out by Blomback and Vestermark.[38] These authors isolated fibrinopeptides from clot supernatants at intervals following addition of thrombin using ion-exchange chromatography. They confirmed Bettelheim's observations concerning the relative rates of peptide release and were able to show that a linear correlation existed between the quantity of fibrin formed and the quantity of fibrinopeptide A released. No such correlation was found between fibrin formation and fibrinopeptide B release. These critical findings by Blomback and Vestermark were later confirmed by Abildgaard[39] in experiments with human fibrinogen and thrombin.

The reaction of fibrinogen with thrombin is first order, as determined by the appearance of N-terminal glycine[33,34] and also by release of fibrinopeptide A. Because release of fibrinopeptide B occurs so slowly relative to release of fibrinopeptide A, the reaction velocity (V_{max}) of thrombin with fibrinogen is essentially a measure of A peptide release.[34,40,75]

Hogg and Blombäck[53] reported that the V_{max} for thrombin proteolysis of human fibrinogen is 0.2 nmol/sec/U thrombin, using data derived from quantitative N-terminal analysis. Comparable V_{max} values were obtained by Bando et al.[76] for the bovine thrombin-fibrinogen reaction. By directly measuring fibrinopeptide A release with more sensitive immunologic techniques. Nossel et al.[77] have reported the V_{max} for this reaction to be about 0.8 nmol/sec/V thrombin. The Michaelis constant (Km) reported by these workers for the human fibrinogen-thrombin reaction is about 3 μM, or about 60% of the value reported by Bando et al.[76] for the bovine fibrinogen-thrombin reaction. One explanation for these discrepancies is that the measurements by Nossel et al.[77] were carried out in systems that contained much lower concentrations of thrombin (2×10^{-2} to 2×10^{-5} U/mℓ) than did those of the other investigators. Kinetic studies carried out by quantitative N-terminal analysis require the use of much higher concentrations of thrombin.[53, 76]

2. Soluble Fibrin (Fibrin Monomer)

Polymerization of fibrin to produce an insoluble mass occurs rapidly under physiologic conditions. However, the spontaneous polymerization of soluble fibrin can be inhibited by alterations in the pH or ionic strength of its solvent. Ehrenpreis et al.[78] demonstrated that fibrin could easily be maintained in solution in 1 *M* NaBr at pH 5.3, but it would readily polymerize when dialyzed against an appropriate buffer system. Dilute acid solutions[79] and 3 *M* urea[80] have also been used to prepare solutions of intact fibrin for use in physiologic studies, but stronger acid solutions and high concentrations of chaotropic substances produce irreversible denaturation. Chemical modification of fibrinogens by acetylation[81] or maleilation[82] renders the protein nonclottable, even though the fibrinopeptides are releasable by thrombin. However, modification of free amino groups of fibrinogen by amidination, which preserves the charge of these amino groups, does not alter clottability.[83,84]

Shainoff et al.[85,86] demonstrated that fibrin forms stable, soluble complexes with fibrinogen. These workers observed that fibrin will remain in solution provided that a 5:1 ratio of fibrinogen to fibrin is maintained. The theory advocated by Blombäck and associates,[5] that fibrinogen contains separate polymerizing sites in the amino-terminal (E) and carboxy-terminal (D) domains, readily explains this phenomenon. Fibrinogen, being in excess, will saturate the available E domain binding sites in fibrin. Because the E domain binding site of fibrinogen is blocked by the fibrinopeptides, further propagation of this complex is inhibited. Extending this reasoning further, any proteolytic fragment of fibrinogen with an intact D domain polymerizing site will form soluble complexes with fibrin. Experimental evidence exists to support this hypothesis. Blomback et al.[5] and Kudryk et al.[30] found that high molecular weight (100,000) plasmin fragment D binds to both immobilized fibrin and to immobilized thrombin-treated disulfide knot (DSK) fragments of fibrinogen.

In contrast, Smith and Bang[87] and Latallo et al.[88] have analyzed mixtures of fibrinogen, plasmin digestion fragments, and thrombin by exclusion gel chromatography.

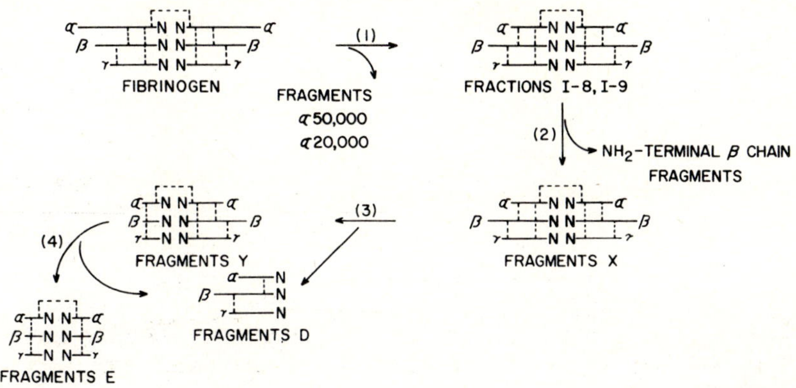

FIGURE 5. Lysis of human fibrinogen by plasmin. (Adapted from Pizzo, S. V., Schwartz, M. L., Hill, R. L., et al., *J. Biol. Chem.*, 247, 636, 1972.)

These workers concluded that only fibrinogen and clottable early plasmin digestion fragments larger than fragment Y are incorporated into soluble fibrin complexes. Nonclottable plasmin fragments Y, D, and E were not incorporated. Differences exist between these solution experiments and the affinity chromatographic studies discussed earlier which may account for these discrepancies. First, the amount of soluble fibrin that could be employed in the solution experiments is quite limited as compared to the amounts of thrombin-altered fibrinogen or fibrin that could be made available in the affinity experiments. Since differences were noted by Matthias et al.[89] in the rates at which different plasmin digestion fragments were adsorbed to immobilized fibrin, the relative concentrations of constituents could clearly affect the composition of the complex formed. In addition, studies by Matthias and Heene[90] on immobilized fibrin prepared with reptilase suggest that the availability of the polymerizing site protected by fibrinopeptide B is required for adsorption of plasmin degradation products to immobilized fibrin. It is not clear from the experiments described by Latallo et al.[88] how much fibrinopeptide B was removed in generating their fibrin complexes.

Soluble fibrin complexes may be precipitated from solution by addition of either ethanol or protamine sulfate, both of which tend to alter their solubility. This phenomenon, designated paracoagulation, has been used by a number of investigators to measure circulating fibrin complexes generated in vivo. Paracoagulation assays employing ethanol or protamine sulfate will be discussed in detail below.

B. Derivatives Resulting from Plasmin Action

Most workers agree that plasmin proteolysis occurs in a sequential fashion, with the initial attack at the COOH-terminal portions of the α chains, followed by cleavage of peptide bonds in the β and γ chains.[10,91-98] Large, clottable, fibrinogenlike molecules (e.g., fractions I-8, I-9,[99-101] fragment X) are produced first; these are then further degraded through a family of nonclottable intermediates (fragments Y). The end results of plasmin digestion are relatively stable core products (fragments D and E) and single-chain derived polypeptide fragments. Pizzo et al.[10] have proposed a general scheme to account for the generation of these fragments (Figure 5). In addition to these specific pieces, a larger number of peptides of molecular weight 5000 to 15,000 daltons is also released during various stages of digestion.

Knowledge of the structural chemical and immunologic characteristics of the D and E core fragments as well as several of the smaller peptide plasmin digestion products has proceeded apace. Space will not permit more than a brief overview of this new information, and only those fragments whose in vivo measurements are of actual or potential clinical interest will be discussed.

1. Multiple-Chain Derivatives

a. Thrombin-Clottable Derivatives

Fraction I-8 — Mosseson et al.[97] have advanced the hypothesis that substantial amounts of coagulable catabolic intermediates of fibrinogen exist in the circulation under physiologic circumstances. Comparison of so-called high-solubility fibrinogen fractions (I-8, I-9) with the fibrinogen fractions regarded as typical for "normal" fibrinogen (I-4) showed that the molecular weight of fraction I-8 differed from fraction I-4 by 54,000 daltons. Since NH_2-terminal analysis and studies of fibrinopeptide release showed no substantial differences between these two fractions, it was postulated that the size difference was due to cleavage occurring in the COOH-terminal regions of the molecule. The molecular weight difference between fractions I-4 and I-8 can be almost entirely accounted for by the release of fragment α 50,000 (see below) from the COOH-terminal two-thirds of the Aα chain, and a 27-residue peptide representing the Aα COOH-terminus.[98] Although it is difficult to exclude the possibility that some degradation of fibrinogen occurred during the process of isolation and analysis,[102] Mosesson[92,103] and Sherman et al.[104,105] have theorized that fibrinogenolysis may be a major pathway for physiologic fibrinogen catabolism; the evidence this theory is based on is the demonstration in normal animals that fraction I-4 is partly catabolized by conversion to fraction I-8, accounting for 25% of the turnover of the fraction I-4 pool.[104]

Fragment X — Fragment X is a family of heterogeneous intermediates, thought to represent the first stage beyond the "high-solubility" fractions I-8 and I-9. Fragment X is thrombin clottable and is thought to exert anticoagulant effects by interfering with soluble fibrin polymerization.[106] Inferences based on the molecular size of its component chains suggest that the NH_2-terminal region of the Bβ chain as well as the COOH-terminal two-thirds of the Aα chain have been removed.[95-97]

b. Nonthrombin-Clottable Derivatives

Fragment Y — Further plasmin degradation of fragment X results in a heterogeneous family of fragments no longer thrombin clottable. Analysis of component polypeptide chains and fibrinopeptide content[20] are consistent with the interpretation by Marder and Budzynski[91,107] and by others[10,17,96] that fragment D is asymmetrically cleaved from fragment X, resulting in fragment Y. Alternative interpretations of these findings have been proposed.[4,15] Although nonclottable, fragment Y possesses potent anticoagulant properties and is thought to interfere both with fibrin polymerization[12,106] and the action of thrombin or fibrinogen.[108,109]

Fragment D — Fragment D is a heterogeneous family of plasmin-induced derivatives representing remnants of the COOH-terminal portion of the fibrinogen molecule. Molecular weight estimates, as determined by nonreduced SDS acrylamide gel electrophoresis or by diffusion studies, range from 80,000 to 115,000 daltons.[9,10,13,19,21,110,111] Analysis of fibrinogen fragment D on disc gel electrophoresis following reduction and alkylation reflects a monomeric structure in which constituent α, β, and γ chain remnants are covalently bound via disulfide bridges. Most molecular, weight estimations for α and β chain remnants are 12,000 to 14,000 and 40,000 to 45,000 daltons, respectively,[10,13,21,94] and considerable heterogeneity is seen in the γ chain remnants, accounting for the molecular weight variations seen in the D fragment species as a whole.[10,13,94,111] Thus the presence of high molecular weight γ chain segments of 42,500 daltons reflects "early" fragment D species[10,13], but γ remnants of 23,000 to 39,000 daltons are thought to represent later fragment D species.[94,110,111-112]

Collen et al.[13] reported isolation of a relatively homogeneous species of fragment D (~ 100,000 daltons) from human fibrinogen by a combination of affinity chromatography and gel filtration. Sequence analysis of the reduced and alkylated γ remnant showed overlap with γ chain sequences known to occur in both plasmin-derived fragment E[113] and in CNBr-derived NH_2-terminal DSK (N-DSK).[114] Recently, Henschen and Lottspeich[278] and Gårdlund[11] have described the sequence of the portion of the β chain linking these two fragments. The contiguity of plasmin fragment D with plasmin fragment E along the length of the γ and β chains has therefore been unequivocally demonstrated.[11,13,22,113,114,278]

Fragment D-D — Activated Factor XIII is a transamidase that catalyzes the formation of γ-glutamyl-e-lysyl bonds in fibrin,[115-117] rendering the latter insoluble in solvents such as 5 *M* urea and 1% monochloracetic acid. Studies by several investigators have localized fibrin cross-linking sites to the carboxy-terminal portions of the γ chains[18,19,118,119] and of the α chains.[119,120]

Analysis of plasmin digests of highly cross-linked fibrin by SDS acrylamide gel electrophoresis[18,19] showed the presence of a unique fragment, approximately twice the size of fragment D, derived from plasmin digestion of fibrinogen. Further investigations have shown that this product, termed fragment D-D, arises from the isopeptide γ chain linkages catalyzed by Factor XIIIa. Chen and Doolittle[118] and Sharp et al.[121] have isolated and structurally characterized this γ chain cross-linking site from CNBr digests of fibrin prepared from purified human fibrinogen. Fragment D-D (189,000 daltons)[122] essentially consists of two covalently linked fibrinogen fragments D.

Measurement of fragment D-D in the circulation is of potential clinical interest because its presence signifies lysis of cross-linked fibrin as distinct from fibrinogenolysis and it may also serve as an index of Factor XIIIa activity.

Fragment E — Fragment E is a 50,000-dalton piece derived from stage 2 or stage 3 plasmin digests of fibrinogen.[12,91] Virtually all available data derived from compositional analysis[11,22,112,113,123,124] indicate the origins of fragment E to be the dimeric amino-terminus of the fibrinogen molecule. As mentioned earlier, the sequence of fragment E has been completely determined;[11] the structure of this fragment may be defined as $(A\alpha 1\ \text{Ala-81 Lys})_2\ (B\beta\ 54\ \text{Lys-121 Leu})_2\ \gamma\ 1\ \text{Tyr-58 Lys})_2$.

Plasmin digestion of fibrin gives rise to a core fragment E that, except for the absence of the fibrinopeptides, appears similar in size and structure to fragment E derived from fibrinogen.[18] This finding is explained by the carboxy-terminal locations of the cross-linking sites on the γ chain and of the α chains as well. Presumably, levels of circulating fragment E in blood could reflect both fibrin and fibrinogenolysis.

2. Single-Chain Derivatives

a. Aα Chain Plasmin Fragments

Approximately 12 to 20% of the Aα chain's total mass is represented in the plasmin core fragments D and E. The remaining 80 to 86% appear in plasmic digests as mid-chain- and carboxy-terminal-origin peptides of varying lengths. Some of these comprise what has been termed degradation products A, B, and C, representing Aα chain fragments with molecular weights in the 11,000 to 20,000 dalton range. These have been consistantly found as end-products of fibrinogenolysis along with core fragments D and E.[8,10,96] Although numerous intermediate Aα chain derivatives have been described within a range of 11,000 to 48,000 daltons (References 4, 15, 92, 96, 97 inter alia), the majority of these fragments cannot be reliably retrieved from digests because they are susceptible to further plasmic digestion. By careful control of time, temperature, and other conditions of enzymatic digestion, it had been possible for several

TABLE 1

Cyanogen Bromide and Plasmin Derivatives of Fibrinogen (A α Chain Presumed to be Components of α 50,000)

Fragment	Synonym	Derivation	Mol wt	Ref.
Hi2-DSK	FcB-3	CNBr	28,000	14, 128, 279
H	Hi2-Met,A	Plasmin	20,000	3, 120, 125, 127, 128
Hi2-Ala	—	Plasmin	23,000	120, 126, 128

investigators to isolate some of these transient Aα chain peptides in quantities sufficient for their chemical[120,125,126] and immunologic[126-128] characterization.

Recent structural studies of the carboxy-terminal regions of the α chains by Cottrell and associates[282] have precisely localized the cross-linking sites involved in Factor XIII-catalyzed α chain polymerization.

Since the attack by plasmin on fibrinogen is believed to be directed initially at the carboxy-terminal region of the Aα chain,[10,93-98] measurement of circulating α chain fragments is of potential value as an index of early plasmin action. That several of these fragments reportedly contain acceptor sites involved in α chain cross-linking further enhances the potential of such measurements.

α50,000 — Hessel[126] reported the isolation and characterization of a unique family of fragments with a mean molecular weight of 50,000 daltons from 10 min plasmin digest of human fibrinogen. That these fragments were derived from the Aα chain was demonstrated by their reactivity with antisera to the Aα chain and by the failure of these fragments to react with antisera to the Bβ or γ chains. Hessel's studies[126] indicate that the family of plasmin-resistant 20,000 to 25,000-dalton α chain remnants that she and other investigators (See References 8, 10, 15, 93, 95, 120, 125, 129 inter alia) have observed in terminal plasmin digests of fibrinogen may in fact be derived by further breakdown of α50,000 (Table 1). Peptides isolated from CNBr digests of α50,000 show sequence homology with plasmin fragments H[125] and Hi2-Ala,[120, 126] as well as with CNBr fragment Hi2-DSK, a 28,000-dalton peptide derived from Aα chains[14] (Table 1). These findings, as well as COOH-terminal analyses of α50,000,[126] locate this fragment within the COOH-terminal two thirds of the Aα chain proximal to the COOH-terminus.

α20,000 — In separate reports, Harfenist and Canfield,[125] Hessel,[126] and Takagi and Doolittle[120] described isolation and chemical characterization of a family of plasmin-resistant peptides of Aα chain origin arising in the course of early fibrinogenolysis by plasmin. The chemical compositions and properties of these fragments appear quite similar, and Edman degradation analysis shows considerable overlap in terms of sequence of amino terminal regions. These products are probably similar to plasmin fragment A described by Nussenzweig et al.[8] in 1961. Fragment H was isolated by Harfenist et al.[125] from 1.25-hr plasmin digests of human fibrinogen incubated at 0°C. Its amino-terminal sequence appears identical to fragment A isolated by Takagi and Doolittle[120] from 10-min plasmin digests. An early plasmin-derived fragment similar to H and A, termed Hi2-Met was also reported by Blombäck et al.[128] Molecular weight estimates for both fragments H and A are similar ($\sim$ 20,000 daltons), as are amino acid compositions. Fragments H and A appear to differ from fragment Hi2-Ala described by Hessel[126] in that the latter extends an additional 9 residues further toward the amino-terminus of the Aα chain. The 9-residue amino-terminal extension of Hi2-Ala is plasmin cleavable and has been shown by Takagi and Doolittle[120] to possess one α chain cross-linking acceptor site, the second acceptor located more toward the COOH-terminal in the A fragment. The amino-terminal sequence of fragments H and

A differs from fragment Hi2-DSK isolated from CNBr cyanogen bromide digests of fribrinogen by Blombäck et al.[14] only by the absence of amino-terminal methionine in the latter. Hi2-DSK (28,000 daltons) is larger than fragments H and A, extending further toward the COOH-terminal region of the Aα chain.

NH_2-terminal B chain fragments — In contrast to the NH_2-terminal region of the Aα chain, which is relatively resistant to plasmin action, the NH_2-terminal region of the Bβ chain contains ten plasmin-susceptible bonds.[130] Analysis of peptide fragments released during the initial stages of plasmin attack on human fibrinogen was shown by Lahiri and Shainoff[129] to consist in part of NH_2-terminal segments of the Bβ chain. Release of fibrinopeptide B-containing fragments appeared complete following 90 min of digestion of 45 mg of fibrinogen with 2.4 units of plasmin at 37°C. That release of fibrinopeptide B-containing fragments coincided with early plasmin action of fibrinogen was confirmed by other workers.[95,131] Studies by Mills and Karpatkin[93,95] suggest that plasmin proteolysis of the COOH-terminal portion of the Aα chain seems to precede proteolysis of the NH_2-terminal portion of the Bβ chain.

C. Circulating Derivatives Resulting from Other Enzymes

1. Snake Venoms

Arvin is a commercial preparation of partially purified coagulant fraction from the Malayan pit viper (*Ancistrodon rhodostoma*).[132] Parenteral injection of Arvin into man and laboratory animals results in defibrination, presumably through the direct action of Arvin on plasma fibrinogen. This procedure has been termed therapeutic defibrination and has been used in the treatment of patients with thromboembolic disorders.[133-137]

Studies by Ewart et al.,[138] showed that Arvin contains both a thrombin-like coagulant enzyme, which cleaves only fibrinopeptide A from fibrinogen, and a less specific protease fraction, capable of degrading fibrinopeptide A as well as other proteins. Unlike thrombin, Arvin does not activate Factor XIII.[139] Other thrombin-like snake venoms (e.g., Defibrase, derived from *Bothrops atrox* have also been applied clinically as defibrinating agents.[140])

2. Leukocyte Proteases

Several neutral proteases distinct from plasmin have been derived from leukocytes that are capable of cleaving fibrinogen and fibrin under physiologic conditions.[141,142] These neutral proteases include elastases,[143-146] collagenases,[147-149] and chymotrypsin-like enzymes.[150,151] Studies by Plow and Edgington[152] show that leukocyte proteases degrade fibrinogen into nonclottable fragments that are clearly different from plasmin-derived fragments. The fragments generated exhibit anticoagulant activity by interfering with fibrin polymerization.

Detailed immunochemical studies by Bilezikian and Nossel[153] of the cleavage of the NH_2-termini of the Aα and Bβ chains by crude leukocyte proteases have shown that the fibrinopeptides themselves were not cleaved, but that larger dialyzable fragments containing these peptides were removed. It is possible that leukocyte proteases function in normal[154] and pathologic[151,155] processes involving degradation of fibrinogen and fibrin as well as other clotting factors. Egbring and associates[156] have presented evidence that leukocyte elastase circulates in the plasma of patients with acute leukemia and septicemia, where it is measurable immunologically as a complex bound to α antitrypsin. Of ten patients with acute myelogenous or acute myelomonocytic leukemia who were found to have circulating elastase-antitrypsin complexes, all had elevated fibrin(ogen) degradation products, and seven showed a decrease in Factor XIII activity below 50%. These data suggest that proteolytic enzymes released from blast cells proteolyze fibrinogen and certain clotting factors and may be in part responsible for the coagulopathies noted in patients with these disorders.

IV. CLINICAL ASSAYS FOR MEASUREMENT OF THROMBIN-DERIVED PROTEOLYSIS PRODUCTS

A. Determinations of Soluble Fibrin-Fibrinogen Complexes

Early studies by Blombäck and associates[5, 32] had shown that soluble intermediate products are produced during the conversion of fibrinogen to fibrin. The potential physiologic significance of the formation of fibrin-fibrinogen complexes was demonstrated by Shainoff and Page,[157] who found soluble intermediate fibrin-fibrinogen complexes in the blood of rabbits treated with endotoxin. These complexes consisted of fibrinogen with fibrin lacking only fibrinopeptide A and were also cold precipitable (cryofibrin). When the level of cryofibrin in the rabbits' circulation exceeded 26% of the plasma fibrinogen, the cryofibrin dissociated into fibrinogen and fibrin in equimolar proportions, the fibrin then precipitating from solution.[85] Soluble fibrin-fibrinogen complexes have been presumed to be formed in various disease states, particularly disseminated intravascular coagulation, and several assays have been proposed to detect and quantitate these complexes in clinical blood samples.

1. Paracoagulation Assays

Fibrinogen is a large protein of limited solubility in aqueous media. Alteration of solubility by varying salt concentration,[34] either through the addition of organic solvents such as ethanol[158] and dimethylformamide[159] or the addition of charged substances such as protamine sulfate, various dyes, lysozyme, and other compounds,[160-163] has been used to precipitate fibrinogen and certain of its derivatives. It follows that macromolecular complexes formed between fibrinogen, soluble fibrin, and various degradation products will be less soluble than fibrinogen itself and may be collected or quantitated by differential precipitation techniques. The term paracoagulation was first applied by Derechin,[164,165] who observed that when human plasma in which plasminogen had been activated by streptokinase was clotted with thrombin, and the resulting clot dissolved, addition of quantities of protamine sulfate or toluidine blue insuffient to precipitate fibrinogen from solution led to reclotting of the mixture.

Although Bomchil and Derechin were aware of the potential applicability of the paracoagulation phenomenon to the diagnosis of clinical disorders such as intravascular clotting associated with fibrinolysis,[166] the first attempts to study paracoagulation systematically and to develop assays based on this principle were carried out several years later by others.[161,162,167-169] Those studies seem to indicate the following:

1. Protamine sulfate, in final concentrations of less than 0.09% does not precipitate fibrinogen, plasmin-derived fibrinogen proteolysis products, or their mixture from plasma.[162,170] "Early" fibrin degradation products cause paracoagulation , whereas "late" fibrin degradation products lose this capability.[163,169-171]
2. As clotting proceeds in normal whole blood, paracoagulation induced by addition of protamine sulfate gradually increases and then decreases, finally disappearing once all the fibrinogen in the plasma sample has been clotted.[170] Soluble fibrin complexes added in vitro to normal plasma are also precipitable by low concentrations of protamine sulfate.[162,169-173]

Several paracoagulation assays with protamine sulfate[162,170,171,174,175] and ethanol[176-178] as precipitating agents have been described. Variables such as incubation time and temperature,[70] fibrinogen level,[179] anticoagulant used to collect the blood sample, and brand of protamine sulfate[170,173,175] seem to be of critical importance.

The ethanol gelation test is reportedly insensitive to early fibrin degradation products[173,177] and is said to respond primarily to soluble fibrin.[176,177] Studies by Yudelman et al.[180] showed that at room temperature, ^{125}I-labeled soluble fibrin was only slightly more readily precipitable by ethanol than was ^{125}I-fibrinogen. In contrast, ^{125}I-fibrin was markedly more sensitive to precipitation by protamine sulfate at room temperature than was ^{125}I-fibrinogen. From these data, it would seem that the plasma protamine paracoagulation assay is preferable to assays employing ethanol.

The sensitivity of the plasma protamine paracoagulation test is difficult to assess since few quantitative data are available in the literature. Reportedly, the assay is sensitive to 0.02 to 0.05 mg/mℓ of fibrin dissolved in plasma[170,171] and 5 to 10 mg/mℓ of early fibrin degradation products.[171] The plasma protamine paracoagulation test appears to be a qualitative assay of limited specificity and sensitivity whose principal clinical usefulness may be as an adjunctive screening test for disseminated intravascular coagulation.

2. Gel Exclusion Chromatography

In addition to differential precipitation, gel sieving methods may be used for identification of macromolecular complexes of fibrinogen in circulating blood. Agarose gel chromatography for identification of complexes of higher molecular weight than native fibrinogen formed in vitro, first described by Sasaki et al.,[86] has been applied to studies of clinical blood samples by Fletcher and associates.[181-184] The technique used by Fletcher et al. employs relatively short (15 to 30 cm) Bio-gel® A-5M columns; elution conditions are carefully controlled, and the fibrinogen in eluates is determined immunologically by an automated system.[183] The proportion of fibrinogen-related antigen eluting before and after a fibrinogen standard is analyzed using a computer program. Use of longer gel columns increases the time required for analysis but provides substantially greater resolution.[185,186]

A critical problem with chromatographic analysis of macromolecular fibrinogen complexes in clinical samples has been specificity, since the complexes are likely to represent products of intact and plasmin-degraded fibrin, fibrinogen, and other proteins.[1,187] Recent in vitro data compiled by Bang and associates[187] suggest that plasmin fragment X derived from fibrin polymerizes to form soluble macromolecular complexes. Furthermore, components of early plasmin fibrin digest mixtures copolymerize with fibrinogen in the absence of thrombin to yield soluble complexes with molecular weights of 500,000 to 700,000 daltons. In addition, these early fibrin digest fragments (? fibrin fragment X) can polymerize with newly forming fibrin. Complex formation between components of early plasmin fibrin digests and fibrinogen, as well as incorporation of these components into fibrin clots, has also been shown by these investigators to occur in vivo.[188] These observations suggest that components of early fibrin digests, in addition to being capable of paracoagulation, have other properties in common with soluble fibrin and may play a similar physiologic role.

3. Affinity Methods

Matthias and co-workers[31,89,90,91,277] prepared stabilized, insoluble derivatives of human fibrinogen by immobilizing the protein to CNBr-activated Sepharose 6B. It was found that when thrombin-treated plasma was passed through columns containing immobilized fibrinogen, the fibrin was absorbed and could be eluted with buffers containing 1 *M* NaCl or 2 *M* NaBr. Similar results were observed when plasma samples from a patient with disseminated intravascular coagulation were chromatographed by this affinity system.[277] Yudelman et al.[180] found that affinity chromatography with fibrinogen Sepharose columns provided better discrimination between radiolabeled fibrinogen and fibrin than either the protamine sulfate or the ethanol paracoagulation assay. However, in view of the recent studies of Chang and Bang[187,188] on complex formation between early fibrin degradation products and fibrinogen, it is unlikely that the affinity method can distinguish between soluble fibrin and early plasmin-fibrin digestion product complexes in plasma samples.

Sepharose-fibrinogen affinity chromatography has not been widely applied to studies of clinical plasma samples, probably because the method is time consuming and not readily adaptable to studies on a large number of samples. Recently, Kisker and associates[189] have proposed a simplified affinity assay in which insoluble immune complexes of fibrinogen and antifibrinogen antiserum are used to absorb soluble fibrin complexes from plasma samples. The feasibility of such an approach awaits further study.

B. Measurement of Fibrinopeptides A and B

Measurement of fibrinopeptides A and B released from fibrinogens in solution has been carried out indirectly by techniques such as quantitative NH_2-terminal analysis (References 5, 32 to 34, 39, 131, 190 to 192 inter alia), or directly by electrophoretic and chromatographic method (References 38, 62, 157, 193 to 196 inter alia). More sensitive radioimmunoassay procedures have been developed for measurement of fibrinopeptide A in human plasma by Nossel et al.[65,197] and others,[124,198-202] and also for quantitation of fibrinopeptide B.[40] Quantitation of fibrinopeptide A immunoreactivity in canine plasma has also been reported.[72] The assay procedures reported are all quite similar: competitive binding radioimmunoassay systems are used with antisera prepared by immunizing rabbits with native or synthetic fibrinopeptides conjugated to proteins such as albumin. Tracers are prepared by radioiodination of tyrosyl analog of the fibrinopeptides, since all mammalian fibrinopeptide A and certain B peptides (including human) do not contain tyrosine in their primary structure.[34]

1. Immunochemistry

Fibrinogen and fragments of the fibrinogen molecule containing fibrinopeptide A react to variable degrees with antifibrinopeptide A antisera, and thus require processing procedures for removal of fibrinogen and fibrinopeptide A-containing fibrinogen fragments from plasma samples prior to assay. To achieve this, plasma samples have been subjected to ultrafiltration,[65,124] dialysis[198,202] or deproteinization with agents such as ethanol[72,197,200] or trichloracetic acid.[201]

Nossel and co-workers[203,204] examined the immunoreactivity of 14 antisera to human fibrinopeptide A, prepared by immunizing rabbits with this peptide conjugated to albumin carrier protein. Several different procedures were used, including water-soluble carbodiimide, glutaraldehyde, and toluene diisocyanate. It was found that all the antisera tested showed comparable reactivity to free human fibrinopeptide A in solution, but disparate reactivities were observed when fibrinogen and fragments of the fibrinogen molecule containing fibrinopeptide A were tested. Based on the reactivity of the antisera to fibrinogen fragments containing fibrinopeptide A, the antisera could be divided into three categories: group I could readily distinguish free fibrinopeptide A from fragments of fibrinogen with the fibrinopeptide A sequence, whereas groups II and III could distinguish the free peptide from its parent molecule less well or not at all. One group I antiserum (R2) could distinguish free fibrinopeptide A (Aα 1-16) from the smallest plasmin derived fragment (Aα 1-23) that might be present by an order of 100-fold difference in immunoreactivity.[203] The hypothesis was advanced that in the

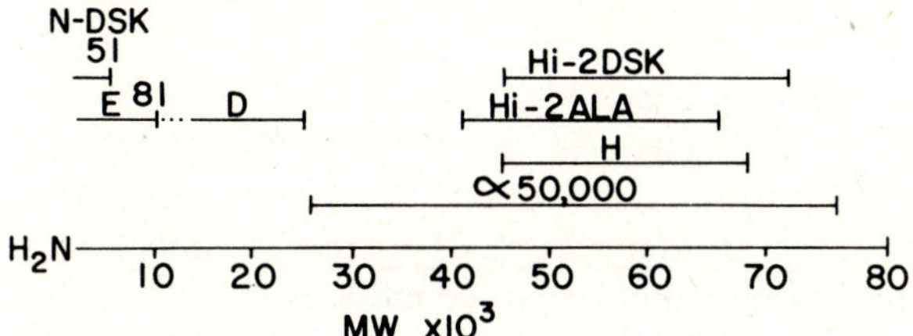

FIGURE 6. Localization of Aα chain remnants of various plasmic and cyanogen bromide-derived fragments of fibrogen. (Courtesy of Dr. R. E. Canfield.)

group I, but not in the group II and III antisera, antigenic determinants were hidden in the larger fibrinopeptide A-containing fragments of the fibrinogen molecule, suggesting that the immunoreactive sites on the fibrinopeptide molecule detectable by these groups of antisera differed as well.

Wilner and associates[70] compared the reactivities of a group I antiserum (R2) and of a group II antiserum (R33) with synthetic COOH-terminal homologs of human fibrinopeptide A (Figure 6). It was found that the antigenic determinants of R2 antiserum specificity resided within the COOH-terminal ten residues of the fibrinopeptide A molecule, and the Phe 8, Asp 7, and Arg 16 contributed to R2 immunoreactivity. The antigenic determinants required for R33 specificity were clearly different and seemed to include residues in the more hydrophilic NH_2-terminal half of the fibrinopeptide molecule as well. These studies demonstrate that by the use of specific immunologic reagents and techniques, assays could be developed that are both sensitive and specific and are clearly capable of distinguishing the products of thrombin proteolysis from those of plasmin proteolysis in clinical blood samples.

2. *In Vitro Studies*

When the assays were used to study the in vitro rates at which fibrinopeptides A and B were cleaved by various enzymes from fibrinogen, thrombin cleaved fibrinopeptide A much faster than fibrinopeptide B. Plasmin cleaved fragments containing fibrinopeptide B more rapidly than peptides that contained fibrinopeptide A.[40] Trypsin, snake venoms, and proteases derived from leukocytes demonstrated specific cleavage patterns.[40, 153] Studies on the rates of fibrinopeptide cleavage by thrombin from congenitally abnormal fibrinogen New York I showed that at low enzyme levels, only 1 mol each of fibrinopeptides A and B were released, whereas all the fibrinopeptides could be released at higher thrombin concentrations.[205] These findings suggest the presence of circulating equimolar concentrations of thrombin-sensitive and thrombin-insensitive species of fibrinogen.

3. *In Vivo Studies*

Elevated plasma levels of fibrinopeptide A have been found in patients with disseminated intravascular coagulation, deep venous thrombosis associated with pulmonary embolism, acute infections such as cellulitis and lobar pneumonia, systemic lupus erythematosus, renal-transplant rejection, and aortic aneurysm.[65, 197-202, 206-208] However, the interpretation of these elevated levels is unclear at the present time.

Relatively little is known about the metabolism of the fibrinopeptides in vivo. Studies by Nossel and co-workers[197] have shown that at elevated plasma levels, the half-life for removal of human fibrinopeptide A from the circulation is about 3 min. Mean fibrinopeptide A levels in normal subjects are estimated to be 0.6 pmo/mℓ with a range of 0.1 to 1.5 pmd/mℓ. Normal fibrinopeptide B levels have not been determined.

Only a small fraction of fibrinopeptide A estimated to be cleared from the circulation is recoverable as immunoreactivity in urine.[206] Structurally intact fibrinopeptides could not be recovered from the urine of experimental animals defibrinated by endotoxin[157] or thrombin infusions,[196] suggesting that the peptides are rapidly metabolized rather than directly excreted. Incubation of human fibrinopeptides with normal human serum results in slow conversion of fibrinopeptide A to AY (i.e., loss of NH_2-terminal alanine) and cleavage of COOH-terminal arginine from the fibrinopeptide B.[193] Human fibrinopeptide A immunoreactivity is stable in plasma for periods up to 4 hr following withdrawal of the blood sample.[209]

Studies in animal models on the transport of fibrinopeptide A from extravascular sites into the circulation[210] show that the resulting peak peptide levels obtained following intravenous injection of purified human fibrinopeptide A are 21 times the peak levels obtained following intramuscular injection of a comparable dose. Acute inflammation increases the absorption of fibrinopeptide A from extravascular sites, but the peak fibrinopeptide A levels achieved following intravenous injection are still 13 times greater than the peak levels obtained following injection of an equivalent dose of peptide into an acutely inflamed muscle. These findings suggest that intravascular thrombin action is far more effective in elevating plasma fibrinopeptide A levels than is extravascular thrombin action, and elevations in peptide levels are likely to reflect intravascular events.

Nossel and associates[77] have found that the fibrinopeptide A level rises gradually in blood samples collected in polypropylene syringes and added at regular intervals to tubes containing anticoagulant. The rate of fibrinopeptide A generation measured in this manner in normal subject is less than 0.5 pmol/mℓ/min, while in patients with disseminated intravascular coagulation or those receiving Factor IX concentrate (Proplex®) infusions, the rate of generation is usually in excess of 1.0 pmol/mℓ/min. Generation curves similar to those observed in clinical samples with increased rates of fibrinopeptide A generation can be simulated by the addition of small quantities of thrombin to systems containing purified fibrinogen in buffer solutions. These findings suggest that small quantities of thrombin and other active clotting intermediates circulate in the blood of patients with certain thrombotic disorders.

C. Clinical Assays for Measurement of Plasmin-Derived Proteolysis Products

1. General Tests

The estimation of plasmin-derived proteolysis products of fibrin(ogen) in clinical blood samples has, for the most part, relied on the use of tests that are relatively nonspecific and semiquantitative. Assays in common use in clinical laboratories for detecting plasmin-derived fibrin(ogen) degradation products include the following:

a. Thrombin and Reptilase Time Tests

These tests[211-213] are based on the observation that nonclottable fibrinogen or derivatives of fibrin(ogen) resulting from enzymatic proteolysis by plasmin or other enzymes inhibit clot formation following addition of thrombin or reptilase to the test plasma.[108,213,214] The anticoagulant effect of these fibrin(ogen) fragments appears to result from either inhibition of fibrin polymerization in the plasma sample[214] or competitive inhibition of thrombin cleavage of fibrinopeptide due to substrate excess. Reptilase, a thrombin-like enzyme derived from the venom of *Bothrops atrox*,[215] is not inhibited by heparin and may be used in place of thrombin to distinguish the anticoagulant effect of heparin from that of the fibrin(ogen) fragments.[213] In vitro studies show that these tests are more sensitive in detecting early plasmin-derived fragments of fibrinogenolysis than they are in detecting the smaller terminal end-stage fragments.[12,106,213]

b. Staphylococcal Clumping Test

Hawiger and co-workers[216] developed a rapid assay for detecting either nonclottable fibrinogen or large proteolysis fragments of fibrinogen or fibrin in serum samples based on the ability of fibrinogen to clump certain strains of bacteria. Further investigations into the mechanism of the clumping reaction showed that the staphylococci bound to the COOH-terminal portions of the Aα and Bβ chains. Plasmin-derived fragment E and the N-DSK region did not bind.[217] As with the thrombin time and reptilase time tests, the staphylococcal clumping test performed on in vitro samples is more sensitive to increased levels of early plasmin digests of fibrin(ogen) than to terminal plasmin digest.[218,219]

c. Measurements of Fibrinogen-Related Antigens

A variety of immunologic methods, including hemagglutination inhibition,[220,221] counter immunoelectrophoresis,[222] latex agglutination,[223] and radioimmunoassay,[224,225] have been used to detect fibrinogen immunoreactivity in serum samples using antisera specific for native fibrinogen. These assays, particularly the tanned red cell hemagglutination inhibition immunoassay (TRCHII) of Merskey et al.,[220,221] have had wide use in clinical laboratories as a method for detecting fibrin(ogen) degradation products resulting from plasmin action. Although the immunologic measurement of fibrinogen-related antigen in serum as an index of plasmin proteolysis products offers better sensitivity in comparison to either the thrombin time test or the staphylococcal clumping test, the tests are at best semiquantitative. In studies on the immunochemical expression of native fibrinogen antigens by various plasmin-derived cleavage fragments, Plow and Edington[225] found more than 1000-fold difference in immunoreactivity between fibrinogen and terminal digest fragments D and E. Fragment X, representing 80% of the parent fibrinogen molecule, expressed only 36% of the native antigens recognizable by antisera prepared against native fibrinogen.

Several groups of investigators have recently attempted to develop laboratory tests that would be both quantitative and specific for plasmin proteolysis and could distinguish early from late plasmin action and fibrinogenolysis from fibrinolysis. These new assays all rely on the measurement of specific plasmin cleavage products by immunologic means.

2. Assays of Early Plasmin Cleavage Products

a. Fragment H Radioimmunoassay

Harfenist and co-workers[127] have described a radioimmunoassay for an early plasmin cleavage fragment derived from the COOH-terminal end of the Aα chain which these investigators have called fragment H. As stated above, this fragment is probably identical to fragments A and Hi2-Met described by other workers. In vitro studies, with purified reagent systems showed that fragment H immunoreactivity was released by plasmin action on fibrinogen, but not as a result of thrombin action. Maximal release of fragment H immunoreactivity seemed to correlate with the generation of fragment X. Studies on early plasmin digests of fibrinogen showed that fragment H immunoreactivity was released as part of larger Aα chain fragments of 35,000 to 50,000 daltons, and that these larger species were secondarily degraded to H. Studies on sera derived from three normal individuals showed H immunoreactivity levels of 100 to 300 pmol/mℓ. Clinical studies employing this assay are presently in progress.

b. Hi2-DSK Radioimmunoassay

Gollwitzer and Timpl[279] and Blombäck and associates[128] have described a radioimmunoassay for measurement of Hi2-DSK immunoreactivity. Fragment Hi2-DSK[14] is a 28,000-dalton CNBr-derived fragment from the COOH-terminal two thirds of the Aα chain, partially overlapping both fragments H and Hi2-Ala. Blombäck et al.[128] used antiserum prepared against fragment Hi2-DSK and found that no immunologic distinction could be made between Hi2-DSK, H, Hi2-Ala, α50,000, and alkylated Aα chains. Following addition of purified fragments α50,000 to samples of human serum, oligomers of α50,000 could be detected in gel filtration experiments, suggesting that this radioimmunoassay might be useful in detecting α chain polymer fragments arising due to lysis of cross-linked fibrin.

c. Fibrinopeptide B Radioimmunoassay

The potential of measuring fibrinopeptide B immunoreactivity as an index of early plasmin action has been explored only to a very limited extent. Bilezikian and co-workers[40] have shown that, following addition of purified plasmin to fibrinogen dissolved in buffer, fragments of fibrinogen containing fibrinopeptide B were rapidly released into the supernatant. Release of fibrinopeptide B-containing fragments was essentially completed within 2 hr following the addition of plasmin (0.1 U/mℓ). No release of fibrinopeptide A could be detected during this 2-hr digestion period. The size, composition, and rate of release of fragments of this Bβ chain containing fibrinopeptide B as a result of early plasmin action is uncertain and remains to be more fully investigated. Data reported by Takagi and Doolittle[22] suggest that fragment Bβ 1-42 may be cleaved initially. Studies by Nossel et al.[283] suggest that this fragment is released during saline-induced abortions coincident with early fibrin(ogen)olysis.

3. Assays of Late Plasmin Cleavage Products

a. Fragment D

In a series of elegant studies, Plow and associates[225,226-228] have explored the detailed immunochemistry of terminal plasmin digest fragment D arising during the course of fibrinogenolysis. The hypothesis was advanced that the immunoreactivity of fibrinogen could be altered as a result of plasmic cleavage, due to the unmasking of previously unavailable antigenic determinants. These "neoantigenic" determinants appeared to be best expressed in fragment D and secondarily fragment E, but they were not expressed to any significant extent in the intact fibrinogen molecule.[225] Subpopulations of antibodies specific for the cleavage-associated neoantigenic determinants of the fragment D (fg-Dneo) were collected by absorption of antisera prepared against these fragments with intact native fibrinogen. Immunochemical determinations were carried out by a double-antibody radioimmunoassay system, whereby immunoreactivity could be expressed in terms of 50% competitive inhibition and relative binding affinity, as estimated from the slope of the assay curve. Using this assay system, fg-Dneo was found in fragments X, Y, and D, but not in fragment E or fibrinogen.[225] Elevated levels of fg-Dneo were found in plasma samples from patients with presumed disseminated intravascular coagulation.[225] The sensitivity of the fg-Dneo radioimmunoassay reported by Plow and Edgington currently exceeds 10 pmol if the assay procedure is performed under nonequilibrium conditions.[229] A comparable assay system for quantitation of fg-Dneo immunoreactivity has also been reported by Gordon and associates[230,231]

In contrast to immunologic assays employing antisera to fibrinogen, which may be affected by nonclottable fibrinogen or excessive anticoagulation, the assays for fg-Dneo provide a direct index of circulating proteolyzed fibrin(ogen) in plasma, and may therefore prove clinically advantageous. Extensive clinical studies using this assay system remain to be carried out.

b. D-D Dimer

Although it has been reported that fibrin- and fibrinogen-derived plasmin degradation products could be distinguished by differences in fg-Dneo radioimmunoassay inhibition curve slopes,[232,233] a direct measurement of fibrinolysis as distinct from fibrinogenolysis would be of considerable clinical interest. In a preliminary report, Budzynski and co-workers[234,284] described a radioimmunoassay procedure for measurement of fragment D-D derived from plasmin digests of cross-linked fibrin. These investigators report some cross-reactivity of their assay system with fragment D, and further work is required to characterize the specificity of their assay system.

c. Fragment E

Immunologic assays specific for the NH_2-terminal regions of the fibrinogen molecule have been developed by several groups of investigators (see References 13, 230, 231, 235 to 238) with antisera specific for either plasmin-derived fragment E, or the CNBr-derived N-DSK, which bears considerable structural homology with fragment E.

Despite their structural similarity, antisera prepared with N-DSK as immunogen showed only limited reactivity with the plasmin-derived fragment.[235,238] These findings suggest that significant conformational differences exist between N-DSK and fragment E which are expressed as differences in immunoreactivity.

Edgington[236,239,240] have studied the effects of plasmin fibrinogenolysis on the immunoreactivity of certain determinants located in the γ chain remnant (γ36-53)[240] of fragment E. These determinants, called Fg-E_{NEO}, are sequestered in intact fibrinogen but became progressively exposed as fibrinogenolysis proceeded. Measurement of these determinants may provide a dynamic index of the extent of plasmin cleavage.

V. SIGNIFICANCE OF MEASUREMENTS IN CLINICAL STATES

A. Disseminated Intravascular Coagulation (DIC)

Disseminated intravascular coagulation (DIC) is a major intermediary mechanism in the pathophysiology of a variety of diverse clinical disorders; it frequently presents as an acquired hemorrhagic diathesis, the bleeding manifestations of which may be severe.[241-245] The clinical diagnosis of DIC rests on the demonstration of accelerated fibrinogen catabolism as evidenced by increased levels of fibrin(ogen) degradation products and decreased fibrinogen levels. These changes are often accompanied by decreased levels of other clotting factors and reduced numbers of platelets. Although the mechanism by which episodes of DIC are triggered is presently unknown, the hemorrhagic manifestations appear to be due to excessive plasma procoagulant and fibrin(ogen)olytic activity. Therefore, the principal clinical applications for measurement of circulating fibrinogen derivatives have been in the diagnosis and management of clinical DIC states. Indeed, the introduction by Mersky and co-workers[220,221] of the first sensitive method for estimation of fibrin(ogen) degradation products provided a major stimulus both for studying the mechanism of DIC and for further development for new assays for measurement of circulating fibrinogen derivatives.

The general tests for measuring derivatives resulting from plasmin action have been significant adjuncts for confirming the diagnosis of DIC.[246,247] In a review of cases of clinical DIC diagnosed in a 2½-year period, Colman and co-workers[247] found that measurements of fibrin(ogen) degradation products by means of a commercial latex agglutination assay (Fi test) was elevated in 92% of patients in whom DIC was suspected based on abnormal coagulation screening tests and clinical findings. In studies comparing the various general assays used clinically to identify fibrin(ogen) degradation products in serum samples. Marder and co-workers[219] found that the TRCHII as described by Mersky and colleagues provides better sensitivity than either the immune diffusion or flocculation tests. The TRCHII was found capable of detecting 0.5 to 1.0 μg/mℓ of stage 1 and 2 plasmin digests of fibrinogen and about 2 μg/mℓ of stage 3 digests. These differences in sensitivity did not appear to deter significantly the general usefulness of the various clinical "split product" assays as confirmatory tests in the diagnosis of DIC.

Thomas and co-workers[248] studied ten patients with diagnosed DIC; an excellent correlation was found between qualitative elevations in fibrin(ogen) degradation products measured by the TRCHII, the staphylococcal clumping test, and the latex agglutination assay. However, immune diffusion assays were positive only in those patients with marked elevations in fibrin(ogen) degradation products as measured by the other three tests. Similar findings were reported in the studies of Carvalho et al.,[249] who noted that despite differences in sensitivity and specificity, the latex agglutination assay appeared qualitatively to be as useful as the staphylococcal clumping test in detecting elevations in fibrin(ogen) degradation products in the sera of 17 patients with DIC.

The plasma paracoagulation assays have been advocated by several groups of investigators as useful adjunctive tests in the diagnosis of DIC. Seaman[174] reported his experience with the plasma protamine paracoagulation assay during a 1-year period, during which time almost 3000 specimens were tested. Eight patients fulfilling clinical and laboratory criteria for DIC were found to have abnormal protamine paracoagulation assays. No patients who displayed other clinical and laboratory evidence for DIC had negative protamine paracoagulation assays. Similarly, Niewiarowski and Gurewich[171] reported six patients with clinical and laboratory evidence for DIC who had elevated protamine paracoagulation assays. Comparable findings were reported by Breen and Tullis,[177] who used ethanol in place of protamine as the paracoagulating agent in five cases of clinically documented DIC. However, a significant number of false-positive results has been reported by other investigators with the protamine and ethanol paracoagulation tests. Palester-Chlebowczyk et al.[250] found an incidence of 2 positive protamine gelation assays in 36 normal subjects. Kidder and associates[170] performed the plasma protamine paracoagulation assay during an 11-month period on 1500 plasma samples from patients with a variety of clinical disorders, including obstetrical complications, infections, neoplasms, and shock. Of the 44 patients in this group found to have positive test results, DIC could be adequately documented in 30 patients based on other laboratory findings. In contrast to the findings reported by Palester-Chlebowczyk et al.,[250] no abnormal protamine gelation test results were obtained in 62 normal subjects tested, including pregnant and postpartum patients.

Elevations in plasma fibrinogen levels (≥ 600 mg/dℓ) have been associated with false-positive results in the ethanol gelation test,[173,251] but not with the protamine paracoagulation assay.[170,171] Hedner and Nilsson[252] reported negative protamine sulfate paracoagulation assays in 12 of 13 postoperative patients with laboratory evidence of DIC. A positive ethanol gelation test was found in only four of these patients. Similarly, Margolis[253] found negative ethanol gelation tests in eight children with laboratory and clinical findings consistent with DIC.

Thus it appears that the paracoagulation assays with either ethanol or protamine sulfate are neither completely sensitive nor specific as a conformatory test for DIC. Based on the previous discussion of the lack of specificity of the ethanol and protamine paracoagulation tests, it seems unlikely that these assays can distinguish between DIC and "primary fibrinolysis", as has been claimed by several investigators.[171,177]

Although some clinical application has been made of many of the newer assays, including affinity chromatography and some of the specific plasmin-derived fragment assays, in patients with DIC, insufficient numbers of studies have been carried out to warrant review at this time. These newer methods may be applied in the study and definition of the pathophysiology of DIC, as well as being used as an additional aid in its clinical diagnosis. Mention has been made of the discovery by means of the fibrinopeptide A radioimmunoassay of proteolytic thrombin-like activity in blood samples of certain patients with DIC,[77] and it is likely that other specific cleavage product assays will be of use in elucidating the role of specific enzymes in the pathogenesis of this disorder.

B. Venous Thrombosis and Pulmonary Embolism

Methods used to definitely diagnose deep venous thrombosis and pulmonary embolism include angiographic and radionuclide imaging procedures. Ancillary diagnostic tests, including ^{125}I-fibrinogen scanning, and physical procedures, such as impedance plethysmography, ultrasound, and thermography, may also be of value under certain clinical circumstances.[254] In an attempt to define hemostatic alterations associated with deep venous thrombosis and pulmonary thromboembolism, measurements of circulating fibrinogen derivatives in patients with these disorders have been carried out by several investigators. Elevations in fibrin(ogen) degradation products,[255-258] in plasmin-derived fragment E,[259,260] and abnormalities in plasma paracoagulation assays[175,256,258] have been reported; however, studies by other workers have failed to confirm these findings.

Gallus and associates[261] found no useful correlation between clinically asymptomatic venous thrombosis diagnosed by radiolabeled fibrinogen scan and protamine sulfate, ethanol gelation, and fibrin(ogen) degradation product assays. Light and Bell[262] found elevated fibrin(ogen) degradation products in only 6 of 35 patients with pulmonary embolism. Lahnborg and Bergström[263] found no correlation between elevations in fibrin(ogen) degradation products and pulmonary thromboembolism. The significance of these changes and the reasons for differences reported by various investigators is not clear but may be related to whether or not the patients were symptomatic at the time the thrombotic episodes were diagnosed. In studies by Gurewich and associates[256] of patients with venous thrombosis diagnosed by venography, 25 of 29 symptomatic patients gave positive results with the protamine sulfate paracoagulation test, whereas only 4 of 17 asymptomatic patients showed positive results with this assay. In an experimental study employing animal models, Cade and associates[264] found that dogs that were embolized with autologous blood clot containing ^{125}I-labeled fibrin developed increased levels of fibrin(ogen) degradation products as measured by the TRCHII assays. This increase in fibrin(ogen) degradation products consisted principally of nonradioactive products and was therefore related to lysis of fibrinogen or fibrin not related to the original embolus. Heparin markedly inhibited the rise in degradation products following embolization, suggesting that elevations in fibrin(ogen) degradation products seen in association with pulmonary embolism may be derived from clotting occurring post-embolization as well as lysis of the original embolus.

Yudelman and associates[208] have measured fibrinopeptide A levels in patients with deep venous thrombosis with and without associated pulmonary embolism. In 24 patients with positive lung scans and/or venography, fibrinopeptide A levels were elevated to mean levels of 6.2 pmol/mℓ. In ten patients suspected of having deep venous thrombosis or pulmonary embolism who had negative venography and/or lung scans and no other associated disease, fibrinopeptide A levels were within the normal range (mean 1.1 pmol/mℓ).

Fletcher and co-workers[184] have studied the correlation between deep venous thrombosis occurring in postoperative patients, diagnosed by radiolabeled fibrinogen scanning, and the presence of increased amounts of circulating high molecular weight fibrin(ogen) complexes, as measured using their gel exclusion chromatographic procedure. A significant correlation was found between positive leg scans and abnormal gel chromatographic data. Of 27 patients with positive leg scans on the first postoperative day, 22 were found to have elevated levels of high molecular weight fibrinogen complexes. Conversely, elevations in high molecular weight fibrinogen complexes were found in 6 of 26 patients whose leg scans were normal on the first postoperative day. Although a correlation does exist between these data and the presence of venous thrombosis, the significant numbers of false-positive and false-negative findings limit the usefulness of chromatography as a diagnostic procedure in this disorder.

C. Renal Disease

Measurements of fibrin(ogen) degradation products have been proposed as an index of the survival of human renal allografts. Braun and Merrill[265] reported that urinary fibrin(ogen) degradation products were absent in 62 specimens from 15 patients without rejection 2 weeks following transplantation, but were present in 7 patients undergoing rejection. In patients with reversible rejection, the appearance of urinary degradation products could be abolished by immunosuppression. The etiology of these degradation products is thought to be a localized reaction within the graft rather than generalized DIC.[266]

Elevations in urinary fibrin(ogen) degradation products may also result from infection[267] and various disease states associated with glomerular damage.[268] The latter conditions must be ruled out if urinary degradation product measurement is to be useful as an index of renal allograft rejection.

Cronlund et al.[201] found that patients with active systemic lupus erythematosis who had evidence of nephritis had higher plasma levels of fibrinopeptide A than patients with active systemic lupus erythematosis without active nephritis. Plasma fibrinopeptide A levels were found to correlate directly with serum DNA-binding activity and inversely with serum C3 levels. Unlike plasma fibrinopeptide A levels, measurements of urinary fibrin(ogen) degradation products were found by Marchesi and co-workers[269] to correlate poorly with these indices of lupus activity and could not be used to gauge the progress of glomerular damage in individual patients.

D. Other Clinical States

Elevations in circulating high molecular weight fibrin(ogen) complexes have been reported in a wide array of diverse disorders, including cerebrovascular disease, myocardial infarction, and following major surgery, to name a few examples.[270] The rationale for such elevations in circulating fibrinogen derivatives is unknown.

Elevations of fibrin(ogen) degradation products have been reported in patients with fulminant liver failure[271] or cirrhosis.[272] The mechanism for these increased levels of degradation products is not clear. Although it has been postulated that the elevated levels were a result of abnormal fibrinolysis due to poor hepatic clearance of plasminogen activator,[273] more recent studies suggest that increased degradation products are associated with DIC.[271,272,274]

VI. FUTURE APPLICATIONS

A. Management of Anticoagulant Therapy

The potential for the use of plasma fibrinopeptide A measurements to regulate anticoagulant therapy was demonstrated in recent studies by Yudelman and associates.[208] Fibrinopeptide A levels were measured serially in patients with confirmed thromboembolism who were treated with heparin. In 12 of 15 patients there was a marked drop in fibrinopeptide A levels within the first 15 min following the initial dosage of heparin, and in eight patients the levels became normal within 30 min. Daily fibrinopeptide A levels were measured in ten patients on anticoagulant therapy. In four patients the levels remained normal and these patients experienced no new symptoms. In the remaining patients, episodic elevations in fibrinopeptide A levels were associated with either recurrence of symptoms or the appearance of new lesions on pulmonary scan. Recurrent symptoms and elevation in fibrinopeptide A levels often coincided with either suboptimal anticoagulation or a change from heparin to oral anticoagulation. These findings suggest that plasma fibrinopeptide A levels may provide a valid index for gauging the clinical effectiveness of anticoagulant regimens, and is therefore worth further clinical investigation.

B. Assessment of Hemostatic Compatibility of Biomedical Devices

Veenhof[280] found elevated plasma fibrinopeptide A levels in patients undergoing hemodialysis. Substantially higher levels were found in samples obtained from the venous line leaving the membrane than in samples taken from the arterial line. These findings suggest that the dialysis membrane itself may have been contributing to the observed elevations in plasma fibrinopeptide A levels.

By means of a radioimmunoassay specific for canine fibrinopeptide A,[72] Casarella and Wilner[275] studied the in vivo procoagulant effects of three angiographic guidewires of different compositions in a canine model that closely simulated the use of these wires in humans. Differences were observed in the amount of fibrinopeptide A generated as well as the in vivo insertion time required for maximal fibrinopeptide A generation. Fibrinopeptide A generation due to insertion of these guidewires could be suppressed by means of low-dose (40 U/kg) heparin therapy. In related work with a canine model system used to study the in vivo clot-promoting activities of five commercially available angiographic catheters, these investigators[276] found a direct correlation between the amount of fibrin thrombus deposited in the catheter lumen over a 30-min period, as judged by scanning electron microscopy, and the mean plasma canine fibrinopeptide A level averaged over the same 30-min period. It was judged possible to classify the relative clot-promoting activity of individual catheters by the mean level of fibrinopeptide A generated during the 30-min test period. These studies demonstrate the feasibility of using specific and sensitive assays for circulating derivatives of fibrinogen as an index of the promoting activity of biomedical devices. A significant advantage is that the use of these assays permits devices to be dynamically tested under conditions and time spans closely approximating their actual clinical application. Studies of the mechanisms by which biomedical devices exert their thrombogenic effects represents a broad area of application for these newer assay procedures.

VII. SUMMARY

Fibrinogen plays a pivotal role in both the humoral and cellular mechanisms involved in hemostasis. In performing its hemostatic function, fibrinogen in turn is acted on by several independent enzyme systems that either modify its structure or cleave specific fragments of the molecule into the surrounding milieu. Measurements of enzymatically modified fibrinogen or its proteolysis products represent a means whereby the action of these specific enzymes can be quantitated both in vitro and in vivo. Advances in such techniques as protein purification, affinity chromatography, peptide synthesis, and radioimmunoassay technology permit the translation of recently acquired primary structural data on this important protein into sensitive and specific assays for its circulating derivatives. These assay systems are important tools for probing mechanisms of hemostasis and thrombosis.

ACKNOWLEDGMENTS

I would like to thank Dr. N. Bang, Dr. R. E. Canfield, Dr. H. L. Nossel, Dr. M. Mosesson, and J. Sobel for their many helpful suggestions and comments. The technical assistance of R. MacAvoy in preparing this manuscript is gratefully acknowledged.

REFERENCES

1. **Mosher, D. F.,** Cross-linking of cold-insoluble globulin by fibrin-stabilizing factor, *J. Biol. Chem.,* 250, 6614, 1975.
2. **Patterson, J. C.,** The pathology of venous thrombi, in *Thrombosis,* Sherry, S., Brinkhous, K. M., Genton, E., and Stengle, J. M., Eds., National Academy of Sciences, Washington, D.C., 1969, 321.
3. **Doolittle, R. F.,** Fibrinogen and fibrin, in *The Plasma Proteins,* Vol. 2, 2nd ed., Putnam, F. W., Ed., Academic Press, New York, 1975, 109.
4. **Mosesson, M. W. and Finlayson, J. S.,** The search for the structure of fibrinogen, *Prog. Hemostasis Thromb.,* 3, 61, 1976.
5. **Blombäck, B., Hogg, D. H., Gårdlund, B. et al.,** Fibrinogen and fibrin formation, *Thromb. Res.,* 8 (Suppl. 2), 329, 1976.
6. **Murano, G.,** The molecular structure of fibrinogen, *Semin. Thromb. Hemostasis,* 1, 1, 1974.
7. **Doolittle, R. F., Goldbaum, D., and Doolittle, L. R.,** Amino acid sequence studies on human fibrinogen: arrangement of interchain disulfide bonds, *Thromb. Haemostasis,* 38 (Abstr.), 26, 1977.
8. **Nussenzweig, V., Seligmann, M., Pelmont, J. et al.,** Les produits de dégrédation du fibrinogéne humain par la plasmine. I. Séparation et proprietés physico-chimiques, *Ann. Inst. Pasteur (Paris),* 100, 377, 1961.
9. **Marder, V. J., Shulman, N. R., and Carroll, W. R.,** High molecular weight derivatives of human fibrinogen produced by plasmin. I. Physicochemical and immunological characterization, *J. Biol. Chem.,* 244, 2111, 1969.
10. **Pizzo, S. V., Schwartz, M. L., Hill, R. L. et al.,** The effect of plasmin on the subunit structure of human fibrinogen, *J. Biol. Chem.,* 247, 636, 1972.
11. **Gårdlund, B.,** Human fibrinogen — amino acid sequence of fragment E and of adjacent structures in the Aα and Bβ chains, *Thromb. Res.,* 10, 689, 1977.
12. **Marder, V. J. and Budzynski, A. Z.,** Data for defining fibrinogen and its plasmic degradation products, *Thromb. Diath. Haemorrh.,* 33, 199, 1975.
13. **Collen, D., Kudryk, B., Hessel, B. et al.,** Primary structure of human fibrinogen and fibrin. Isolation and partial characterization of chains of fragment D, *J. Biol. Chem.,* 250, 5808, 1975.
14. **Blombäck, B., Blombäck, M., Finkbeiner, W. et al.,** Enzymatic reduction of disulfide bonds in fibrinogen by the thioredoxin system. I. Identification of reduced bonds and studies on reoxidation process, *Thromb. Res.,* 4, 55, 1974.
15. **Mosesson, M. W., Finlayson, J. S., and Galanakis, D. K.,** The essential covalent structure of human fibrinogen evinced by analysis of derivatives formed during plasmic hydrolysis, *J. Biol. Chem.,* 248, 7913, 1973.
16. **Marder, V. J.,** Physicochemical studies of intermediate and final products of plasmin digestion of human fibrinogen, *Thromb. Diath. Haemorrh. Suppl.,* 39, 187, 1970.
17. **Mills, D. A.,** A molecular model for the proteolysis of human fibrinogen by plasmin, *Biochim. Biophys. Acta,* 263, 619, 1972.
18. **Pizzo, S. V., Schwartz, M. L., Hill, R. L. et al.,** The effect of plasmin on the subunit structure of human fibrin, *J. Biol. Chem.,* 248, 4574, 1973.
19. **Pizzo, S. V., Taylor, L. M., Jr., Schwartz, M. L. et al.,** Subunit structure of fragment D from fibrinogen and cross-linked fibrin, *J. Biol. Chem.,* 248, 4584, 1973.

20. **Budzynski, A. Z., Marder, V. J. and Shainoff, J. R.,** Structure of plasmic degradation products of human fibrinogen. Fibrinopeptide and polypeptide chain analysis, *J. Biol. Chem.*, 249, 2294, 1974.
21. **Ferguson, E. W., Fretto, L. J., and McKee, P. A.,** A re-examination of the cleavage of fibrinogen and fibrin by plasmin, *J. Biol. Chem.*, 250, 7210, 1975.
22. **Takagi, T. and Doolittle, R. F.,** Amino acid sequence studies on plasmin-derived fragments of human fibrinogen: amino terminal sequence of intermediate and terminal fragments, *Biochemistry*, 14, 940, 1975.
23. **Milhalyi, E., Weinberg, R. M., Towne, D. W. et al.,** Proteolytic fragmentation of fibrinogen. I. Comparison of the fragmentation of human and bovine fibrinogen by trypsin or plasmin, *Biochemistry*, 15, 5372, 1976.
24. **Shrager, R. I., Milhalyi, E., and Towne, D. W.,** Proteolytic fragmentation of fibrinogen. II. Kinetic modeling of the digestion of human and bovine fibrinogen by plasmin or trypsin, *Biochemistry*, 15, 5382, 1976.
25. **Siegel, B. M., Mernan, J. P., and Scheraga, H. A.,** The configuration of native and partially polymerized fibrinogen, *Biochim. Biophys. Acta*, 11, 329, 1953.
26. **Hall, C. E. and Slayter, H. S.,** The fibrinogen molecule: its size, shape, and mode of polymerization, *J. Biophys. Biochem. Cytol.*, 5, 11, 1959.
27. **Mosesson, M. W.,** Fibrinogen structure after spraying on mica: assessing the electron microscopic basis for a trinodular model, *Thromb. Res.*, 8, 737, 1976.
28. **Marguerie, G. and Stuhrmann, H. B.,** A neutron small angle scattering study of bovine fibrinogen, *J. Mol. Biol.*, 102, 143, 1976.
29. **Donovan, J. W. and Mihalyi, E.,** Conformation of fibrinogen: calorimetric evidence for a three-nodular structure, *Proc. Natl. Acad. Sci. U.S.A.*, 71, 4125, 1974.
30. **Kudryk, B., Collen, D., Woods, K. R. et al.,** Evidence for localization of polymerization sites in fibrinogen, *J. Biol. Chem.*, 249, 3322, 1974.
31. **Heene, D. L. and Matthias, F. R.,** Adsorbtion of fibrinogen derivatives on insolubilized fibrinogen and fibrinmonomer, *Thromb. Res.*, 2, 137, 1973.
32. **Blombäck, B. and Lauren, T. C.,** N-Terminal and light scattering studies on fibrinogen and its transformation to fibrin, *Ark. Kemi*, 12, 137, 1957.
33. **Blombäck, B.,** Studies on the action of thrombic enzymes on bovine fibrinogen as measured by N-terminal analysis, *Ark. Kemi*, 12, 321, 1958.
34. **Blombäck, B.,** Fibrinogen to fibrin transformation, in *Blood Clotting Enzymology*, Seegers, W. H., Ed., Academic Press, New York, 1967, 143.
35. **Kudryk, B., Blombäck, B., and Blombäck, M.,** Fibrinogen Detroit. An abnormal fibrinogen with non-functional NH_2-terminal polymerization domain, *Thromb. Res.*, 9, 25, 1976.
36. **Mammen, E. F., Prasad, A., Barnhart, M. I. et al.,** Congenital dysfibrinogenemia: Fibrinogen Detroit, *J. Clin. Invest.*, 48, 235, 1969.
37. **Bettleheim, F. R.,** The clotting of fibrinogen. I. Fractionation of peptide material liberated, *Biochim. Biophys. Acta*, 19, 121, 1956.
38. **Blombäck, B. and Vestermark, A.,** Isolation of fibrino-peptides by chromatography, *Ark. Kemi*, 12, 173, 1958.
39. **Abildgaard, U.,** N-Terminal analysis during coagulation of purified human fibrinogen, fraction I, and plasma, *Scand. J. Clin. Lab. Invest.*, 17, 529, 1965.
40. **Bilezikian, S. B., Nossel, H. L., Butler, V. P., Jr. et al.,** Radioimmunoassay of human fibrinopeptide B and kinetics of fibrinopeptide cleavage by different enzymes, *J. Clin. Invest.*, 56, 438, 1975.
41. **Shainoff, J. R. and Dardik, B. N.,** Fibrinopeptide B and aggregation of fibrinogen, *Thromb. Haemostasis*, 38 (Abstr.), 191, 1977.
42. **Laurent, T. C. and Blomback, B.,** On the significance of the release of two different peptides from fibrinogen during clotting, *Acta Chem. Scand.*, 12, 1875, 1958.
43. **Osbahr, A. J., Gladner, J. A., and Laki, K.,** Studies on the physiological activity of the peptide released during fibrinogen-fibrin conversion, *Biochim. Biophys. Acta*, 86, 535, 1964.
44. **Blombäck, B., Blombäck, M., and Olsson, P.,** Synthetic peptides with anticoagulant and vasodilating activity, *Scand. J. Clin. Lab. Invest. Suppl.*, 107, 59, 1969.
45. **Bayley, T., Clements, J. A., and Osbahr, A. J.,** Pulmonary and circulatory effects of fibrinopeptides, *Circ. Res.*, 21, 469, 1967.
46. **Colman, R. W., Osbahr, A. J., and Morris, R. E., Jr.,** New vasoconstrictor, bovine peptide-B released during blood coagulation, *Nature (London)*, 214, 1040, 1967.
47. **Osbahr, A. J.,** Structure-activity relationships of the vasopressor activity of canine peptide A from fibrinogen, *Biochim. Biophys. Acta*, 386, 373, 1975.
48. **Osbahr, A. J. and Custodio, R.,** Action of peptide-B bovine fibrinogen on ATPase activity and super-precipitation of myosin B, *Am. J. Physiol.*, 228, 488, 1975.

49. **Kay, A. B., Pepper, D. S., and McKenzie, R.,** The identification of fibrinopeptide B as a chemotactic agent derived from human fibrinogen, *Br. J. Haematol.,* 27, 669, 1974.
50. **Ittyerah, T. R., Dodgson, K. S., and Curtis, C. G.,** Plasma fibrinogen concentrations after intravenous administration of fibrinopeptides to rats, *Biochem. J.,* 128, 733, 1972.
51. **Kropatkin, M. L. and Izak, G.,** Studies on the hypercoagulable state. The regulation of fibrinogen production in experimental hyper- and hypofibrinogenemia, *Thromb. Diath. Haemorrh.,* 19, 547, 1968.
52. **Hageman, T. C. and Scheraga, H. A.,** Mechanism of action of thrombin on fibrinogen. Reaction of the N-terminal CNBr fragment from the Aα chain of human fibrinogen with bovine thrombin, *Arch. Biochem. Biophys.,* 164, 707, 1974.
53. **Hogg, D. H. and Blombäck, B.,** The specificity of the fibrinogen-thrombin reaction, *Thromb. Res.,* 5, 685, 1974.
54. **Cottrell, B. A. and Doolittle, R. F.,** Amino acid sequences of lamprey fibrinopeptides A and B and characterization of the junctions split by lamprey and mammalian thrombins, *Biochim. Biophys. Acta,* 453, 426, 1976.
55. **Blombäck, B. and Doolittle, R. E.,** The sequence of amino acids at the N-terminal end of bovine fibrinopeptide B, *Acta Chem. Scand.,* 17, 1816, 1963.
56. **Blombäck, B. and Doolittle, R. F.,** Amino acid sequence studies on fibrinopeptides from several species, *Acta Chem. Scand.,* 17, 1819, 1963.
57. **Doolittle, R. F., Schubert, D., and Schwartz, S. A.,** Amino acid sequence studies on artiodactyl fibrinopeptides. I. Dromedary camel, mule deer, and cape buffalo, *Arch. Biochem. Biophys.,* 118, 456, 1967.
58. **Balestrieri, C., Colonna, G., and Irace, G.,** Covalent structure of fibrinopeptides from buffaloes breeding in Italy, *Biochim. Biophys. Acta,* 405, 517, 1975.
59. **Blombäck, B., Blombäck, M., Edman, P. et al.,** Human fibrinopeptides isolation: characterization and structure, *Biochim. Biophys. Acta,* 115, 371, 1966.
60. **Huseby, R. M.,** Conformational structure of the fibrinopeptides released during fibrinogen to fibrin conversion, *Physiol. Chem. Phys.,* 5, 1, 1973.
61. **Teger-Nilsson, A. C. and Blombäck, B.,** Rate of thrombin-fibrinogen reaction in some mammalian species, *Thromb. Res.,* 5, 223, 1974.
62. **Murtaugh, P. A.,** A modified procedure for rapid isolation of fibrinopeptides, *Arch. Biochem. Biophys.,* 163, 784, 1974.
63. **Erickson, B. W. and Merrifield, R. B.,** Solid-phase peptide synthesis, in *The Proteins,* Vol. 2, Neurath, H. and Hill, R. L., Eds., Academic Press, New York, 1976, 255.
64. **Johnson, B. J. and May, W. P.,** Rapid peptide synthesis: synthesis of human fibrinopeptide A, *J. Pharm. Sci.,* 58, 1568, 1969.
65. **Nossel, H. L., Younger, L. R., Wilner, G. D. et al.,** Radioimmunoassay of human fibrinopeptide A, *Proc. Natl. Acad. Sci. U.S.A.,* 68, 2350, 1971.
66. **Andreatta, R. H., Liem, R. K., and Scheraga, H. A.,** Mechanism of action of thrombin on fibrinogen. I. Synthesis of fibrinogen-like peptides, and their proteolysis by thrombin and trypsin, *Proc. Natl. Acad. Sci. U.S.A.,* 68, 253, 1971.
67. **Liem, R. K., Andreatta, R. H., and Scheraga, H. A.,** Mechanism of thrombin on fibrinogen. II. Kinetics of hydrolysis of fibrinogen-like peptides by thrombin and trypsin, *Arch. Biochem. Biophys.,* 147, 201, 1971.
68. **Budzynski, A. Z. and Marder, V. J.,** Solid phase synthesis of human fibrinopeptides A and B, in *Protides of the Biological Fluids,* Peeters, H., Ed., Pergamon Press, Oxford, 1973, 287.
69. **Baligidad, S. K. and Sivanandaiah, K. M.,** The use of O-nitrophenyl-sulphenyl group for N-protection during the synthesis of the protected hexapeptide sequence (5-10) of human fibrinopeptide-A, *Curr. Sci.,* 43, 373, 1974.
70. **Wilner, G. D., Nossel, H. L., Canfield, R. E. et al.,** Immunochemical studies of human fibrinopeptide A using synthetic peptide homologues, *Biochemistry,* 15, 1209, 1976.
71. **Lobo, A. P., Wos, J. D., Yu, S. M. et al.,** Active site studies of human thrombin and bovine trypsin: peptide substrates, *Arch. Biochem. Biophys.,* 177, 235, 1976.
72. **Wilner, G. D. and Birken, S.,** Synthesis and radioimmunoassay of canine fibrinopeptide A, *Thromb. Res.,* 7, 753, 1975.
73. **Wilner, G. D.,** unpublished data.
74. **Svendsen, L., Blombäck, B., Blombäck, M., et al.,** I. Synthetic chromogenic substrates for determination of trypsin, thrombin, and thrombin-like enzymes, *Thromb. Res.,* 1, 267, 1972.
75. **Hageman, T. C. and Scheraga, H. A.,** Mechanism of action of thrombin on fibrinogen. Reaction of N-terminal CNBr fragment from the Bβ chain of bovine fibrinogen with bovine thrombin, *Arch. Biochem. Biophys.,* 179, 506, 1977.

76. **Bando, M., Matsushima, A., Hirano, J. et al.**, Thrombin-catalyzed conversion of fibrinogen to fibrin, *J. Biochem.*, 71, 897, 1972.
77. **Nossel, H. L., Ti, M., Kaplan, K. et al.**, The generation of fibrinopeptide A in clinical blood samples. Evidence for thrombin activity, *J. Clin. Invest.*, 58, 1136, 1976.
78. **Ehrenpreis, S., Laskowski, M., Jr., Donnelly, T. H. et al.**, Equilibria in fibrinogen-fibrin conversion. IV. Kinetics of the conversion of fibrinogen to fibrin monomer, *J. Am. Chem. Soc.*, 80, 4255, 1958.
79. **Sherman, L. A., Harwig, S., and Lee, J.**, In vitro formation and in vivo clearance of fibrinogen: fibrin complexes, *J. Lab. Clin. Med.*, 86, 100, 1975.
80. **Müller-Berghaus, G., Mahn, I., Köveker, G., and Maul, F. D.**, In vivo behavior of homologous urea-soluble ^{131}I-fibrin and ^{125}I-fibrinogen in rabbits: the effect of fibrinolysis inhibition, *Br. J. Haematol.*, 33, 61, 1976.
81. **Caspary, E. A.**, Studies on the acetylation of human fibrinogen, *Biochem. J.*, 62, 507, 1956.
82. **Kloczewiak, M., Wegrzynowicz, Z., Matthias, F. R. et al.**, Studies on chemically modified fibrinogen, *Thromb. Hemostasis*, 35, 324, 1976.
83. **Fuller, G. M. and Doolittle, R. F.**, The formation of crosslinked fibrins: evidence for the involvement of lysine-e-amino groups, *Biochem. Biophys. Res. Commun.*, 25, 694, 1966.
84. **Phillips, H. M. and York, J. L.**, Bovine fibrinogen. I. Effects of amidination on fibrin monomer aggregation, *Biochemistry*, 12, 3637, 1973.
85. **Shainoff, J. R. and Page, I. H.**, Significance of cyrofibrin in fibrinogen-fibrin conversion, *J. Exp. Med.*, 116, 687, 1962.
86. **Sasaki, T., Page, I. H., and Shainoff, J. R.**, Stable complex of fibrinogen and fibrin, *Science*, 152, 1069, 1966.
87. **Smith, G. F. and Bang, N. U.**, Formation of soluble fibrin polymers. Fibrinogen degradation fragments D and E fail to form soluble complexes with fibrin monomer, *Biochemistry*, 11, 2958, 1972.
88. **Latallo, Z. S., Mattler, L. E., Bang, N. U. et al.**, Analysis of soluble fibrin complexes by agarose gel chromatography and protamine sulfate gelatin, *Biochim. Biophys. Acta*, 420, 69, 1976.
89. **Matthias, R. F., Heene, D. L., and Konradi, E.**, Behavior of fibrinogen and fibrinogen degradation products (FDP) towards insolubilized fibrinogen and fibrinmonomer, *Thromb. Res.*, 3, 657, 1973.
90. **Matthais, R. F. and Heene, D. L.**, Comparative adsorbtion studies between fibrinogen and its degradation products, and fibrin monomer produced by reptilase and thrombin, *Thromb. Res.*, 3, 745, 1973.
91. **Marder, V. J. and Budzynski, A. Z.**, The structure of fibrinogen degradation products, *Prog. Hemostasis Thromb.*, 2, 141, 1974.
92. **Mosesson, M. W.**, Fibrinogen catabolic pathways: determinations from analyses of the structural features of circulating fibrinogen and of derivatives produced in vitro by the action of plasmin or thrombin, *Semin. Thromb. Hemostasis*, 1, 63, 1974.
93. **Mills, D. and Karpatkin, S.**, Heterogeneity of human fibrinogen: possible relation to proteolysis by thrombin and plasmin as studied by SDS-polyacrylamide gel electrophoresis, *Biochem. Biophys. Res. Commun.*, 40, 206, 1970.
94. **Gaffney, P. J. and Dobos, P.**, A structural aspect of human fibrinogen suggested by its plasmin degradation, *FEBS Lett.*, 15, 13, 1971.
95. **Mills, D. and Karpatkin, S.**, The initial macromolecular derivatives of human fibrinogen produced by plasmin, *Biochim. Biophys. Acta*, 271, 163, 1972.
96. **Furlan, M. and Beck, E. A.**, Plasmic degradation of human fibrinogen. I. Structural characterization of degradation products, *Biochim. Biophys. Acta*, 263, 631, 1972.
97. **Mosesson, M. W., Finlayson, J. S., Umfleet, R. A. et al.**, Human fibrinogen heterogeneities. I. Structural and related studies of plasma fibrinogens which are high solubility catabolic intermediates, *J. Biol. Chem.*, 247, 5210, 1972.
98. **Cottrell, B. A. and Doolittle, R. F.**, The amono acid sequence of a 27-residue peptide released from the α-chain carboxyterminus during the plasmic digestion of fibrinogen, *Biochem. Biophys. Res. Commun.*, 71, 754, 1976.
99. **Mosesson, M. W. and Sherry, S.**, The preparation and properties of human fibrinogen of relatively high solubility, *Biochemistry*, 2, 2829, 1966.
100. **Mosesson, M. W., Alkjaersig, N., Sweet, B. et al.**, Human fibrinogen of relatively high solubility. Comparative biophysical, biochemical and biological studies with fibrinogen of lower solubility, *Biochemistry*, 6, 3279, 1967.
101. **Sherman, L. A., Mosesson, M. W., and Sherry, S.**, Isolation and characterization of the clottable, low molecular weight fibrinogen derived by limited plasmin hydrolysis of human fraction I-4, *Biochemistry*, 8, 1515, 1969.
102. **Collen, D., Semeraro, N., and Verstraete, M.**, The fibrinogenolytic pathway of fibrinogen catabolism: a reply, *Thromb. Res.*, 4, 491, 1974.

103. **Mosesson, M. W.**, The fibrinogenolytic pathway of fibrinogen catabolism, *Thromb. Res.*, 2, 185, 1973.
104. **Sherman, L. A., Fletcher, A. P., and Sherry, S.**, In vivo transformation between fibrinogen of varying ethanol solubilities: a pathway of fibrinogen catabolism, *J. Lab. Clin. Med.*, 73, 574, 1969.
105. **Sherman, L. A.**, Fibrinogen turnover: demonstration of multiple pathways of catabolism, *J. Lab. Clin. Med.*, 79, 710, 1972.
106. **Marder, V. J. and Shulman, N. R.**, High molecular weight derivatives of human fibrinogen produced by plasmin. II. Mechanism of their anticoagulant activity, *J. Biol. Chem.*, 244, 2120, 1969.
107. **Marder, V. J.**, Immunologic structure of fibrinogen and its plasmin degradation products. Theoretical and clinical considerations, in *Fibrinogen*, Laki, K., Ed., Arnold, London, 1968, 339.
108. **Latallo, Z. S., Budzynski, A. Z., Lipinski, B. et al.**, Inhibition of thrombin and fibrin polymerization, two activities derived from plasmin-digested fibrinogen, *Nature (London)*, 203, 1184, 1964.
109. **Triantaphyllopoulos, D. C. and Triantaphyllopoulos, E.**, Evidence of antithrombic activity of the anticoagulant fraction of incubated fibrinogen, *Br. J. Haematol.*, 12, 145, 1966.
110. **Furlan, M., Kemp, G., and Beck, E. A.**, Plasmic degradation of human fibrinogen. III. Molecular model of the plasmin-resistant disulfide knot in monomeric fragment D, *Biochim. Biophys. Acta*, 400, 95, 1975.
111. **Hormann, H.**, A subfraction of fragment D isolated from a plasmin hydrolysate of human fibrinogen, *Hoppe-Seylers Z. Physiol. Chem.*, 356, 1947, 1975.
112. **Gardlund, B., Kowalska-Loth, B., Gröndahl, N. J. et al.**, Plasmic degradation products of human fibrinogen. I. Isolation and characterization of fragments E and D, and their relationship to "disulfide knots," *Thromb. Res.*, *1*, 371, 1972.
113. **Kowalska-Loth, B., Gårdlund, B., Egberg, N. et al.**, Plasmic degradation products of human fibrinogen. II. Chemical and immunological relation between fragment E and N-DSK, *Thromb. Res.*, 2, 423, 1973.
114. **Iwanaga, S., Wallén, P., Gröndahl, N. J. et al.**, On the primary structure of human fibrinogen. Isolation and characterization of N-terminal fragments from plasmic digest, *Eur. J. Biochem.*, 8, 189, 1969.
115. **Lorand, L., Downey, J., Gotoh, T. et al.**, The transpeptidose system which crosslinks fibrin by γ-glutamyl-e-lysine bonds, *Biochem. Biophys. Res. Commun.*, 31, 222, 1968.
116. **Matacić, S. and Loewy, A. G.**, The identification of isopeptide crosslinks in insoluble fibrin, *Biochem. Biophys. Res. Commun.*, 30, 356, 1968.
117. **Pisano, J. J., Finlayson, J. S., and Peyton, M. P.**, Cross-link in fibrin polymerized by factor XIII: e(γ-glutamyl) lysine, *Science*, 160, 892, 1968.
118. **Chen, R. and Doolittle, R. F.**, γ-γ Cross-linking sites in human and bovine fibrin, *Biochemistry*, 10, 4486, 1971.
119. **McDonagh, R. P., McDonagh, J., and Blombäck, B.**, S-Carboxymethyl derivatives of cross-linked and noncrosslinked human fibrin, *Proc. Natl. Acad. Sci. U.S.A.*, 69, 3648, 1972.
120. **Takagi, T. and Doolittle, R. F.**, Amino acid sequence studies of the α chain of human fibrinogen: location of four plasmin attack points and a covalent crosslinking site, *Biochemistry*, 14, 5149, 1975.
121. **Sharp, J. J., Cassman, K. G., and Doolittle, R. F.**, Amino acid sequence of the carboxy-terminal cyanogen bromide fragment from bovine and human fibrinogen γ-chains, *FEBS Lett.*, 25, 334, 1972.
122. **Marder, V. J. Budzynski, A. Z., and Barlow, G. H.**, Comparison of the physiochemical properties of fragment D derivatives of fibrinogen and fragment D-D of cross-linked fibrin, *Biochim. Biophys. Acta*, 427, 1, 1976.
123. **Marder, V. J., Budzynski, A. Z., and James, H. L.**, High molecular weight derivatives of human fibrinogen produced by plasmin. Their NH_2-terminal amino acids and comparison with the "NH_2-terminal disulfide knot," *J. Biol. Chem.*, 247, 4775, 1972.
124. **Budzynski, A. Z., Marder, V. J., and Sherry, S.**, Reaction of plasmic degradation products of fibrinogen in the radioimmunoassay of human fibrinopeptide A, *Blood*, 45, 757, 1975.
125. **Harfenist, E. J. and Canfield, R. E.**, Degradation of fibrinogen by plasmin. Isolation of an early cleavage product, *Biochemistry*, 14, 4110, 1975.
126. **Hessel, B.**, On the structure of the COOH-terminal part of the Aα-chain of human fibrinogen, *Thromb. Res.*, 7, 75, 1975.
127. **Harfenist, E. J., Lauer, R. C., Canfield, R. E. et al.**, Isolation, characterization and radioimmunoassay of a peptide resulting from limited proteolysis of human fibrinogen by plasmin, in 5th Congr. Int. Soc. Thrombosis and Hemostasis, Paris, 1975, Abstr. 390.
128. **Blombäck, M., Blombäck, B., and Holmquist, H.**, Immunological characterization of early fibrinogen degradation products. Radioimmunoassay of fragments released from the Aα chain of fibrinogen, *Thromb. Res.*, 8, 567, 1976.

129. **Lahiri, B. and Shainoff, J. R.**, Fate of fibrinopeptides in the reaction between human plasmin and fibrinogen, *Biochim. Biophys. Acta,* 303, 161, 1973.
130. **Wallén, P.**, Plasmic degradation of fibrinogen, *Scand. J. Haematol. Suppl.,* 13, 3, 1971.
131. **Kierulf, P.**, N-Terminal analysis of "fibrins" from plasmin hydrolyzed fibrinogen. Evidence for lack of fibrinopeptide B, *Thromb. Res.,* 1, 527, 1972.
132. **Esnouf, M. P. and Tunnah, G. W.**, The isolation and properties of the thrombin-like activity from *Ancistrodon rhodastoma* venom, *Br. J. Haematol.,* 13, 581, 1967.
133. **Bell, W. R., Pitney, W. R., and Goodwin, J. F.**, Therapeutic defibrination in the treatment of thrombotic disease, *Lancet,* 1, 490, 1968.
134. **Sharp, A. A., Warren, B. A., Paxton, A. M. et al.**, Anticoagulant therapy with a purified fraction of Malayan pit viper venom, *Lancet,* 1, 493, 1968.
135. **Kakker, V. V., Flanc, C., Howe, C. T. et al.**, Treatment of deep vein thrombosis. A trial of heparin, streptokinase and Arvin, *Br. Med. J.,* 1, 806, 1969.
136. **Pitney, W. R., Holt, P. J. L., Bray, C., et al.**, Acquired resistance to treatment with Arvin, *Lancet,* 1, 79, 1969.
137. **Lowe, G. D. O., Forbes, C. D. and Prentice, C. R. M.**, Plasma-fibrinogen, thromboembolism and hip fractures, *Lancet,* 1, 426, 1977.
138. **Ewart, M. R., Hatton, M. W. C., Basford, J. M. et al.**, The proteolytic action of Arvin on human fibrinogen, *Biochem. J.,* 118, 603, 1970.
139. **Barlow, G. H., Hollerman, W. H., and Lorand, L.**, The action of Arvin on fibrin stabilizing factor (factor XIII), *Res. Commun. Chem. Pathol. Pharmacol.,* 1, 39, 1970.
140. **Asbeck, F., Lechler, E., Martin, M. et al.**, Derivatives of fibrinogen and fibrin during Defibrase therapy: separation of high and low molecular weight derivatives of fibrinogen and fibrin by agarose gel filtration, *Hemostasis,* 3, 340, 1974.
141. **Hermann, G. and Miescher, P. A.**, Differentiation of leukocyte fibrinolytic enzymes from plasmin by the use of plasmatic inhibitors, *Int. Arch. Allergy Appl. Immunol.,* 27, 246, 1965.
142. **Ohlsson, K.**, Properties of leukocyte protease, *Clin. Chim. Acta,* 32, 299, 1970.
143. **Janoff, A. and Scherer, J.**, Mediators of inflammation in leukocyte lysosomes. IX. Elastinolytic activity in granules of human polymorphonuclear leukocytes, *J. Exp. Med.,* 128, 1137, 1968.
144. **Janoff, A.**, Mediators of tissue damage in leukocyte lysosomes. X. Further studies on human granulocyte elastase, *Lab. Invest.,* 22, 228, 1970.
145. **Ohlsson, K. and Olsson, I.**, The neutral proteases of human granulocytes. Isolation and partial characterization of granulocytic elastases, *Eur. J. Biochem.,* 42, 519, 1974.
146. **Janoff, A., Blondin, J., Sandhaus, R. A. et al.**, Human neutrophil elastase: in vitro effects on natural substrates suggest important physiological and pathological actions, in *Proteases and Biological Control,* Cold Spring Harbor Conferences on Cell Proliferation, Vol. 2, Reich, E., Rifkin, D. B., and Shaw, E., Eds., Cold Spring Harbor Laboratory, Cold Spring Harbor, N.Y., 1975, 603.
147. **Lazarus, G. S., Daniels, J. R., Brown, R. S., et al.**, Degradation of collagen by a human granulocytic collagenolytic system, *J. Clin. Invest.,* 47, 2622, 1968.
148. **Ohlsson, K. and Ohlsson, I.**, The neutral proteases of human granulocytes. Isolation and partial characterization of two granulocytic collagenases, *Eur. J. Biochem.,* 36, 473, 1973.
149. **Ohlsson, K.**, Granulocyte collagenase and elastase and their interactions with $\alpha 1$ antitrypsin and $\alpha 2$ macroglobulin, in *Proteases and Biological Control,* Cold Spring Harbor Conferences on Cell Proliferation, Vol. 2, Reich E., Rifkin, D. B., and Shaw, E., Eds., Cold Spring Harbor Laboratory, Cold Spring Harbor, N.Y., 1975, 591.
150. **Schmidt, W. and Havemann, K.**, Isolation of elastase-like and chymotrypsin-like neutral proteases from human granulocytes, *Hoppe-Seylers Z. Physiol. Chem.,* 355, 1077, 1974.
151. **Schmidt, W., Egbring, R. E., and Havemann, K.**, Effect of elastase-like and chymotrypsin-like neutral proteases from human granulocytes on isolated clotting factors, *Thromb. Res.,* 6, 315, 1975.
152. **Plow, E. F. and Edgington, T. S.**, An alternative pathway for fibrinolysis. I. The cleavage of fibrinogen by leukocyte proteases at physiologic pH, *J. Clin. Invest.,* 56, 30, 1975.
153. **Bilezikian, S. B. and Nossel, H. L.**, Unique pattern of fibrinogen cleavage by human leukocyte proteases, *Blood,* 50, 21, 1977.
154. **Riddle, J. M. and Barnhardt, M. I.**, Ultrastructural study of fibrin dissolution via emigrated polymorphonuclear neutrophils, *Am. J. Pathol.,* 45, 805, 1964.
155. **Mersky, C.**, Defibrination syndrome or ...?, *Blood,* 41, 599, 1973.
156. **Egbring, R., Schmidt, W., Fuchs, G. et al.**, Demonstration of granulocytic proteases in plasma of patients with acute leukemia and septicemia with coagulation defects, *Blood,* 49, 219, 1977.
157. **Shainoff, J. R. and Page, I. M.**, Cofibrins and fibrin-intermediates as indicators of thrombin activity in vivo, *Circ. Res.,* 8, 1013, 1960.
158. **Blomback, B. and Blomback, M.**, Purification of human and bovine fibrinogen, *Ark. Kemi,* 10, 415, 1956.

159. **Blombäck, B., Blombäck, M., and Holmberg, E.,** A new method for fractionation of proteins, *Acta Chem. Scand.*, 20, 2317, 1966.
160. **Mylon, E., Winternitz, M. C., and de Sütö-Nagy, G. J.,** The determination of fibrinogen with protamine, *J. Biol. Chem.* 143, 21, 1942.
161. **Kopéc, M., Kowalski, E., and Stachurska, J.,** Studies on paracoagulation. Role of antithrombin VI, *Thromb. Diath. Haemorrh.*, 5, 285, 1960.
162. **Lipinski, B. and Worowski, K.,** Detection of soluble fibrin monomer complexes in blood by means of protamine sulfate test, *Thromb. Diath. Haemorrh.*, 20, 44, 1968.
163. **Stewart, G. J. and Niewiarowski, S.,** Aggregation of fibrinogen and its degradation products by basic proteins. An electron microscopic study, *Thromb. Diath. Haemorrh.*, 25, 566, 1971.
164. **Derechin, M.,** Paracoagulacion fibrinolytica. Nuevo fenomeno vinculado a la fibrinolisis, *Prensa Med. Argent.*, 40, 2763, 1953.
165. **Derechin, M.,** Caracteres généraux de la paracoagulation fibrinolytique, *Rev. Hematol.*, 10, 35, 1955.
166. **Bomchil, G. and Derechin, M.,** Fibrinolyse hémorrhagique mortelle par gasrectomie. Prevues diagnostiques basées sur la paracoagulation fibrinolytique, *Rev. Hematol.*, 10, 41, 1955.
167. **Kowalski, E., Budzynski, A. Z., Kopéc, M. et al.,** Studies on the molecular pathology and pathogenesis of bleeding in severe fibrinolytic states in dogs, *Thromb. Diath. Haemorrh.*, 17, 65, 1964.
168. **Lipinski, B., Wegrzynowicz, Z., Budzynski, A. Z. et al.,** Soluble unclottable complexes formed in the presence of fibrinogen degradation products (FDP) during fibrinogen-fibrin conversion, and their potential significance in pathology, *Thromb. Diath. Haemorrh.*, 17, 65, 1967.
169. **Latallo, Z. S., Wegrzynowicz, Z., Budzynski, A. Z. et al.,** Effect of protamine sulfate on the solubility of fibrinogen, its derivatives, and other plasma proteins, *Scand. J. Haematol. Suppl.*, 13, 151, 1971.
170. **Kidder, W. R., Logan, L. J., Rapaport, S. I. et al.,** The plasma protamine paracoagulation test: Clinical and laboratory evaluation, *Am. J. Clin. Pathol.*, 58, 675, 1972.
171. **Niewiarowski, S. and Gurewich, V.,** Laboratory identification of intravascular coagulation. The serial dilution protamine sulfate test for the detection of fibrin monomer and fibrin degradation products, *J. Lab. Clin. Med.*, 77, 665, 1971.
172. **Kowalski, E.,** Fibrinogen derivatives and their biologic activities, *Semin. Hematol.*, 5, 45, 1968.
173. **Gurewich, V.,** Ethanol gelation and protamine sulfate. Comparison and critique, *Thromb. Diath. Haemorrh.*, 29, 733, 1973.
174. **Seaman, A. J.,** The recognition of intravascular clotting: the plasma protamine paracoagulation test, *Arch. Intern. Med.*, 125, 1016, 1970.
175. **Gurewich, V. and Hutchinson, E.,** Detection of intravascular coagulation by a serial-dilution protamine sulfate test, *Ann. Intern. Med.*, 75, 895, 1971.
176. **Godal, H. C. and Abildgaard, U.,** Gelation of soluble fibrin in plasma by ethanol, *Scand. J. Haematol.*, 3, 342, 1966.
177. **Breen, F. A., Jr. and Tullis, J. L.,** Ethanol gelation: a rapid screening test for intravascular coagulation, *Ann. Intern. Med.*, 69, 1197, 1968.
178. **Breen, F. A. Jr. and Tullis, J. L.,** Ethanol gelation test improved, *Ann. Intern. Med.*, 71, 433, 1969.
179. **Slaastad, R. A., Godal, H. C., and Kierulf, P.,** The amount of fibrin necessary to give a positive ethanol gelation test at various fibrinogen levels, *Scand. J. Haematol.*, 15, 153, 1975.
180. **Yudelman, I., Spanondis, K., and Nossel, H. L.,** Comparative behavior of ^{125}I-fibrinogen and ^{125}I-fibrin in solution, *Thromb. Res.*, 5, 495, 1974.
181. **Fletcher, A. P., Alkjaersig, N., O'Brien, J. et al.,** Blood hypercoagulability and thrombosis, *Trans. Assoc. Am. Physicians*, 83, 159, 1970.
182. **Fletcher, A. P. and Alkjaersig, N.,** Blood hypercoagulability, intravascular coagulation and thrombosis: new diagnostic concepts, *Thromb. Diath. Haemorrh. Suppl.*, 45, 389, 1971.
183. **Fletcher, A. P., Alkjaersig, N., Roy, L. et al.,** Early detection of blood hypercoagulable states and early thromboembolic lesions in man, in *Advances in Automated Analysis*, 1972 Technicon International Congress, Vol. 4, Mediaid, Tarrytown, N.Y., 1973, 31.
184. **Fletcher, A. P., Alkjaersig, N. K., O'Brien, J. R. et al.,** Fibrinogen catabolism in the surgically-treated patient and in those with postoperative venous thrombosis. Correlation of plasma fibrinogen chromatographic findings with ^{125}I-labeled fibrinogen scan findings, *J. Lab. Clin. Med.*, 89, 1349, 1977.
185. **Vermylen, J., Donati, M. B., and Verstraete, M.,** The identification of fibrinogen derivatives in plasma and serum by agarose gel filtration, *Scand. J. Haematol. Suppl.*, 13, 219, 1971.
186. **Donati, M. B., Verhaeghe, R., Culasso, D. E. et al.,** Molecular size distribution of fibrinogen derivatives formed in vitro and in vivo. A chromatographic study, *Thromb. Haemostasis*, 36, 14, 1976.
187. **Bang, N. U.,** personal communication.
188. **Chang, M. L. and Bang, N. U.,** Biological behavior of higher molecular weight products of fibrinolysis, *J. Lab. Clin. Med.*, 90, 216, 1977.

189. **Kisker, C. T., Plummer, G., Taylor, B. et al.**, A method for measurement of fibrin monomer with the use of an immune precipitate of fibrinogen, *J. Lab. Clin. Med.*, 89, 653, 1977.
190. **Bailey, K., Bettelheim, F. R., Lorand, L. et al.**, Action of thrombin in the clotting of fibrinogen, *Nature (London)*, 167, 233, 1951.
191. **Lorand, L. and Middlebrook, W. R.**, The action of thrombin on fibrinogen, *Biochem. J.*, 52, 196, 1952.
192. **Kierulf, P. and Abildgaard, U.**, Studies on soluble fibrin in plasma. I. N-terminal analysis of a modified fraction I (Cohn) from normal and thrombin-induced plasma, *Scand. J. Clin. Lab. Invest.*, 28, 231, 1971.
193. **Teger-Nilsson, A. C. and Blombäck, B.**, Degradation of human fibrinopeptides in serum, *Acta Chem. Scand.*, 21, 307, 1967.
194. **Teger-Nilsson, A. C.**, Studies on tissue thromboplastin, thrombin and fibrinopeptides in intravascular coagulation, *Acta Physiol. Scand. Suppl.*, 319, 26, 1968.
195. **Grondähl, N. J., Miller, S. P., and Teger-Nilsson, A. C.**, Isolation of fibrinopeptide formed during intravascular coagulation in dogs, *Acta Physiol. Scand.*, 76, 369, 1969.
196. **Teger-Nilsson, A. C. and Grondähl, N. J.**, A search for fibrinopeptides in urine during experimental intravascular coagulation in dogs, *Thromb. Res.*, 4, 131, 1974.
197. **Nossel, H. L., Yudelman, I., Canfield, R. E. et al.**, Measurement of fibrinopeptide A in human blood, *J. Clin. Invest.*, 54, 43, 1974.
198. **Gerrits, W. B. J., Flier, O. T. N., and van der Meer, J.**, Fibrinopeptide A immunoreactivity in human plasma, *Thromb. Res.*, 5, 197, 1974.
199. **Budzynski, A. Z. and Marder, V. J.**, Determination of human fibrinopeptide A by radioimmunoassay in purified systems and in the blood, *Thromb. Diath. Haemorrh.*, 34, 709, 1975.
200. **Kockum, C.**, Radioimmunoassay of fibrinopeptide A. Clinical applications, *Thromb. Res.*, 8, 225, 1976.
201. **Cronlund, M., Hardin, J., Burton, J. et al.**, Fibrinopeptide A in plasma of normal subjects and patients with disseminated intravascular coagulation and systemic lupus erythematosis, *J. Clin. Invest.*, 58, 142, 1976.
202. **Hofmann, V. and Straub, P. W.**, A radioimmunoassay technique for the rapid measurement of human fibrinopeptide A, *Thromb. Res.*, 11, 171, 1977.
203. **Canfield, R. E., Dean, J., Nossel, H. L. et al.**, Reactivity of fibrinogen and fibrinopeptide A-containing fibrinogen fragments with antisera to fibrinopeptide A, *Biochemistry*, 15, 1203, 1976.
204. **Nossel, H. L., Butler, V. P., Jr., Wilner, G. D. et al.**, Specificity of antisera to human fibrinopeptide A used in clinical fibrinopeptide A assays, *Thromb. Haemostasis*, 35, 101, 1976.
205. **Al-Mondhiry, H. A. B., Bilezikian, S. B., and Nossel, H. L.**, Fibrinogen "New York" — an abnormal fibrinogen associated with thromboembolism: functional evaluation, *Blood*, 45, 607, 1975.
206. **Nossel, H. L.**, Radioimmunoassay of fibrinopeptides in relation to intravascular coagulation and thrombosis, *N. Engl. J. Med.*, 295, 428, 1976.
207. **Nossel, H. L., Butler, V. P., Jr., Canfield, R. E. et al.**, Potential use of fibrinopeptide A measurements in the diagnosis and management of thrombosis, *Thromb. Diath. Haemorrh.*, 33, 426, 1975.
208. **Yudelman, I. M., Nossel, H. L., and Kaplan, K. L.**, Fibrinopeptide A (FPA) levels in venous thrombosis and pulmonary embolism before and during anticoagulant therapy, *Clin. Res.*, 25 (Abstr.), 352A, 1977.
209. **Qureshi, G. D. and Nossel, H. L.**, Stability studies of human fibrinopeptide A as measured by radioimmunoassay, *Proc. Soc. Exp. Biol. Med.*, 140, 1069, 1972.
210. **Wilner, G. D., Chatpar, P., Te, A. et al.**, Effects of extravascular clotting on fibrinopeptide A levels in blood, *J. Lab. Clin. Med.*, 91, 205, 1978.
211. **Latallo, Z.**, Critical evaluation of the thrombin time test, in *Proc. 8th Congr. Eur. Soc. Haemotology*, Karger, S. Basel, 1961-1962, 423.
212. **Biggs, R., Ed.**, *Human Blood Coagulation, Hemostasis and Thrombosis*, Oxford, Blackwell, 1972.
213. **Arnesen, H., Kierulf, P., and Godal, H. C.**, The influence of fibrinogen degradation products on the reptilase-time of plasma, *Scand. J. Haematol.*, 11, 360, 1973.
214. **Alkjaersig, N., Fletcher, A. P., and Sherry, S.**, Pathogenesis of the coagulation defect developing during pathological plasma proteolytic ("fibrinolytic") states. II. The significance, mechanism and consequences of defective fibrin polymerization, *J. Clin. Invest.*, 41, 917, 1962.
215. **Stocker, K. and Barlow, G. H.**, The coagulant enzyme from *Bothrops atrox* venom (Batroxobin), *Methods Enzymol.*, 45, 214, 1976.
216. **Hawiger, J., Niewiarowski, S., Gurewich, V. et al.**, Measurement of fibrinogen and fibrin degradation products in serum by staphylococcal clumping test, *J. Lab. Clin. Med.*, 75, 93, 1970.
217. **Hawiger, J., Hammond, D. K., and Timmons, S.**, Human fibrinogen possesses binding site for staphylococci on Aα and Bβ polypeptide chains, *Nature (London)*, 258, 643, 1975.

218. **Niewiarowski, S., Nandi, M., Colman, R. W. et al.**, Electrophoretic pattern and reactivity of fibrinogen degradation products (FDP) in three assays, *Scand. J. Haematol. Suppl.*, 13, 129, 1970.
219. **Marder, V. J., Matchett, M. O., and Sherry, S.**, Detection of serum fibrinogen and fibrin degradation products. Comparison of six techniques using purified products, and application in clinical studies, *Am. J. Med.*, 51, 71, 1971.
220. **Mersky, C., Kleiner, G. J., and Johnson, A. J.**, Quantitative estimation of split products of fibrinogen in human serum, relation to diagnosis and treatment, *Blood*, 28, 1, 1966.
221. **Mersky, C., Lalezari, P., and Johnson, A. J.**, A rapid, simple, sensitive method for measuring fibrinolytic split products in human serum, *Proc. Soc. Exp. Biol. Med.*, 131, 871, 1969.
222. **Ferguson, A. C., Kennedy, H., Ank, B. J. et al.**, Detection of fibrin degradation products: A comparison of counter immunoelectrophoresis and two hemagglutination-inhibition methods, *Am. J. Clin. Pathol.*, 62, 861, 1974.
223. **Allington, M. J.**, Detection of fibrin(ogen) degradation products by a latex clumping method, *Scand. J. Haematol. Suppl.*, 13, 115, 1971.
224. **Catt, K. J., Hirsh, J., Castelan, D. J. et al.**, Radioimmunoassay of fibrinogen and its proteolysis products, *Thromb. Diath. Haemorrh.*, 20, 1, 1968.
225. **Plow, E. F. and Edgington, T. S.**, Immunobiology of fibrinogen. Emergency of neoantigenic expressions during physiologic cleavage in vitro and in vivo, *J. Clin. Invest.*, 52, 273, 1973.
226. **Plow, E. F., Hougie, C., and Edgington, T. S.**, Neoantigenic expressions engendered by plasmin cleavage of fibrinogen, *J. Immunol.*, 107, 1496, 1971.
227. **Plow, E. F. and Edgington, T. S.**, Molecular events responsible for modulation of neoantigenic expression: the cleavage-associated neoantigen of fibrinogen, *Proc. Natl. Acad. Sci. U.S.A.*, 69, 208, 1972.
228. **Plow, E. F. and Edgington, T. S.**, The number of D and E regions in the fibrinogen molecule, *Proc. Natl. Acad. Sci. U.S.A.*, 71, 158, 1974.
229. **Plow, E. F. and Edgington, T. S.**, Is fibrinolysis a continuous low level mechanism in normal adults? *Thromb. Haemostasis*, 38 (Abstr.), 62, 1977.
230. **Gordon, Y. B., Martin, M. J., Landon, J. et. al.**, The development of radioimmunoassays for fibrinogen degradation products: Fragments D and E, *Br. J. Haematol.*, 29, 109, 1975.
231. **Gordon, Y. B., Martin, M. J., McNeile, E., et al.**, Specific and sensitive determination of degradation products by radioimmunoassay, *Lancet*, 2, 1168, 1973.
232. **Edgington, T. S.**, Fibrinogen and fibrin degradation products: their differentiation, *Thromb. Diath. Haemorrh.*, 34, 671, 1975.
233. **Plow, E. F. and Edgington, T. S.**, Discriminating neoantigenic differences between fibrinogen and fibrin derivatives, *Proc. Natl. Acad. Sci. U.S.A.*, 70, 1169, 1973.
234. **Budzynski, A. Z., Marder, V. J., and Parker, M. E.**, Radioimmunoassay of fragment D-D, a distinctive plasmic derivative of crosslinked human fibrin, *Circulation*, 54 (Abstr.,), 480, 1976.
235. **Kudryk, B., Reuterby, J., and Blombäck, B.**, Immunochemical studies on human fibrinogen and its fragments. Cross-reactivity of NH_2-terminal "disulfide knot" and related structures as determined by radioimmunoassay, *Eur. J. Biochem.*, 46, 141, 1974.
236. **Plow, E. F. and Edgington, T. S.**, A cleavage-associated neoantigenic marker for a γ chain site in the NH_2-terminal aspect of the fibrinogen molecule, *J. Biol. Chem.*, 250, 3386, 1975.
237. **Chen, J. P. and Shurley, H. M.**, A simple efficient production of neoantigenic antisera against fibrinolytic degradation products: radioimmunoassay of fragment E, *Thromb. Res.*, 7, 425, 1975.
238. **Qureshi, G. D., Butler, V. P., Jr., Harfenist, E. J. et al.**, Immunochemistry of the thrombin-altered NH_2-terminal disulfide knot of human fibrinogen, *Thromb. Res.*, 6, 357, 1975.
239. **Edgington, T. S. and Plow, E. F.**, Conformational and structural modulation of NH_2-terminal regions of fibrinogen and fibrin associated with plasmin cleavage, *J. Biol. Chem.*, 250, 3393, 1975.
240. **Plow, E. F. and Edgington, T. S.**, Localization and characterization of the cleavage-associated neoantigen in the E domain of fibrinogen, *Thromb. Hemostasis*, 38, 27, 1977.
241. **Lasch, H. G., Krecke, H. J., Rodriguez-Erdman, F. et al.**, Verbrauchs Koagulopathie (Pathogenese und therapie), *Folia Haematol.*, 61, 325, 1961.
242. **McKay, D. G.**, *Disseminated Intravascular Coagulation*, Harper & Row, New York, 1965.
243. **Verstraete, M., Vermylen, C., Vermylen, J. et al.**, Excessive consumption of blood coagulation components as cause of hemorrhagic diathesis, *Am. J. Med.*, 38, 899, 1965.
244. **Hardaway, R. M.**, *Syndromes of Disseminated Intravascular Coagulation with Special Reference to Shock and Hemorrhage*, Charles C Thomas, Springfield, Ill., 1966.
245. **Minna, J. D., Robboy, S. J., and Colman, R. W.**, *Disseminated Intravascular Coagulation in Man*, Charles C Thomas, Springfield, Ill., 1974.
246. **Deykin, D.**, The clinical challenge of disseminated intravascular coagulation, *N. Engl. J. Med.*, 283, 636, 1970.
247. **Colman, R. W., Robboy, S. J., and Minna, J. D.**, Disseminated intravascular coagulation (DIC): an approach, *Am. J. Med.*, 52, 679, 1972.

248. **Thomas, D. P., Niewiarowski, S., Myers, A. R. et al.,** A comparative study of four methods for detecting fibrinogen degradation products in patients with various diseases, *N. Engl. J. Med.,* 283, 663, 1970.
249. **Carvalho, A. C. A., Ellman, L. L., and Colman, R. W.,** A comparison of the staphlococcal clumping test and an agglutination test for detection of fibrinogen degradation products, *Am. J. Clin. Pathol.,* 62, 107, 1974.
250. **Palester-Chlebowczyk, M., Strzyzewska, E., Sitkowski, W. et al.,** Preliminary results of the protamine sulphate test in plasma of various patients, *Scand. J. Haematol. Suppl.,* 13, 183, 1971.
251. **Godal, H. C.,** Discussion 19-26, *Scand. J. Haematol. Suppl.,* 13, 203, 1970.
252. **Hedner, U. and Nilsson, I. M.,** Parallel determinations of FDP and fibrin monomers with various methods, *Thromb. Diath. Haemorrh.,* 28, 268, 1972.
253. **Margolis, C. Z.,** Ethanol gelation test, *N. Engl. J. Med.,* 284, 53, 1971.
254. **Hirsh, J. and Gallus, A. S.,** Diagnosis of venous thromboembolism: limitations and applications, in *Diagnosis and Prevention of Venous Thromboembolic Disease,* Genton, E. and Hirsh, J., Eds., Grune & Stratton, New York, in press.
255. **Ruckley, C. V., Das, P. C., Leitch, A. G. et al.,** Serum fibrin/fibrinogen degradation products associated with postoperative pulmonary embolus and venous thrombosis, *Br. Med. J.,* 4, 395, 1970.
256. **Gurewich, V., Hume, M. and Patrick, M.,** The laboratory diagnosis of venous thromboembolic disease by measurement of fibrinogen/fibrin degradation products and fibrin monomer, *Chest,* 64, 585, 1973.
257. **Rickman, F. D., Handin, R., Howe, J. P. et al.,** Fibrin split products in acute pulmonary embolism, *Ann. Intern. Med.,* 79, 664, 1973.
258. **Bynum, L. J., Crotty, C., and Wilson, J. E.,** III, Use of fibrinogen-fibrin degradation products and soluble fibrin complexes for differentiating pulmonary embolism from nonthromboembolic lung disease, *Am. Rev. Respir. Dis.,* 114, 285, 1976.
259. **Cooke, E. D., Gordon, Y. B., Bowcock, S. A. et al.,** Serum fibrin(ogen) degradation products in diagnosis of deep vein thrombosis and pulmonary embolism after hip surgery, *Lancet,* 2, 51, 1975.
260. **Butler, M. J., Gordon, Y. B., Irving, M. H. et al.,** Serum levels of fibrin(ogen) degradation fragment E antigen in the diagnosis of deep vein thrombosis after abdominal and inguinal surgery, *Thromb. Res.,* 8, 167, 1976.
261. **Gallus, A. S., Hirsh, J., and Gent, M.,** Relevance of preoperative and postoperative blood tests to postoperative leg-vein thrombosis, *Lancet,* 2, 805, 1973.
262. **Light, R. W. and Bell, W. R.,** LDH and fibrinogen-fibrin degradation products in pulmonary embolism, *Arch. Intern. Med.,* 133, 372, 1974.
263. **Lahnborn, G. and Bergstrom, K.,** Clinical and haemostatic parameters related to thromboembolism and low-dose heparin prophylaxis in major surgery, *Acta Chir. Scand.,* 141, 590, 1975.
264. **Cade, J., Hirsh, J., and Regoeczi, E.,** Mechanisms for elevated fibrin/fibrinogen degradation products in acute experimental pulmonary embolism, *Blood,* 45, 563, 1975.
265. **Braun, W. E. and Merrill, J. P.,** Urine fibrinogen fragments in human renal allografts. A possible mechanism of renal injury, *N. Engl. J. Med.,* 278, 1366, 1968.
266. **Colman, R. W., Braun, W. E., Busch, G. J. et al.,** Coagulation studies in the hyperacute and other forms of renal-allograft rejection, *N. Engl. J. Med.,* 281, 685, 1969.
267. **Whitworth, J. H., Fairley, K. F., McIvor, M. A. et al.,** Urinary fibrin-degradation products and the site of urinary infections, *Lancet,* 1, 234, 1973.
268. **Cortes, P., Potter, E. V., and Kwaan, H. C.,** Characterization and significance of urinary fibrin degradation products, *J. Lab. Clin. Med.,* 82, 377, 1973.
269. **Marchesi, S. L., Aptekar, R. G., Steinberg, A. D. et al.,** Urinary fibrin split products in lupus nephritis. Correlation with other parameters of renal disease, *Arthritis Rheum.,* 17, 158, 1974.
270. **Bang, N. U. and Chang, M. L.,** Soluble fibrin complexes, *Semin. Thromb. Hemostasis,* 1, 91, 1974.
271. **Rake, M. O., Flute, P. T., Shilkin, K. B. et al.,** Early and intensive therapy of intravascular coagulation in acute liver failure, *Lancet,* 2, 1215, 1971.
272. **Coleman, M., Finlayson, N., Bettigole, R. E. et al.,** Fibrinogen survival in cirrhosis: Improvement by "low dose" heparin, *Ann. Intern. Med.,* 83, 79, 1975.
273. **Fletcher, A. P., Biederman, O., Moore, D. et al.,** Abnormal plasminogen-plasmin system activity (fibrinolysis) in patients with hepatic cirrhosis: its cause and consequences, *J. Clin. Invest.,* 43, 681, 1964.
274. **Tytgat, G. N., Collen, D., and Verstraete, M.,** Metabolism of fibrinogen in cirrhosis of the liver, *J. Clin. Invest.,* 50, 1690, 1971.
275. **Casarella, W. J. and Wilner, G. D.,** Guide wire thrombogenicity measured by fibrinopeptide A radioimmunoassay, *Am. J. Roentgenol.,* 128, 363, 1977.
276. **Wilner, G. D., Casarella, W. J., Fenoglio, C. et al.,** In vivo fibrinopeptide A generation induced by angiographic catheters, *Thromb. Hemostasis,* 38 (Abstr.,), 73, 1977.

277. **Matthias, F. R., Reinicke, R., and Heene, D. L.**, Affinity chromatography and quantitation of soluble fibrin from plasma, *Thromb. Res.*, 10, 365, 1977.
278. **Henschen, A. and Lottspeich, F.**, Amino acid sequence linking plasmic fragments E and D in the β chain of human fibrin, *Z. Physiol. Chem.*, 357, 1801, 1976.
279. **Gollwitzer, R. and Timpl, R.**, Isolation and immunological characterization of a disulfide loop region in human fibrinogen α-chain, *FEBS Lett.*, 58, 269, 1975.
280. **Veenhof, C. H. N.**, Blood and Artificial Kidney. Clinical and Experimental Studies, Ph.D. thesis, University of Amsterdam, The Netherlands, 1976.
281. **Shainoff, J. R. and Dardik, B. N.**, Fibrinopeptide B and aggregation of fibrinogen, *Science*, 204, 200, 1979.
282. **Cottrell, B. A., Strong, D. D., Watt, K. W. K., and Doolittle, R. F.**, Amino acid sequence studies on the α chaine of human fibrinogen. Exact location of cross-linking acceptor sites, *Biochemistry*, 18, 5405, 1979.
283. **Nossel, H. L., Wasser, J., Kaplan, K. L., La Gamma, K. S., Yudelman, I., and Canfield, R. E.**, Sequence of fibrinogen proteolysis and platelet release after intrauterine infusion of hypertonic saline, *J. Clin. Invest.*, 64, 1371, 1979.
284. **Budzynski, A. Z., Marder, V. J., Parker, M. E., Shames, P., Brizuela, B. S., and Olexa, S. A.**, Antigenic markers on fragment DD: a unique plasmic derivative of human crosslinked fibrin, *Blood*, 54, 794, 1979.

INDEX

A

B

C

D

E

F

G

H

I

K

L

M

N

O

P

R

S

T

U

V

W